WALKING MANHATTAN

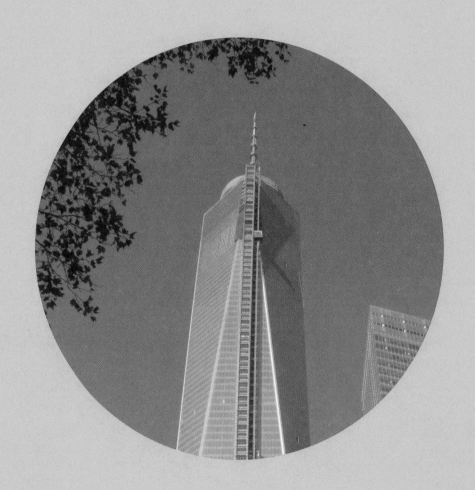

WALKING MANHATTAN

30 Strolls Exploring Cultural Treasures, Entertainment Centers, and Historical Sites in the Heart of New York City

Ellen Levitt

 WILDERNESS PRESS ... *on the trail since 1967*

Walking Manhattan: 30 Strolls Exploring Cultural Treasures, Entertainment Centers, and Historical Sites in the Heart of New York City

Copyright © 2015 by Ellen Levitt

Editor: Adrienne Onofri
Project editor: Ritchey Halphen
Cover and interior photos: Copyright © by Ellen Levitt, except where noted
Cartographer: Scott McGrew
Cover and interior design: Larry B. Van Dyke and Lisa Pletka
Proofreaders: Emily C. Beaumont, Rebecca Henderson
Indexer: Sylvia Coates

Cataloging-in-Publication Data is available from the Library of Congress.

ISBN: 978-0-89997-763-8; eISBN: 978-0-89997-764-5

Manufactured in the United States of America

Published by: **WILDERNESS PRESS**
An imprint of Keen Communications, LLC
PO Box 43673
Birmingham, AL 35243
800-443-7227; fax 205-326-1012

Visit **wildernesspress.com** for a complete listing of our books and for ordering information. Contact us at **info @wildernesspress.com, facebook.com/wildernesspress1967,** or **twitter.com/wilderness1967** with questions or comments.

Distributed by Publishers Group West

Cover photos: *Front, clockwise from top left:* statue of Washington and Lafayette, near Morningside Park; Empire State Building, Midtown; trinkets for sale, Chinatown; Apollo Theater and West 125th Street, Central Harlem; Little Red Lighthouse, Inwood; Trump Unisphere, Central Park West. *Back, top to bottom:* 455 Central Park West (former New York Cancer Hospital); 1 World Trade Center, Financial District; Low Memorial Library, Columbia University.

Frontispiece: 1 World Trade Center

SAFETY NOTICE Although Wilderness Press and the author have made every attempt to ensure that the information in this book is accurate at press time, they are not responsible for any loss, damage, injury, or inconvenience that may occur to anyone while using this book. You are responsible for your own safety and health while following the walking trips described here. Always check local conditions, know your own limitations, and consult a map.

acknowledgments

I INTERVIEWED AND SPOKE WITH a number of people while working on this book. Special thanks are extended to Howard Dankowitz, Jessica and Michelle Dankowitz, Janet Dankowitz, Ben Levitt, Willie DeVries, Mindy Braunstein Weinblatt, Mark Weinblatt, Georgette Asherman, Kenny Chin, Sherryl Feinblum Eluto, Jacqui and Barry Elkayam, Cheryl Mamiye Shayo, Leah Krakowski, Cindy Mazer, Nora Walsh-DeVries and Joan Walsh, Josh Sayer, Frank Jump, Charles Bowe, Elliot Schechter, Patrick Lam, Renee Limongelli Natoli, Julian Voloj, Mario Perez, Nico Collazo, Erik Lieber, Neil Abraham, Dan Evans, Ed Foxxe, Arthur Swerdloff, and Ron Schweiger.

Thanks also to staff members at the New York City Municipal Archives, the New-York Historical Society, the Museum of the City of New York, the New York Public Library, and the Brooklyn Public Library, as well as my former colleagues at Murry Bergtraum High School, Manhattan Comprehensive Night High School, and Abraham Lincoln High School.

If I neglected to acknowledge you, please let me know (nicely). A bibliography of my main print and online sources is at the back of the book.

—*Ellen Levitt*

author's note

AT THE PROUD AGE OF 50, I have done many things in Manhattan, for I have lived my whole life in New York City. I am a native and resident of Brooklyn, but I've spent an enormous amount of my time in Manhattan (certainly more than in Queens, the Bronx, or Staten Island, although I have enjoyed being in them as well).

Should anyone doubt my street cred, I proffer the following incomplete list of things I've done in Manhattan—many positive, some not:

1. Visited museums, the zoo, and national and local monuments.
2. Watched dance performances (ballet, modern, and so on). *(continued)*

3. Went to concerts (rock, jazz, classical, ethnic, and so on).
4. Attended services at synagogues and a few churches.
5. Conducted research for my books.
6. Gave walking tours.
7. Attended parades.
8. Marched in parades.
9. Went on dates.
10. Applied for and received a marriage license.
11. Ate at restaurants.
12. Stood on long lines to pick up license plates.
13. Paid, and fought, parking tickets.
14. Took the test for a city tour-guide license—and passed.
15. Visited family and friends.
16. Took boat rides.
17. Attended funeral services.
18. Watched Broadway, off-Broadway, and off-off-Broadway plays and musicals.
19. Participated in a charity bike ride (the Five Boro, once).
20. Cheered on teams at professional and school basketball and hockey games.
21. Went to the circus.
22. Shopped.
23. Attended professional-development sessions and workshops for teachers.
24. Taught at two high schools and worked as a teaching assistant for a Hunter College course.
25. Worked full-time jobs as a magazine associate editor and at a nonprofit group.
26. Worked part-time jobs as an office assistant, salesperson, and more.
27. Worked student internships at a cable TV station, a synagogue, and a public relations firm.
28. Went bowling, swimming, wall climbing, rowing, hiking, and ice skating.
29. Walked by someone who had a gun and was nabbed by cops . . . but didn't realize it until my friend informed me.

30. Walked by or sat near celebrities—and spoke with a few of them: Andy Warhol, Keith Hernandez, Allen Ginsberg, Jerome Robbins, Quentin Crisp, Hilly Kristal (of CBGB fame), and others.

31. Exhibited photographs at the 4th Street Photo Gallery, CB's 313, 14th Street Y, and other galleries.

32. Attended school as a college undergraduate and a doctoral student.

33. Snapped photographs by myself and with students.

34. Visited and read in libraries (circulating and research).

35. Strolled through street fairs of various types.

36. Checked out or joined rallies and protests (Occupy Wall Street among them).

37. Played piano, guitar, percussion, etc.

38. Sang with choirs and glee clubs.

39. Had my foot run over by a bike messenger.

40. Shoved another bike messenger who nearly knocked me down.

41. Drove my car, parked my car, found my car towed once.

42. Walked aimlessly; rode the subway, PATH trains, and buses; took taxis.

43. Lost items (some of which were found).

Whew!

Yet I don't know it all when it comes to Manhattan. Researching this book helped me to learn so much more about this amazing island. I am humbled by how much one can do and learn here and still never fully grasp its deep importance. Manhattan has changed vastly over the years, even during my lifetime. But there are many trends that resonate, many themes that are constantly being reworked, and many places that people go to time and again. I hope this book will introduce you to places both well known and obscure. I implore you to do more reading and traveling of your own.

This book is intended for many people: newcomers who want to see the main attractions and old-timers who want a fresh look, repeat visitors who want to see something they missed previously, people who will be here for a limited time working or attending school, and anyone else who has a sense of wonderment and a thirst for adventure.

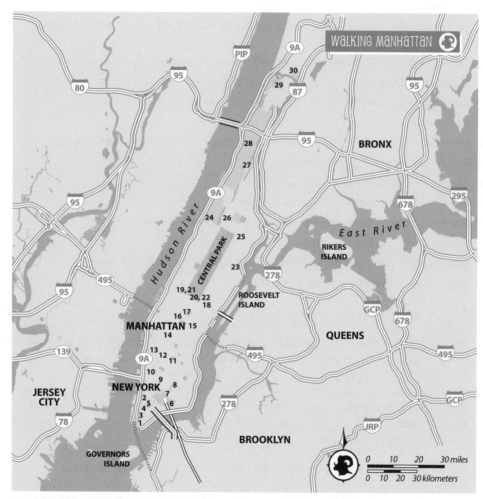

NUMBERS ON THIS LOCATOR MAP CORRESPOND TO WALK NUMBERS.

Table of Contents

INTRODUCTION

LET'S FACE IT: When people think of New York City, most often they're thinking of Manhattan, the most densely populated of the five boroughs that constitute this city. As a lifelong resident of Brooklyn, I bow my head in deference to Manhattan as the capital, the lifeline, the cultural core, the economic engine overall.

The Lenape Indians referred to this long, thin piece of land as *Manna-hata,* or "island of many hills." During colonial times, the Dutch and then the British had control over Manhattan. Some parts sustained much damage during the American Revolution, but once the war for independence was won, New York became the first capital of the nation.

Through the years, Manhattan has been a center of commerce and finance, education and scholarship, entertainment and culture, innovation and research. It has seen destruction in the form of fires, terrorist attacks, storms, power outages, looting, and accidents of many types—car, rail, and construction among them. Meanwhile, the infrastructure of Manhattan is astounding: from bridges to alleys, skyscrapers to pop-up shops, along with commercial and residential edifices, religious and educational sites, parks and playgrounds. Automobiles, buses, trains, boats, and helicopters arrive and depart daily (but not airplanes; the nearest airports are in Queens and New Jersey).

Some walking advice:

- Wherever you go, don't be scared—but do be aware of your surroundings, as well as the time of day.

- It's always helpful to carry certain items, such as a pack of tissues (in case a bathroom stall is out of paper), a pen, a piece of identification, a small umbrella, and a few bandages (you'd be surprised how often you might need these).

- Stay alert to traffic, be it cars and trucks, bikes and strollers, workers with deliveries, or distracted pedestrians. Some New Yorkers jaywalk; if you do, be very careful—and don't assume that everyone obeys traffic lights and the right-of-way. *(continued)*

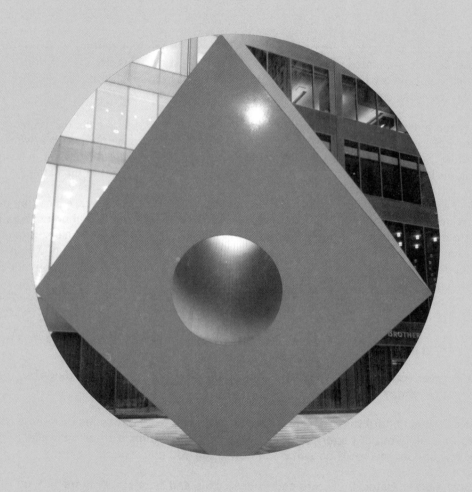

Manhattan's outdoor sculptures—such as Noguchi's The Cube—*can amuse and inspire.*

- Use landmarks to visually orient yourself. Skyscrapers like the Empire State Building are excellent for this.

- When you need a bathroom, among the best places to look for decent, accessible facilities are department stores, libraries, large houses of worship that are open, and hotels. If you're visiting a museum or touristy site and it has a bathroom, you might want to use it while you're there. Other places to find restrooms, although they may not be as pleasant, are parks, certain major subway stations, and portable johns in various locations.

- Look out for broken pavement, construction hazards, dog or horse messes, and other conditions on sidewalks and roads that could cause accidents or unfortunate situations.

- If the street musicians you pass are at least pretty good, give them some coins (or more, if you're feeling generous).

- It may seem that every other New Yorker is preoccupied by a cell phone or handheld device, but you don't want to do that. To experience Manhattan, you need to see, hear, and smell things.

Have a good time, a meaningful time, a *memorable* time walking Manhattan!

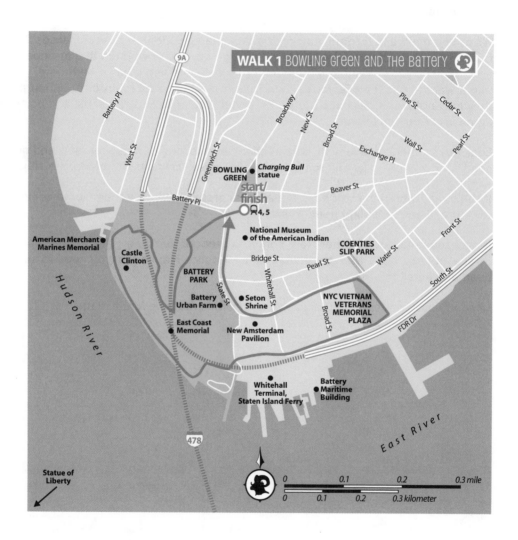

WALK 1 BOWLING GREEN AND THE BATTERY

9A

Battery Pl

West St

Greenwich St

Broadway

New St

Broad St

Pine St

Cedar St

Wall St

Exchange Pl

Pearl St

BOWLING GREEN

Charging Bull statue

Battery Pl

start/finish

4, 5

Beaver St

National Museum of the American Indian

COENTIES SLIP PARK

Front St

American Merchant Marines Memorial

Castle Clinton

BATTERY PARK

Bridge St

Whitehall St

Pearl St

Water St

South St

Hudson River

State St

Battery Urban Farm

Seton Shrine

NYC VIETNAM VETERANS MEMORIAL PLAZA

Broad St

FDR Dr

East Coast Memorial

New Amsterdam Pavilion

478

Whitehall Terminal, Staten Island Ferry

Battery Maritime Building

East River

Statue of Liberty

0   0.1   0.2   0.3 mile
0   0.1   0.2   0.3 kilometer

1 BOWLING GREEN AND THE BATTERY: FERRIES, FINANCE, FUN

BOUNDARIES: Battery Park, Bowling Green, Coenties Slip, ferry terminals
DISTANCE: 2 miles
SUBWAY: 4 or 5 to Bowling Green, 1 to South Ferry, or R to Whitehall St.

The southernmost section of Manhattan is one of the borough's most exciting districts. Weekdays (and often weekends, too) find so many people walking around here, going to and from work, checking out tourist sights, attending cultural events. Densely packed streets hold a mix of skyscrapers and older, shorter buildings in this area, which is surrounded by water and has multiple ferry terminals. Many New Yorkers forget how important the docks and waterfront have been to the Big Apple over the years—and still are. You're likely to see the Staten Island, Liberty Island, or Governors Island ferry boats sail by, and perhaps historical-replica ships operating pleasure cruises. This part of Manhattan presents a jumble of history and culture, commerce and green space. It's an appropriate locale to start exploring Manhattan—even if you think you've seen it all.

● The Bowling Green station of the 4 and 5 trains has one entrance that's a sloped, glass-paneled modern construction and another that's an old-fashioned brick structure resembling a quaint house. If you got off at Whitehall Street or South Ferry, walk north on Whitehall to the small park called Bowling Green. This space was used as a cattle market and a parade ground before it became a park in the 1730s—and yes, they had lawn bowling here long ago. Bowling Green is Manhattan's oldest park, and anti-British protests took place here during colonial times.

A grand building stands along the south end of the park: the former US Custom House, now home to the National Museum of the American Indian, the George Gustav Heye Center. Its interior is sumptuous, with bold staircases and fixtures. Architect Cass Gilbert designed the Beaux Arts building, Daniel Chester French created the outdoor sculptures, and in the rotunda inside are murals by Reginald Marsh. The National Archives at New York City are located on the third floor.

To your right, when your back is to the Custom House, is 2 Broadway, a glass high-rise (designed by the firm headed by Emery Roth) with a modernist mural at the entrance. To your left is "Number One" on Broadway, the impressive United States Lines–Panama Pacific Lines Building, with stately crests above entrance level. A memorial plaque on its corner refers to the Revolutionary War. Just past it, going up Broadway, see the stately Bowling Green Offices, built in 1895–98 in a style its architects, William and George Audsley, described as "Hellenic Renaissance." To the right of the offices is the Cunard Line Building at 25 Broadway, across from the iconic bronze *Charging Bull* statue by Arturo Di Modica. The bull may be a familiar part of the tableau here, but it caused a stir in 1989, when Di Modica surreptitiously installed it a bit farther uptown, in front of the New York Stock Exchange. At the time it seemed like a huge joke, but the statue has become so popular that tourists and partiers flock to it and jockey for the best camera angle. But don't overlook a much older piece a few yards south of the bull: the tall Evacuation Day flagpole, with its moderately worn plaque. November 25, 1783, is the day the British left New York City after the Revolutionary War.

● Head back toward the Custom House and cross Broadway into Battery Park. Many people wander into Battery Park only to get to the Statue of Liberty ferry. But there are many interesting and touching things to view here, including the battered golden sphere that was rescued from the World Trade Center plaza. The Battery Urban Farm, open spring through fall, showcases plants and vegetables growing right in the park. A swooping eagle statue heads the solemn East Coast Memorial, honoring World War II military men. The *Immigrants* statue is a dramatic depiction of newcomers to America. The Norwegian Veterans Monument, the American Merchant Marines Memorial (particularly haunting because of the "drowning" figure), the Eternal Flame, the Korean War Memorial, and others provide mini–history lessons with emotional punch.

● Walk to the round sandstone fort, Castle Clinton, and go inside. This building has served many functions over the generations—military protection, an entertainment venue, the processing center (then dubbed Castle Garden) for immigrants entering the country by boat, the city's aquarium—and now it's where you depart for the Statue of Liberty or Ellis Island. It also has a nifty museum.

Even if you don't get over to the Statue of Liberty, take some time to gaze at her. She has meant a great deal to so many people for several generations. She is a symbol and major monument of not only New York City but also the United States.

● Facing the water and Lady Liberty, walk to your left and you'll come upon the Whitehall Terminal, Manhattan's home for the Staten Island Ferry. Now may be the time for you to take a ferry over to the least populated of the five boroughs of New York City. The ride is fun, and both the Manhattan and Staten Island terminals have things to see and do (as well as copious bathroom stalls). Fine photo ops await your ride.

● To the north of the Whitehall Terminal, the New Amsterdam Pavilion has artistic-looking metal benches, pretty plantings, and a few intriguing pieces that reflect on the early European history of this city. There is a miniature map of the colonial settlement that you can touch, a few plaques, and stones engraved with historic messages (although those are worn and a bit hard to read). Walk to your right and you'll see the Battery Maritime Building. It's of a much older and more elegant style than the modern Staten Island Ferry building. From late spring through early autumn, you can catch a ferry to Governors Island here.

● Cross over to South Street, but be careful of the traffic racing to and from the highway. You will get a nice view of the river from here. Walk away from the Battery on South Street for about two blocks until you get to a sunken plaza with a large glass structure you can walk through, as well as a flower bed, plaques, and a sitting area. This is the New York City Vietnam Veterans Memorial Plaza. I find this one of the most stirring sites in all of Manhattan. Get up close to the pale-green glass, and you will see segments of letters sent to and from people who served in the military during the Vietnam War. Some have mundane messages; others reflect the horror they have seen and the fears they harbor. "Don't ask questions; when I come home if I feel like talking about it I will, but otherwise don't ask," reads one fragment. "Mom, I'd give just about anything for a hot bath, some clean clothes, and a cold drink. . . . Love, Ray," reads another.

● Cross at Water Street to little Coenties Slip Park. This pedestrian walkway showcases an odd metal sculpture and a floor design worth a few minutes of contemplation. If you walk to the northern end of this small space, look to your left at a black-glass high-rise and you will see two or even three other buildings reflected on the glass.

● Back at Water Street, go to your right for a few blocks until it turns into State Street. At #8 (also listed as #7 in some sources), an interesting curved building is The National Shrine of St. Elizabeth Ann Seton, a church and exhibit dedicated to the first

US-born Catholic saint. Proceed to #17 and you will see two cheery, comical statues, yellow and red. These were created by the late pop artist Keith Haring (and even display his etched signature).

● Continue on State Street for a few blocks (one block is a bit lengthy) until you reconnect with the start of Broadway. You can catch the train a few blocks north at Bowling Green.

POINTS OF INTEREST

National Museum of the American Indian/US Custom House nmai.si.edu, 1 Bowling Green, 212-514-3700

Bowling Green nycgovparks.org/parks/bowling-green, Broadway and Whitehall Street

Charging Bull **Statue** chargingbull.com, Broadway and Morris Street

Battery Park nycgovparks.org/parks/battery-park, State Street and Battery Place

Castle Clinton nps.gov/cacl, Battery Park

Whitehall Terminal, Staten Island Ferry siferrry.com, 212-344-7220

New York City Vietnam Veterans Memorial Plaza vietnamveteransplaza.com, 55 Water St., 212-471-9496

Coenties Slip Park Between Water and Pearl Streets

The National Shrine of St. Elizabeth Ann Seton setonheritage.org, 7 State St., 212-269-6865

route summary

1. Walk around Bowling Green and up Broadway to the bull statue.
2. Go back to the south end of Bowling Green and cross Broadway into Battery Park.
3. Make a circuit around the park.
4. Facing the water, walk left to the ferry terminals.
5. Cross and walk right on South Street to the NYC Vietnam Veterans Memorial Plaza.
6. Cross Water St. into Coenties Slip.
7. Walk west on Water Street, which turns into State Street.
8. Walk right on State Street until it merges with Broadway.

connecting the walks

Walk north on Broadway three blocks for the start of Walk 3 (Wall Street/Financial District), or walk about nine blocks to Fulton Street for Walk 4 (City Hall and South Street Seaport).

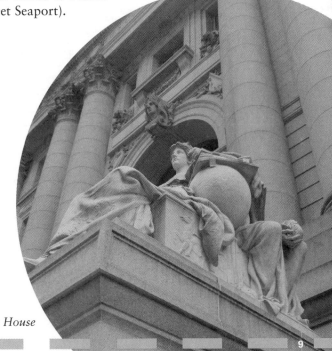

Neoclassical grandeur at the old Custom House

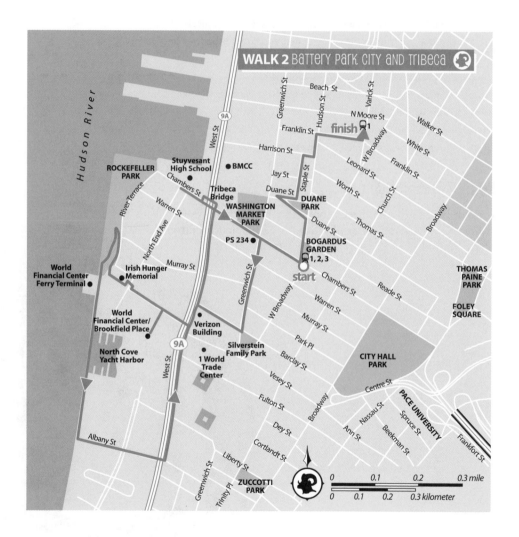

WALK 2 BATTERY PARK CITY AND TRIBECA

Hudson River

9A

Greenwich St
Beach St
Hudson St
Varick St
N Moore St
Franklin St
Walker St
finish

ROCKEFELLER PARK

Stuyvesant High School
BMCC

Harrison St
White St
W Broadway
Franklin St

Chambers St

Tribeca Bridge
Jay St
Leonard St
Church St
Broadway

WASHINGTON MARKET PARK
Duane St
Staple St
Worth St

DUANE PARK

Warren St
River Terrace
North End Ave

PS 234
Duane St
Thomas St

BOGARDUS GARDEN
1, 2, 3

THOMAS PAINE PARK

World Financial Center Ferry Terminal
Irish Hunger Memorial
Murray St
start
Chambers St
Reade St

FOLEY SQUARE

World Financial Center/ Brookfield Place
Verizon Building
W Broadway
Warren St
Murray St

9A

Silverstein Family Park
Park Pl
CITY HALL PARK

North Cove Yacht Harbor
1 World Trade Center
Barclay St
Vesey St
Centre St
PACE UNIVERSITY

West St

Fulton St
Broadway
Nassau St
Spruce St
Beekman St
Frankfort St

Dey St
Ann St

Albany St
Cortlandt St

Greenwich St
Liberty St

Trinity Pl
ZUCCOTTI PARK

0   0.1   0.2   0.3 mile
0   0.1   0.2   0.3 kilometer

10

2 Battery Park City and Tribeca: The Bold and the Beautiful

BOUNDARIES: **Albany St., River Terrace, Franklin St., Varick St.**
DISTANCE: **2 miles**
SUBWAY: **1, 2, or 3 to Chambers St.**

A peaceful yet invigorating feeling imbues Battery Park City, an area bordered by the Hudson River and teeming with high-rise buildings, many of them of fairly recent vintage. Exciting, even intimidating in scale and concentration, much of the neighborhood has a futuristic feel. Its buildings are certainly in striking contrast to the older structures that prevail in the nearby Financial District (see next walk). "BPC" also has the busy and bold World Financial Center, full of shops and offices, exhibition space, and public sculpture.

Battery Park City was badly scarred by the events of September 11, 2001. The community was essentially built on landfill, much of it excavated from the site that became the World Trade Center, so there was more sadness imbued in the landscape. But BPC has bounced back in many ways, and a lot of rebuilding has been done.

This walk also strolls through part of Tribeca ("triangle below Canal"), dominated by buildings far older than Battery Park City's. See the contrasts and enjoy the multiple views of this West Side neighborhood.

● From the subway station, walk west along Chambers Street, named for John Chambers, a colonial-era lawyer who was involved in the 1735 trial of newspaper editor John Peter Zenger; the case is considered an important early test of freedom of the press and civil rights.

Look at 160 Chambers. It's an odd juxtaposition: This onetime firehouse is now . . . a nail salon? Dating to 1862, the building has served as a police station, hospital, firehouse (hence the ENGINE 29 sign), lumberyard, apartments, and service businesses.

- Cross Greenwich Street and make a left. Here is PS 234, a cheery elementary school with an innovative design, a nautical motif, pretty plantings, and a comical sculpture by Tom Otterness called *Frog and Bee.* After Murray Street, the sleek glass building on your right, 75 Park Place, is home to a couple of city agencies, including the Office of Management and Budget.

- Walk another block; at Park Place is a big reddish-brown building with the silver letters BMCC and CUNY affixed to it. This is Fiterman Hall, part of the Borough of Manhattan Community College, a well-regarded school in the City University of New York system. (The rest of the campus lies farther up Greenwich Street between Chambers and Harrison Streets; you'll pass it later on.)

- Walk to Barclay Street to see Silverstein Family Park, a more-or-less triangle that is both somber and frivolous—the inscription THIS PARK IS DEDICATED TO THOSE WHO SURVIVED SEPTEMBER 11, 2001 rings a fountain, in the middle of which is a bulbous red statue by Jeff Koons. The park is in the footprint of the 7 World Trade Center building, destroyed on 9/11; a new 7 WTC was built a block away. Real estate magnate Larry Silverstein is a native son who founded Silverstein Properties, which had acquired the World Trade Center shortly before the terrorist attacks.

- Go right on Barclay to #101, the Bank of New York Mellon Corporation building— glass, glass, and steel for 25 stories. It was closed for several months after 9/11. Then check out the big sign for District Council 37, a city-employee union whose headquarters are located here at 125 Barclay.

- At West Street you have a futuristic and almost shocking sight: the huge, modern skyscrapers of Battery Park City, seemingly piled on top of each other. Don't cross over yet, but ogle 200 West St., the Goldman Sachs tower that was opened in 2010. On your left, the older skyscraper is 140 West St., long known as the Verizon Build- ing but constructed in 1920 for the New York Telephone Company. This Art Deco structure has some creative details, especially at the main entrance (delicate foliage and a bell for "Ma Bell"). The 9/11 attacks caused major damage, but the structure has been restored. Look to the left, past the Verizon Building, to see the new 1 World Trade Center—from here, the view is dizzying.

● Go left and, at Vesey Street, turn right, crossing West Street carefully. As you walk, you'll see a few eateries and the Regal movie theater. Vesey ends at North End Avenue, a street solely within the boundaries of Battery Park City. Cross North End to see something drastically different from all the high-rises around here: the Irish Hunger Memorial.

Resembling an overgrown ruin, this open-air museum is meant to raise awareness of the Great Irish Famine, which spurred much immigration to the United States and especially to New York City. The remnants of an authentic stone cottage were brought over to be part of the installation; the cottage was donated by the descendants of the family who originally lived in it. Stones bear the names of Irish counties; the landscaping comprises both soil and native plants imported from Ireland. A figure-eight walkway runs among the exhibits, and a walled entranceway is replete with quotes. Standing at the top of the memorial, which was finished in 2002, affords you prime views of the neighborhood as well as the Hudson River and even New Jersey (to be specific, Jersey City).

● Walk out of the memorial to see the New York Mercantile Exchange. Use either the path or the River Terrace sidewalk to enter Nelson A. Rockefeller Park, which has an innovative playground and well-thought-out landscaping. The outer edge is buffeted by waves. Walk for about two or three blocks and then double back.

● Go left and pass the World Financial Center ferry terminal and then the North Cove Yacht Harbor, along with an inviting plaza area with seating and tables, some modernist sculptures, and animals scurrying about. Go right, up to the fence at the water's edge of the promenade, and gaze upon the Statue of Liberty,

A dazzling view of 1 World Trade Center

Ellis Island, and the Verrazano-Narrows Bridge. It can be quite peaceful here, in jarring contrast to the bustling streets and highway just a few minutes' walk away.

● Admire the boats, then walk toward the large, glass-vaulted building. This is the World Financial Center's Winter Garden Pavilion—go inside. Completed in 1988, this Cesar Pelli–designed structure was extensively damaged on 9/11 but has been restored with great care. It hosts art exhibits and concerts. The Winter Garden is a fun stroll, what with its excellent views and trees in the main area. You can walk into Brookfield Place, which has luxury shops (including Saks Fifth Avenue) and casual-to-high-end restaurants.

● Within the World Financial Center, ask to be directed outside to the Hudson River Greenway. Take the greenway right (south) two blocks to Albany Street and cross to the east side of West Street. Turn left (north) on West.

● Note the imposing mansard-roofed skyscraper at 90 West. Completed in 1907, the Gothic building was designed by Cass Gilbert, who also designed the Woolworth Building and the former Custom House in lower Manhattan. Continuing down West, past the two entrances for the 9/11 Memorial (see next walk), at Liberty Street and then Fulton Street, you'll see the American Express Tower (formerly 3 World Financial Center) to your left; you also get another great view of 1 World Trade Center at the corner of West and Vesey.

● Keep walking along West Street until you reach Chambers Street, and take the Tribeca Bridge, a pedestrian overpass that crosses West Street/NY 9A. On the other side of the highway is Stuyvesant High School, one of the most prestigious and selective public high schools in the United States. Since the 1992–93 school year, "Stuy" has occupied this 10-story building, featuring an elegant recessed entrance and many windows that afford a lot of natural light.

● Take the Tribeca Bridge (for nice views) or carefully cross West Street (less physical effort) to walk on Chambers Street. Notice the murals painted in bright colors along the curbs of the sports courts—they were painted by children under the auspices of the organization CITYarts. To your left after the murals, a wide path with a checker-board design leads to the main campus of BMCC.

- Walk farther on Chambers to see Washington Market Park, which has a cute gazebo in its center as well as a colorful playground.

- After crossing Greenwich Street, make a left on Hudson Street. Bogardus Garden is a small, pretty green space on the triangle between Hudson and West Broadway.

- Cross Reade Street and make a left at Duane Street. There are some charming buildings here: #168 has a pretty roofline design that includes two circular windows; #172, an early-1870s building with semielliptical cast-iron arches in front, is unusually elaborate. Duane Park, an attractive triangle of benches and plantings, was the first open space that the City of New York acquired specifically for use as a public park, so it's older than both Central Park and Union Square.

- At the far west edge of the park, Duane Street splits to form a Y—make a hard right at the fork to walk on the upper part of Duane.

- Make a left onto Staple Street, a narrow, two-block-long road with an overhead walkway connecting the buildings on either side. Years ago this was a hospital complex, but now it's residential.

- Walk north to Harrison Street, where Staple ends, and go right to Hudson Street. At #6 Harrison is the original New York Mercantile Exchange, from 1884. Made of brick and granite, this red building with white accents looks like a schoolhouse and bears its name over the main entrance.

- Turn left on Hudson and walk one block to Franklin Street. Look at the building on the left that's white for the two lowest floors and then tan, with columns and pilasters to spare. This 1892 creation is the Powell Building; one of its tenants is the pricey Japanese restaurant Nobu.

- Make a right onto Franklin, a cobblestoned street that has several historic cast-iron buildings to ogle. At the corner of Varick Street, cast a side glance rightward to the New York Law School, a glass building one block over at Leonard Street.

- From here you can take the 1 train at Franklin Street. The downtown entrance is on the corner at Varick and Franklin; the uptown entrance, an attractive glass kiosk of a vaguely retro design, is across the street on a small island bordered by Varick and West Broadway.

POINTS OF INTEREST

PS 234 ps234.org, 292 Greenwich St., 212-233-6034

Silverstein Family Park 7 World Trade Center, bounded by Greenwich Street, West Broadway, and Barclay Street

Irish Hunger Memorial bpcparks.org/whats-here/parks/irish-hunger-memorial, Vesey Street and North End Avenue, 212-267-9700

Nelson A. Rockefeller Park River Terrace between Vesey and Chambers Streets

World Financial Center/Brookfield Place brookfieldplaceny.com, 200 Vesey St., 212-417-7000

Stuyvesant High School stuy.edu, 345 Chambers St., 212-312-4800

Borough of Manhattan Community College bmcc.cuny.edu, 199 Chambers St., 212-220-8000

Washington Market Park washingtonmarketpark.org, Greenwich Street between Chambers and Duane Streets

Bogardus Garden bogardusgarden.org, bounded by Hudson Street, West Broadway, and Reade Street

Duane Park nycgovparks.org/parks/duane-park, between Duane and Hudson Streets

ROUTE SUMMARY

1. Start at the Chambers Street subway station and walk west.
2. Make a left on Greenwich Street.
3. Go right on Barclay Street.
4. Turn left on West Street.
5. Go right on Vesey Street.
6. Cross North End Avenue into the Irish Hunger Memorial and Rockefeller Park.
7. Walk along river to the World Financial Center and enter the Winter Garden Pavilion.
8. Walk two blocks south of the World Financial Center on the Hudson River Greenway.
9. At Albany Street, cross to the east side of West Street and head left (north).
10. Cross the Tribeca Bridge to Stuyvesant High School, then double back and walk east on Chambers Street.

11.   At Hudson Street, make a left.

12.   Walk left at Duane Street, then make a hard right on Duane where it forks at the west end of Duane Park.

13.   Turn left on Staple Street.

14.   Turn right on Harrison Street.

15.   Turn left on Hudson Street.

16.   Turn right on Franklin Street.

17.   Take a train at either Franklin and Varick Streets or Varick and West Broadway.

CONNECTING THE WALKS

Walk north on Varick Street about 14 blocks for the start of Walk 10 (West Village). To reach the start of Walk 5 (Civic Center and Chinatown), walk about three blocks east on Franklin Street, then turn right on Broadway and walk about seven blocks to the City Hall subway station, on your left.

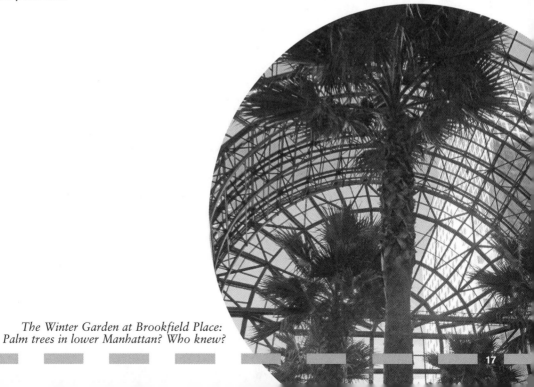

The Winter Garden at Brookfield Place:
Palm trees in lower Manhattan? Who knew?

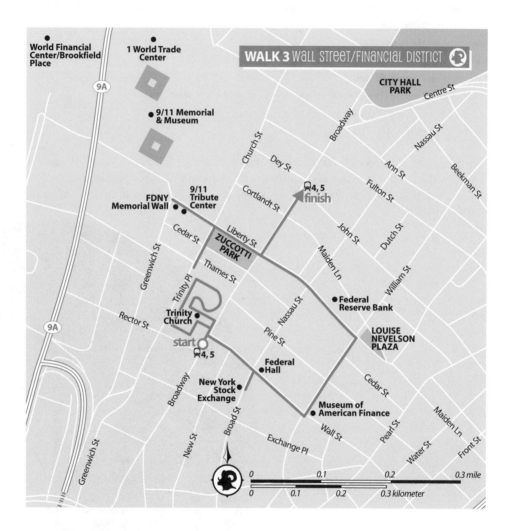

WALK 3 wall street/financial district

World Financial Center/Brookfield Place

1 World Trade Center

CITY HALL PARK

9/11 Memorial & Museum

9A

Church St

Dey St

Broadway

Centre St

Nassau St

Ann St

Beekman St

Cortlandt St

4, 5
finish

Fulton St

FDNY Memorial Wall

9/11 Tribute Center

John St

Dutch St

Cedar St

Liberty St

ZUCCOTTI PARK

Maiden Ln

William St

Greenwich St

Thames St

Trinity Pl

Rector St

9A

Trinity Church

Nassau St

Federal Reserve Bank

LOUISE NEVELSON PLAZA

start
4, 5

Pine St

Cedar St

Federal Hall

Broadway

New St

New York Stock Exchange

Broad St

Museum of American Finance

Wall St

Pearl St

Water St

Maiden Ln

Front St

Greenwich St

Exchange Pl

0   0.1   0.2   0.3 mile

0   0.1   0.2   0.3 kilometer

3 Wall Street/Financial District: risen from the ashes

BOUNDARIES: **Trinity Place, Wall St., William St., Greenwich St.**
DISTANCE: **3 miles**
SUBWAY: **4 or 5 to Wall St.**

Manhattan's Financial District has always been about so much more than the coming and going of fortunes; it is a fascinating place freighted with layers of historical significance. The American Revolution made its mark here. The first capital of the United States was located here. The stock market crashes of 1929 and 1987, along with the economic crisis of 2008, haunt the area. And Tuesday, September 11, 2001, forever changed this neighborhood—more than any other—with the terrorist attacks on the World Trade Center.

Wall Street and its environs are always teeming with activity, but amid the hustle and bustle of workers there is room for the tourist, the pensive walker. A slow, observant walk through the streets will always stay with you. Take special care when you visit Trinity Church, Federal Hall, and the 9/11 Memorial & Museum.

● The subway station on Broadway has more than one exit. If you need to, ask someone to point you to Wall Street and Broadway—or look for the steeple of Trinity Church and walk toward it. There has been a Trinity Church in Manhattan since the late 1690s; the present building, its third, dates to 1846 and was designed by Richard Upjohn. A distinctive feature of this somber brown Gothic Revival structure is the diamond-shaped clock facing south. In addition to the classic statues of saints, note the huge spiderlike sculpture made from a giant sycamore downed on 9/11.

● Walk into the cemetery to the left of the church's main entrance, and roam. There are military memorial stones, including that of Captain James Lawrence, famous for the phrase "Don't give up the ship!" The most eye-catching sight is the statue of stony-faced John Watts, a lawyer and member of the US House of Representatives. Many other tombstones are cracked and hard to read from fading, but the two best-known residents here are steamboat inventor Robert Fulton and Alexander Hamilton.

Walk into the northern section of the churchyard to see the grave of Albert Gallatin (a member of Congress and a founder of New York University), the Astor Cross (the Astor family has a long, prominent history in New York City), the Soldiers' Monument, the Firemen's Memorial Monument, and others. Small patches of herb garden are interspersed.

Go through the church's marvelous main entrance, comprising a carved wooden Christ-and-saints set and brass doors with biblical scenes. Even the ceiling of the vestibule is gorgeous. As you walk around and admire the church interior, you may stumble upon a live musical performance.

- Leave the church and face the other side of Broadway. At #100 is the American Surety Building, an early skyscraper from the 1890s. Among its many features are an ornate entrance and caryatids that seem almost alive. To the right, at #1 Wall Street, is the cavernous Bank of New York (now BNY Mellon) Building. An engraving in the Art Deco tower proudly announces "1930" (the year construction was begun), with contemporary feathered designs carved into the limestone. Look for the plaque titled SITE OF WALL OF NEW AMSTERDAM—yes, Wall Street is named for a long-gone wall built in the 17th century to protect the Dutch settlement that became New York City. The soaring glass entrance of the building is beautiful: The copper-colored walls in the lobby, coupled with the glass outside, make it seem as though the interior were encased in amber.

- Walk on Wall Street to Broad Street and make a right to see the New York Stock Exchange, with its iconic Corinthian-columned facade. It used to have a visitors' gallery, but since 9/11 it's difficult to get in—or even too close—without a major security clearance.

- Turn back to Wall Street and admire Federal Hall, a handsome Greek Revival building with steep steps (a wheelchair-accessible entrance is around the corner). This building has an amazing history: It served first as New York's city hall, then as the first capitol of the fledgling United States. It was also the site of George Washington's inauguration. If you use the main entrance, bid hello to the eagle statue above the clock.

- Upon leaving Federal Hall, walk left to 37 Wall St., the Tiffany & Co. building, a 1907 Beaux Arts treasure originally built for Morgan Guaranty.

- Make a left on William Street. The building at the northwest corner houses the Museum of American Finance. Affiliated with the Smithsonian Institution, it's the only independent museum in the United States dedicated to the history of money, banking, and business. Go one block to Our Lady of Victory Church, a Roman Catholic site also known as the War Memorial Church. It was dedicated in 1947, but its redbrick Georgian Revival design makes it look older. The sanctuary has a stirring half-rose stained-glass window of a sunrise over lower Manhattan, highlighting the Twin Towers that fell on 9/11.

- Continue along William Street until you reach the triangular park at Liberty Street, Louise Nevelson Plaza. Nevelson designed the sculptures and other aspects of the small park, which opened in 1978 and was one of the first plazas in New York City to be named for a woman, and the first to be named for an artist. To the left, along Liberty Street at Nassau Street, is the stern-looking Federal Reserve Bank of New York, built in a subdued Renaissance Revival style. Guided tours are available; among the locations you see is where gold bars are stored in a sub-basement.

- Walk left along Liberty Street. At 55 Liberty stands a 33-story skyscraper built in 1909; it's now a largely residential building called Liberty Tower. Next door to the left is #65, the former Chamber of Commerce building (now a Chinese bank), which has ostentatious round windows on one level and dormer windows higher up. Walk farther, and at Broadway you'll come to the large, dark, modern office building that houses the investment bank Brown Brothers Harriman. The plaza in front is home to the curious red sculpture *The Cube* by Isamu Noguchi.

- Cross Broadway and enter Zuccotti Park. This used to be called Liberty Plaza Park because 1 Liberty Plaza (a.k.a. the US Steel Building) is the large modern building to the right. (I worked a student internship in that building in 1985, for the Financial News Network.) Zuccotti Park, which was the site of the Occupy Wall Street encampment, has a large, bright-red modernist sculpture on the Cedar Street side and a sunken seating area with lush plantings. Walk around, take a rest on a bench, and admire a side view of the ornate building on the left at 115 Broadway, the US Realty Building. Decorating it are a few styles of gargoyles, some of them quite macabre.

- Walk through the park to Trinity Place and check out the statue of a seated businessman rummaging through his briefcase. Called *Double Check,* it was sculpted by J. Seward Johnson. (Note the vintage cassette recorder in the businessman's case.)

- Cross Cedar Street on the south side of Zuccotti Park, and walk on Trinity Place. Across the street, look onto narrow Thames Street. On the next block of Trinity Place, see #86, the former site of the American Stock Exchange, opposite the west side of Trinity Church and its cemetery. Designated as a landmark by the city in 2012, the handsome Art Deco structure has remained vacant since 2008.

- Walk back to Liberty Street, then go left on it. At #120 is the 9/11 Tribute Center, a project of the nonprofit September 11th Families' Association. Its exhibits are powerful, but in my opinion, the tribute at 124 Liberty is even more moving. Here, at the FDNY Ladder Co. 10/Engine Co. 10 firehouse, a 56-foot-long bronze bas-relief sculpture is dedicated to the firefighters who perished during 9/11. Flanking a tableau of the Twin Towers on fire are scenes of firefighters at work on that day, along with inscriptions reading DEDICATED TO THOSE WHO FELL AND TO THOSE WHO CARRY ON and MAY WE NEVER FORGET. The names of the fallen are engraved below the sculpture, flanked by twin Maltese crosses (the traditional fire-service symbol) bearing the number "343"—the total FDNY death toll.

- If you want to visit the site of the original World Trade Center, go across Greenwich Street. If not, look over your shoulder to see the new 1 World Trade Center (formerly named Freedom Tower). This sleek combo of glass, metal, and ingenuity is the tallest building in the western hemisphere and the fourth tallest in the world. Also gaze at the flags of the 9/11 Memorial. Admission is free for the memorial—reflecting pools in the Twin Towers' footprints, with the names of those who died engraved on the pools' perimeters—but there's a charge for the museum on the grounds (see website for details).

- Walk east along Liberty Street until it meets Broadway, then turn left to reach the ultramodern Fulton Street station, a hub bringing together several subway lines.

POINTS OF INTEREST

Trinity Church trinitywallstreet.org, 74 Trinity Pl., 212-602-0800

New York Stock Exchange nyse.com, 18 Broad St., 212-656-3000

Federal Hall nps.gov/feha, 26 Wall St., 212-825-6990

Museum of American Finance mcaf.org, 48 Wall St., 212-908-4110

Louise Nevelson Plaza Bounded by William Street, Maiden Lane, and Liberty Street

Federal Reserve Bank of New York ny.frb.org, 33 Liberty St., 212-720-5000

Zuccotti Park Broadway at Liberty Street

9/11 Tribute Center tributewtc.org, 120 Liberty St., 212-393-9160

FDNY Memorial Wall fdnytenhouse.com/fdnywall, 124 Liberty St.

1 World Trade Center onewtc.com, bounded by West, Vesey, Fulton, and Washington Streets

9/11 Memorial (National September 11 Memorial & Museum) 911memorial.org, 180 Greenwich St., 212-266-5211

route summary

1. Begin at Wall Street and Broadway, and see Trinity Church and its cemetery.
2. Walk on Wall Street to Broad Street and go right.
3. Return to Wall Street and continue in the direction you'd been heading.
4. Walk left on William Street.
5. Walk left at Liberty Street.
6. Cross Broadway and enter Zuccotti Park.
7. Walk left on Trinity Place, then reverse direction.
8. Walk left on Liberty Street to Greenwich Street.
9. Return on Liberty Street to Broadway, then go left to Fulton Street for the train.

connecting the walks

The next walk (City Hall and South Street Seaport) starts where this one ends. For the Civic Center and Chinatown tour (Walk 5), walk north on Broadway almost seven blocks until you reach the City Hall R train station, on your right just past Murray Street.

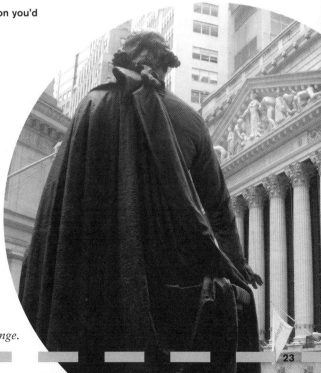

George Washington surveys the Stock Exchange.

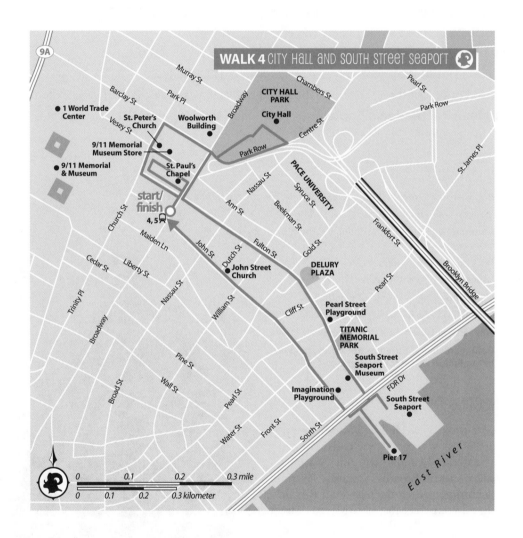

9A

Murray St

Barclay St

Park Pl

Broadway

Chambers St

Pearl St

CITY HALL PARK

City Hall

Park Row

1 World Trade Center

St. Peter's Church

Vesey St

Woolworth Building

Centre St

Park Row

9/11 Memorial Museum Store

St. James Pl

St. Paul's Chapel

PACE UNIVERSITY

9/11 Memorial & Museum

Nassau St

Spruce St

Church St

start/ finish

4, 5

Ann St

Beekman St

Frankfort St

Maiden Ln

John St

Dutch St

Fulton St

Gold St

Brooklyn Bridge

Cedar St

Liberty St

John Street Church

DELURY PLAZA

Trinity Pl

Nassau St

William St

Cliff St

Pearl St

Pearl Street Playground

TITANIC MEMORIAL PARK

Broadway

Pine St

South Street Seaport Museum

FDR Dr

Broad St

Wall St

Pearl St

Imagination Playground

South Street Seaport

Water St

Front St

South St

Pier 17

East River

0   0.1   0.2   0.3 mile

0   0.1   0.2   0.3 kilometer

4 CITY HALL AND SOUTH STREET SEAPORT: CITY HALL AWAITS YOUR CALL

BOUNDARIES: **Broadway, Barclay St., East River, Fulton St.**
DISTANCE: **2.7 miles**
SUBWAY: **A/C/J/2/3/4/5 to Fulton St.**

During the second half of the 1990s, I worked near City Hall. Each day I commuted by train to one of the busiest parts of Manhattan and jockeyed for sidewalk space once I got there. I joined thousands of workers, students, tourists, and fellow New Yorkers who frequented municipal buildings to get licenses, deal with parking tickets, attend court sessions, and conduct research, among other things. I taught at the oddly shaped Murry Bergtraum High School, a large public school with a business theme. It was the best teaching experience of my career.

A built-in bonus of working at MBHS was having City Hall and the South Street Seaport area at my reach. I could easily run errands or shop after school. When I had time on my hands to play tourist, I'd roam the neighborhood, camera in hand (I ran the school's photography club), and admire the architecture and monuments liberally sprinkled about. I had my favorite restaurants and snack shops, and sometimes my colleagues and I would visit one of the bars near the Seaport or stroll to Chinatown to eat congee. If a parade was passing nearby (for the Yankees' World Series win, for example—more on that later), we would stop and watch at some point. Everyone enjoyed scoping out bargains at the discount stores on Fulton Street.

It's hard to believe how spiffy City Hall looks now, its park playing host to rotating outdoor art exhibits, farmers' markets, and other activities. You'll find plenty of other things to see and do around here, though. So don't fight City Hall—have fun at its expense!

● **The Fulton Street subway station is a labyrinthine tangle of platforms, staircases, artwork, shops, and confusion. Whichever train gets you here, look for signs that direct you to an exit on Broadway (if you get out on John Street or Fulton Street, ask for directions to Broadway). As you get some distance from the station, take a look at the "dome" over it. This 2010 addition resembles a Bundt cake pan.**

- Once on Broadway, walk to St. Paul's Chapel, on the north side of Fulton Street. Built in 1766, this is the oldest surviving church building in Manhattan (once upon a time, it was also the tallest building in the city). The brown-and-buff exterior, with its Ionic-columned portico, is kind of somber, but the interior is quite light and airy. The sanctuary has many tributes to 9/11; in the days following the attacks, first responders took refuge here. In addition to prayer and worship, visitors can partake of St. Paul's numerous interactive elements, such as the Pilgrimage Altar (you can contribute your thoughts), the Memorial Altar (remembering 9/11 victims), and other spots to add mementos.

  Remarkable historical artifacts are displayed here as well. The Governor's Box consists of two upholstered chairs with a small wooden border, for use when a governor attends services. George Washington's Pew (actually a replica) is a legendary part of the church; he worshiped here when New York City was the US capital. A beautiful side chapel, trimmed in white and gold, bears the Hebrew word for God on an arch above the altar. Walk outside to the churchyard, which in the wake of 9/11 was heavily covered with debris. Now it offers a monumental view of the new 1 World Trade Center.

- From St. Paul's, make a right on Broadway and then a right on Fulton Street. The 29-story white building on the left, at 195 Broadway, is the old AT&T Building, now owned by Sony. Completed in 1916, it was the site of the first transatlantic phone call.

- Make a right from Fulton onto Church Street and look up, up, up at the new World Trade Center—a triumph over terrorism. Its spire makes it the tallest building in the United States, built to a symbolic 1,776 feet high. New York, and the world, are in awe.

- Continue on Church to Vesey Street. To the left, at #90, is the Federal Office Building and US Post Office. Taking up an entire city block, this Art Deco slab of a building has chiseled eagle decorations. Then turn right onto Vesey. At #20 is the 9/11 Memorial Museum Store, an off-site location that sells souvenirs and also displays artifacts and documentation about that horrific day and its aftermath.

- Next, admire the New York County Lawyers Association, with its six classic pilasters.

- Walk back to Church Street and turn right. Admire more fully the Federal Office Building, festooned with five-point stars, on your left.

● Make a right on Barclay Street, in front of St. Peter's Roman Catholic Church. Near the corner is a cross of silver that resembles a person, and below is a nook with a silver book of names. Both are tributes to 9/11. St. Peter's is the oldest Catholic parish in New York State. This Greek Revival building dates to 1838 and has a covered porch hung with brass lamps; historical markers line the outer wall. The sanctuary walls are mostly white, giving the space a peaceful feel.

● Across the street as you approach Broadway, you will see a magnificent building that fairly drips with detail. There are many faces and gargoyles to be found! Cass Gilbert designed this wonder: the Woolworth Building, the tallest building in the world from 1913 to 1930. The lobby has glittering mosaics and stained glass, but you can't go inside unless you have official business here or you're taking one of the occasional tours of the building.

● Cross Broadway onto Park Row, which curves slightly as it emerges from Barclay Street. Turn left into City Hall Park, often filled with local workers eating lunch. It hosts temporary exhibitions of sculpture and art. Floor plaques (some with maps) explain the history of the area and document the park itself. A restored fountain is a showcase piece here.

Closer to the City Hall building is a statue of patriot Nathan Hale. Take a good look at City Hall, built in 1811 and altered at various times. Its Renaissance Revival style gives it a royal demeanor, but it is so very American, having been in use longer than any other US city hall.

● Exit the park to the right when facing City Hall, and you should see the Brooklyn Bridge. Walk right on Park

Historic ships remind us of Manhattan's past.

Row for two impressive-looking structures with notable histories. Now part of Pace University, 41 Park Row was built in 1889 to house *The New York Times.* The red-and-black edifice at #38 is the Potter Building, built just a few years earlier. It had very advanced fireproofing for its time and is a masterwork of terra-cotta detail.

- Continue along Park Row, which merges into Broadway. Make a left onto Fulton Street. Among the many stores in this stretch are some with unusual architectural details. Notice the accessories shop at #144, which despite its uninteresting contemporary veneer at street level has intriguing turn-of-the-century decorations (a small, elegant pediment flanked by octagonal-shaped lamps) near its curving roofline. At the southwest corner of Nassau Street, 130 Fulton is a lovely Renaissance Revival building from 1893 that's now largely residential. Amid the terra-cotta flourishes, busts of a handsome youth peek out of the colonnade along what was once the highest floor. Unfortunately, a 2005 addition to the top of the building looks tacked on.

- Walk more along Fulton and check out stores, eats, and such. At Gold Street is John J. Delury Sr. Plaza, a small park named for (wait for it) a city sanitation worker. Past Cliff Street, a one-block-long path on your left, is St. Margaret's House, a senior facility at 49 Fulton. The outside exemplifies cloddish postwar construction, but inside the lobbies are brightened with amateur artworks. When I taught at Bergtraum High, I sometimes ate tasty and low-priced lunches at St. Margaret's cafeteria.

- A block up, at Pearl Street, is the cheery Pearl Street Playground, which my daughters used to romp around when they were younger. Across the street is a tall office building with a quirky plaza area. There are seats in primary colors and a setup that resembles convoluted giant monkey bars.

- Turn right onto Water Street to see the large outdoor digital clock on the building at the corner of Water and John Street. It's fun to watch in action. Return to Fulton Street to see Titanic Memorial Park. History buffs and fans of the film will appreciate this pensive patch, with its white lighthouse and rock-filled garden plot.

- Water Street continues on the park's south side, split from the part you just passed by. Here, it's a cobblestone street with old buildings, enhanced to look more like a throwback. The South Street Seaport Museum is located here, along with pieces such as an anchor and tie-posts on the street.

- As you resume walking toward the river on Fulton Street, it too becomes a cobble-stoned walkway. (Hopefully you aren't wearing stilettos.) Along the way, you'll see shops and restaurants housed in redbrick Federal-style buildings.

- Cross carefully at South Street to the fabled South Street Seaport's piers. This is a relaxing, picturesque place to roam. Admire the elevated highway over your shoulder, as well as skyscrapers not far away. A walking and biking path runs under the high-way and along the river.

- Walk toward the water side of Pier 15 to enjoy the East River views and admire the bridges: Brooklyn (closest), Manhattan (middle), and Williamsburg (farthest north). You can also see the Brooklyn neighborhoods of Brooklyn Heights (including the Promenade) and Dumbo, some of Brooklyn's piers, boats upon the water, and more. Next to Pier 17 are a few old-style ships to gaze at and, possibly, go aboard. Check out the 1885 iron sailing ship *Wavetree,* the lightship *Ambrose* from 1908, and others. A new Pier 17 is slated to open in 2016.

- When you finally pull yourself away from this scene, go back across South Street and walk northwest on John Street, passing the Imagination Playground, an interactive play space created by celebrated architect David Rockwell, on your right. John Street follows a mildly wiggly path, and it has many shops to peer into. At #44 is the John Street Church, the oldest Methodist congregation in North America, founded in 1766. The 1846 church house is dark and grim-looking from the outside, but inside it has a homey simplicity: white walls and pews, with plaques on the walls and modestly decorated stained-glass windows. A bit past the church is an entrance to the Fulton Street subway station.

POINTS OF INTEREST

St. Paul's Chapel trinitywallstreet.org/content/st-pauls-chapel, 209 Broadway, 212-602-0800

9/11 Memorial Museum Store tinyurl.com/911museumstore, 20 Vesey St., 212-267-2047

St. Peter's Roman Catholic Church stpetersnyc.org, 22 Barclay St., 212-233-8355

Woolworth Building woolworthtours.com, 233 Broadway, 203-966-9663

City Hall Park and City Hall nycgovparks.org/parks/city-hall-park, Broadway and Park Row at Barclay Street, 212-639-9675

John J. Delury Sr. Plaza Fulton Street between Gold Street and Ryders Alley

Pearl Street Playground Fulton and Pearl Streets

Titanic Memorial Park Fulton Street between Pearl and Water Streets

South Street Seaport Museum southstreetseaportmuseum.org, 12 Fulton St., 212-748-8600

South Street Seaport southstreetseaport.com, Fulton Street and South Street, 212-732-8257

Imagination Playground Bounded by John Street, Front Street, and South Street

John Street Church johnstreetchurch.org, 44 John St., 212-269-0014

route summary

1. Commence at Fulton St. and Broadway, and go into St. Paul's Chapel.
2. Walk right on Broadway.
3. Go right on Fulton Street.
4. Walk right on Church Street.
5. Walk right on Vesey Street.
6. Walk back to Church Street and turn right.
7. Walk right on Barclay Street.
8. At Park Row, enter City Hall Park.
9. Exit the park and make a right on Park Row.
10. Merge onto Broadway.
11. Go left onto Fulton Street, dipping in and out of Water Street to the right.
12. Cross South Street from Fulton to the piers.
13. Make a right across South Street onto John Street.
14. Take the train from the entrance just past John Street Church, or continue up John Street to the subway station on Broadway.

CONNeCTING THe WaLKS

The previous walk (Wall Street/Financial District) can be done in reverse from the start of this one. For the next walk (Civic Center and Chinatown), go north on Broadway almost seven blocks until you reach the City Hall R train station, just past Murray Street on your right.

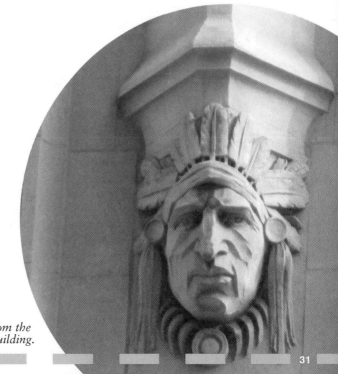

A somber Native American peers out from the Woolworth Building.

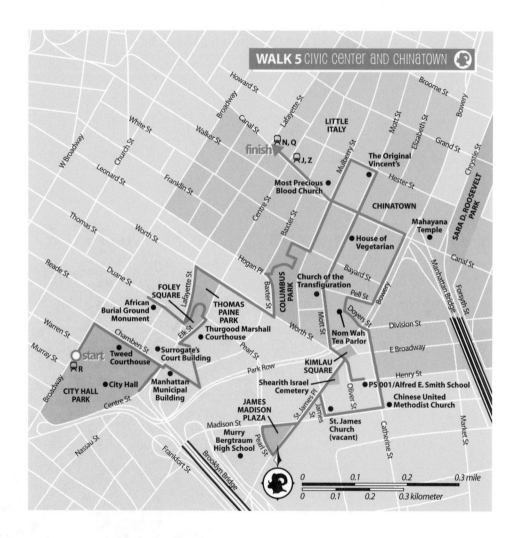

Howard St

Broome St

Bowery

Broadway

Canal St

Lafayette St

LITTLE
ITALY

Mott St

Elizabeth St

Grand St

White St

Walker St

Church St

The Original
Vincent's

Chrystie St

Leonard St

Franklin St

Mulberry St

Hester St

W Broadway

finish

N, Q

J, Z

SARA D. ROOSEVELT PARK

Most Precious ●
Blood Church

CHINATOWN

Mahayana
Temple ●

Centre St

Baxter St

Thomas St

Worth St

● House of
Vegetarian

Canal St

Reade St

Duane St

Hogan Pl

Bayard St

Manhattan Bridge

Forsyth St

Lafayette St

FOLEY
SQUARE

Baxter St

COLUMBUS
PARK

Church of the
Transfiguration

Pell St

Bowery

African ●
Burial Ground
Monument

THOMAS
PAINE
PARK

Elk St

Doyers St

Division St

Warren St

Chambers St

Thurgood Marshall
Courthouse ●

Worth St

Mott St

Nom Wah
Tea Parlor

E Broadway

Murray St

● Surrogate's
Court Building

Pearl St

● Tweed
Courthouse

Park Row

KIMLAU
SQUARE

Henry St

Broadway

start

R

● City Hall

Manhattan
Municipal
Building

Shearith Israel
Cemetery

St. James Pl

Oliver St

● PS 001/Alfred E. Smith School

Chinese United
● Methodist Church

CITY HALL
PARK

Centre St

JAMES
MADISON
PLAZA

James St

St. James
Church
(vacant)

Catherine St

Market St

Madison St

Murry
Bergtraum
High School ●

Pearl St

Nassau St

Frankfort St

Brooklyn Bridge

0   0.1   0.2   0.3 mile

0   0.1   0.2   0.3 kilometer

5 CIVIC CENTER AND CHINATOWN: CULTURE CRAWL

BOUNDARIES: **Broadway, Grand St., Mott St., Murray St.**
DISTANCE: **3.4 miles**
SUBWAY: **R to City Hall**

Manhattan has places that are busy and frenetic interspersed with relatively relaxed and even quiet spots. The Civic Center and Chinatown are two such places, neighboring precincts where people are constantly on the go—walk through either district, and you'll hear dialects of legalese and Chinese spoken loudly—but even in these neighborhoods you can find mellower outposts.

The Civic Center area is dominated by buildings dedicated to public services and agencies, politics, law, and official business of many types; it also provides fascinating lessons in history and culture. Chinatown is lively and gritty, exotic to tourists and many New Yorkers alike.

The energy in both areas is immeasurable, but don't be afraid to stop your stroll. Public parks offer seats for the weary. Slow down to examine artistic details, architectural touches, and more. Check out the wares sold by street vendors, or perhaps pause for some dim sum.

- When you arrive at the City Hall station, ascend the stairs and walk on Broadway with City Hall and City Hall Park to your right. Dispersed throughout parts of the sidewalk are panels with historical and geographical lessons, such as one about the "British Soldiers' Barracks." At Chambers Street, notice an old-fashioned clock clamped to the corner building on your right: THE SUN, IT SHINES FOR ALL is the message delivered along with the time. It's a reference to *The Sun,* a newspaper published from 1833 to 1950.

- Go to the right along Chambers. The building with many stairs, its pediment supported by four classical columns, is the Tweed Courthouse, back-to-back with City Hall. Ah, William Magear Tweed—perhaps the most cartoonishly crooked politico in New York City history. This handsome Italianate building was built with a rapidly rising tab, due to corruption in "Boss" Tweed's time. Now it houses the Department of Education, among other city services.

Back Story: a Tale Out of School

New Yorkers love their Yankees. (Some love the Mets too.) The New York Yankees have won more World Series than any other Major League Baseball team; thus, a heckuva lotta victory parades have been held in the Yankees' honor. One year, some friends and I nearly got swallowed up in one such parade.

The Yanks won the Series in 1998, sweeping the San Diego Padres. At the time, I was teaching at Murry Bergtraum High School in downtown Manhattan, and on the day of the parade, our usually solid student attendance was way down. Enthusiastic students warned us grumpy adults in advance that they would be at the parade, so please don't give homework or tests that day, pleasepleaseplease.

Along with Howard, Nigel, and Robin, three of my cronies from the social studies

department, I hatched a lunchtime plan to go over to the parade—it was, after all, practically at our doorstep. Once there, we realized that we were thick in a throng and we might have a hard time getting back in time to teach our next classes.

We saw a bit of the parade—the crowds being what they were, we heard a lot more than we saw—and then we had to beg the beleaguered police officers on duty to help us get back to Bergtraum. They had us enter the Brooklyn Bridge subway station, walk through the concourse level, and come back up across the street. Of course, there was the one cop who didn't quite buy our story about being teachers trying to make their way back to work. But we did it, returning in time to teach just a handful of kids, who seemed resentful that they too hadn't braved the crowds outside.

● Across the street is a more opulent building, the Emigrant Industrial Savings Bank. Notice the beehive decorations on the main doors. (Other old bank buildings in town have bees and beehive decor, apparently symbolic links to Freemasonry, royalty, and even productivity.) Farther down the block is 31 Chambers St., the Surrogate's Court. Among the city offices and services housed here are the Municipal Archives, records offices, the Department of Cultural Affairs, county courts, and more. The main lobby and staircases are gorgeous Beaux Arts dreams. The outside has fanciful statues and carvings, columns, and a roof that is full of detail and replete with beautiful windows.

● Walk more and behold 1 Centre St., the Manhattan Municipal Building. Many New Yorkers come and go here all the time and don't think much about it—trust me on that. But for five years I walked by it or through it every workday, when I taught at nearby Murry Bergtraum High School, and I did admire its art and architecture. Several city agencies are based here, as are the offices of the Manhattan borough president. First occupied in 1913, this regal C-shaped building of neoclassical design rises 40 stories and is topped by a gilded statue called *Civic Fame* that can be seen from afar. She holds a five-peaked crown, each peak representing one of the five boroughs. The building's south arcade has a ceiling of lovely white Guastavino tiles. (In case you didn't know, any place in New York City that has Guastavino tiling always brags about it.)

● Wander around here a bit, then go back across Centre Street and to the left, into City Hall Park, where you'll encounter the Horace Greeley statue, the Joseph Pulitzer plaque, the quaint domed kiosk entrance of the Brooklyn Bridge subway station, and more. (Sometimes you might see fenced pens of vegetables growing on the grass in this part of the park.) The pedestrian access to the Brooklyn Bridge is next to the Municipal Building. On the other side of the bridge entrances, note a tall, shimmery metallic building in the near distance. That's 8 Spruce St., a.k.a. New York by Gehry, a reference to its architect, Frank Gehry.

Turn around and gaze again at the Surrogate's Court building; try to discern the statues near the top. The pegleg guy is Peter Stuyvesant, governor of the Dutch colony of New Amsterdam from 1647 to 1664. He was roundly disliked in his time but is memorialized in many ways throughout Manhattan.

● Walk back to the Municipal Building and follow the path through the arcade to the spacious plaza area. You'll see a few intriguing sights, such as the Sugar House Prison Window, part of a Revolutionary War–era prison (although there is some debate about that), and the curious red sculpture called *Five in One,* by Bernard Rosenthal. Like the *Civic Fame* statue, it references the five boroughs of New York City, in this case with five giant interlocking disks. Farther ahead on the right is Police Plaza, headquarters for the NYPD.

● Where the pathway through the Municipal Plaza ends, walk left on St. Andrew's Plaza, follow it back to Centre Street (also signed as Foley Square) and turn right. Along this stretch, there are often food kiosks as well as seating areas. On your right, you'll come first to the massive Thurgood Marshall US Courthouse, with its 30-story tower, and then the New York State Supreme Court Building, reminiscent of a Greek temple. neoclassical in design, these buildings are often in the news; trucks and vans from media outlets are usually nearby. The Supreme Court Building should also be familiar to fans of TV's *Law & Order.*

● Across Centre St. from the courts are Thomas Paine Park to the north and Foley Square to the south. Foley Square has a black-marble modernist sculpture called *Triumph of the Human Spirit,* which relates to the nearby African Burial Ground. The horizontal piece is meant to evoke a slave ship, the vertical piece an African antelope mask. This space was originally the Collect Pond, a freshwater source that was drained and filled in (1811). During the Victorian era, the immediate neighborhood was known as the rough and tough Five Points, a breeding ground for gangs that was immortalized in the novel and movie *Gangs of New York.* Hard to believe that this highly bureaucratic district was once so lawless.

● From the south end of Foley Square (more of a triangle, really), walk northwest on Duane Street. The modern building on your right, with the huge glass windows, is the United States Court of International Trade. Just past it is 26 Federal Plaza, the Jacob K. Javits Federal Building. (Javits was a longtime US senator from New York.) If you like 1960s space-age office buildings, you'll love this one.

Evoking a completely different era and mood are the green space and memorial to your left at Elk Street, the African Burial Ground National Monument. In 1991, during excavation for the construction of a government building, hundreds of graves were discovered; research determined the site to have been a major burial ground for enslaved and free blacks from the late 17th century into the 18th century. The current site, comprising a monument, burial mounds, and a visitor center, is supervised by the National Park Service. Granite structures, the Circle of the Diaspora and the Ancestral Chamber, are inscribed with signs and symbols that are significant to different African cultures, such as an Egyptian ankh, a Muslim star and crescent, and a Ghanaian *sankofa.*

● Walk back on Duane Street to Lafayette Street and turn left.

- At Worth Street, lined with even more government buildings, make a right. On your left is the New York City Department of Health building; the geometric metal grill-work over its entrance is a typical Art Deco touch. A freestanding column topped with a stylized eagle flanks each side of the entrance. Then cross Centre Street to see the Louis J. Lefkowitz State Office Building, named for a New York attorney general. Art Deco with a twist, this 1928 building incorporates Egyptian elements into both its exterior ornamentation (such as the sphinxlike gargoyles at the roofline) and its extravagant lobby. A bit farther along Worth on the right side is a newer court building, the Daniel Patrick Moynihan United States Courthouse, named for the late New York senator. It's opposite Columbus Park, an oddly shaped but appealing green space with a playground, sports courts, lots of benches, and an open-air pavilion on its northern end. Nowadays it seems relaxed, dominated by Chinese seniors playing mah-jongg or doing Tai Chi exercises, kids running around, teens shooting hoops. But in the mid-1800s this was Mulberry Bend, the heart of Five Points, rife with slum housing and gang domination.

- Walk on Baxter Street with Columbus Park to your right, passing the New York City Criminal Courts Building on your left, and make a right into the park. Just inside the entrance stands a bronze statue of Dr. Sun Yat-sen, the father of modern China, atop a descriptive black-marble base. Sun was once a New Yorker, having lived in China-town briefly at the turn of the century before returning home to help over-throw the Qing Dynasty and estab-lish the Republic of China.

- Notice the park's cottagelike pavil-ion, built in 1897. For decades, it was a blighted eyesore—and a favorite haunt of the city's pigeons—but it was renovated in 2007.

The stately columns of the Tweed Courthouse

- If you haven't been yanked into a game of checkers, continue on through the park to Mulberry Street and Bayard Street. The redbrick corner building diagonally across from the park, #70, has some cool architectural touches, such as corner windows set on diagonals. It was built as a public school in the early 1900s, but now Chen Dance Center and Chinatown Manpower Project are among the cultural and community tenants here. Walk onto Mulberry with that building to your right and examine a typical Chinatown street: fish store, tchotchkes and souvenirs, Chinese and Vietnamese eateries, and much more.

- Cross Canal Street carefully; it gets crowded here, and some drivers jump the traffic lights. Farther up Mulberry Street, the ethnic pride shifts to Italian. This was traditionally the heart of Little Italy, but over the years Chinatown has expanded and the Italian presence has diminished. Still, pause a moment to see the Church of the Most Precious Blood, set back from the street on your left. (If it looks plain and drab, that's because this is the rear of the church—the main entrance, on Baxter Street, would look right at home in Italy.) An arched gate announces the church's name; a colorful Statue of Liberty mural is painted on the side wall of the building next door. Most Precious Blood is a focal point of Little Italy's annual Feast of San Gennaro, an 11-day street fair held in late September.

  As you might expect, this block also has numerous Italian restaurants and pastry shops. The building at 121 Mulberry bears the inscription ANNA ESPOSITO 1926 near the roofline, along with a pretty sunburst decoration. (The Espositos, one of Little Italy's leading families, built #121.) Also notice the WELCOME TO HISTORIC LITTLE ITALY banners on streetlight poles. Red, white, and green streamers are strung from one side of the street to the other on Mulberry and other streets around here, reflecting the colors of the Italian flag.

- At Hester Street, make a right and you'll notice a greater concentration of Italian establishments. On the right, at Mott Street, is The Original Vincent's. Established in 1904, this red-sauce joint is one of the oldest restaurants in the area, and it has a nifty neon sign.

- The rest of Mott Street, however, is much more Chinese in character. Turn right on Mott; past Canal Street, at #68, is House of Vegetarian, one of the better-regarded vegan ethnic restaurants in Manhattan. (Try the turnip cake. My younger daughter and I love it.) At 64 Mott is the Eastern States Buddhist Temple. Housed in a storefront, it's far less splashy than other area temples but is nonetheless dominated by the color red. Look left at Bayard Street and you'll see The Original Chinatown Ice Cream Factory, the place for unusual ice-cream flavors such as red bean or lychee.

- Walk farther on Mott Street to where it bends at Pell Street. Here, on your right, are the Church of the Transfiguration, a Catholic congregation, and its companion school building. Built in the Georgian style, the church dates to 1801 (it was originally a Lutheran congregation) and features Manhattan schist as well as brownstone; an octagonal copper-clad tower was added in 1868. Inside, the church is beautiful and light, with a fresco of the Last Supper painted on the ceiling above the altar. Most of Transfiguration's parishioners are Chinese, so you'll see signs in both Chinese and English.

- As you walk along Mott and other streets in the vicinity, don't forget to notice the Eastern decorative touches on the buildings: human faces, sunbursts, floral swirls, shells, and such. Sometimes there are political touches, too, such as the Taiwanese flags hanging over Hop Lee Restaurant at 16 Mott.

- Mott Street ends at Bowery (also signed as Park Row and Chatham Square) and intersects Worth Street, Oliver Street, and East Broadway. Be vigilant when crossing Bowery, especially if there's no traffic cop on duty. Walk to the pedestrian plaza, Kimlau Square, which consists of a statue, memorial, and small park dedicated to Chinese American servicemen who perished in World War II. (The square is named for Benjamin Ralph Kimlau, a bomber pilot who grew up in New York City and was shot down over New Guinea in 1944.)

- With the park to your left, walk on Oliver Street and stop in front of the Mariners' Temple Baptist Church on Henry Street. It was built in the 1840s, in the Greek Revival style. Turn left on Henry Street; on your right is an old school building, still active, with GRAMMAR SCHOOL NO. 1 inscribed over its entrance. Known today as PS 001 Alfred E. Smith, the school dates to 1897.

- Go back in the direction you came on Henry and then Oliver to St. James Place. At the large intersection, make a left on St. James. Pass a building with a few stores, then come to a tiny cemetery, raised several feet off the ground and fenced in. This is the original cemetery of the Spanish–Portuguese synagogue Shearith Israel, established in 1654. It is the very first Jewish cemetery in the United States and the second-oldest burial ground in Manhattan—only the northernmost section of the cemetery at Trinity Church is older (see Walk 3). This is just a small portion of the original graveyard, situated on land purchased by the congregation from the Roosevelt family. Shearith Israel has two other small cemeteries in Manhattan (see Walk 9, Central Greenwich Village, and Walk 12, Chelsea and Madison Square Park; also see Walk 21, Central Park West, which includes the synagogue itself). This highly historic site is bedraggled now, but pay it respect.

● Walk a couple of blocks down St. James Place, passing James Madison Plaza on your right. Across Pearl Street on your right is a smaller triangular building, Murry Bergtraum High School. I taught here for five years (see Back Story), and it was a very good experience, although the classroom layout took some getting used to.

● Backtrack on St. James Place to James Street, and turn right. At the corner stands a triangle-shaped school building, Hall of St. James School, now used by the Transfiguration School upper campus (you passed Church of the Transfiguration a few blocks back, at Mott and Mosco Streets). Above the entrance, note the logo with the interlocking *S* and *J*.

● Walk south on James Street to see St. James Church, built in 1836. It's the second-oldest Catholic church building still standing in New York City; however, there is currently no active parish here. At the end of James Street you can see the sort-of-X-shaped apartment buildings of the Smith Houses, a public housing project named for Al Smith, a four-term governor of New York.

● Make a left on Madison Street and walk two blocks to Catherine Street. Make another left and admire the neat little brick Chinese United Methodist Church. It has pretty stained-glass windows and a plaque about the Five Points Mission, a Methodist charity established in 1850 (it moved to this site in 1921). As you cross Henry Street, you'll again see PS 001 on your left.

● Walk farther on Catherine and cross Bowery carefully, merging onto Doyers Street, a crooked little thoroughfare with an ugly concrete box of a post office. A bend in the street was known as the "Bloody Angle" decades ago because Chinese gangs (*tongs*) would fight there. At #13 is the Nom Wah Tea Parlor, which has been serving dim sum since 1920.

- Doyers ends at Pell Street; make a right on Pell and walk until you hit Bowery in one block. Across the street is the Confucius Plaza complex. Go left on Bowery, crossing Bayard Street and then walking a lengthier block to Canal Street. To the right you have the Manhattan Bridge, and catty-corner from you is the Mahayana Temple Buddhist Association. It's big and colorful—and housed in a former adult-movie theater.

- Make a left on Canal—which was indeed a canal long ago—and pass a multitude of stores, offices, eateries, sidewalk vendors . . . a bit dizzying perhaps, but definitely an experience. You can catch the subway where Canal intersects Centre Street or Lafayette Street.

POINTS OF INTEREST

Surrogate's Court Building nycourts.gov/courts/1jd/surrogates, 31 Chambers St., 646-386-5000

Manhattan Municipal Building manhattanbp.nyc.gov, 1 Centre St., 212-669-8300

City Hall Park and City Hall nycgovparks.org/parks/city-hall-park, Broadway and Park Row at Barclay Street, 212-639-9675

Thurgood Marshall US Courthouse ca2.uscourts.gov, 40 Foley Square, 212-857-8500

New York State Supreme Court nycourts.gov, 60 Centre St., 646-386-3600

African Burial Ground National Monument nps.gov/afbg, 290 Broadway, 212-637-2019

Columbus Park nycgovparks.org/parks/columbus-park-m015, bounded by Mulberry Street, Baxter Street, Worth Street, and Bayard Street

Church of the Most Precious Blood tinyurl.com/mostpreciousblood, 109 Mulberry St., 212-226-6427

The Original Vincent's tinyurl.com/originalvincents, 119 Mott St., 212-226-8133

House of Vegetarian 68 Mott St., 212-226-6572

The Original Chinatown Ice Cream Factory chinatownicecreamfactory.com, 65 Bayard St., 212-608-4170

Church of the Transfiguration transfigurationnyc.org, 29 Mott St., 212-962-5157

Kimlau Square nycgovparks.org/parks/kimlau-square, bounded by Park Row/Chatham Square/Bowery, Oliver Street, and East Broadway

PS 001 Alfred E. Smith tinyurl.com/ps001alfredesmith, 8 Henry St., 212-267-4133

Chatham Square Cemetery, Congregation Shearith Israel shearithisrael.org/content/chatham-square-cemetery, 55 St. James Place

Murry Bergtraum High School for Business Careers tinyurl.com/bergtraumhs, 411 Pearl St., 212-964-9610

Chinese United Methodist Church cumc-nyc.org, 69 Madison St., 212-267-6464

Nom Wah Tea Parlor nomwah.com, 13 Doyers St., 212-962-6047

Mahayana Temple Buddhist Association mahayana.us, 113 Canal St., 212-925-8787

route summary

1. Walk up Broadway from City Hall station.
2. Walk right on Chambers Street to the Manhattan Municipal Building, across Centre Street.
3. Cross Centre Street to explore City Hall Park, then return to the Municipal Building.
4. Walk through the arcade/plaza of the Municipal Building and, where the walkway ends, turn left on St. Andrew's Plaza.
5. Follow St. Andrew's Plaza back to Centre Street, and turn right.
6. Go northeast on Centre Street into Foley Square and Thomas Paine Park.
7. From the south end of Foley Square, walk northwest on Duane Street to Elk Street.
8. Double back on Duane Street and make a left on Lafayette Street.
9. Make a right on Worth Street.
10. Go left on Baxter Street with Columbus Park on your right; enter the park in the middle of the block.
11. Go north on Mulberry Street out of the park.
12. Go right on Hester Street.
13. Go right on Mott Street.
14. Where Mott ends, cross Bowery to Kimlau Square, then go south on Oliver Street.
15. Make a left on Henry Street, walk halfway down the block, then go back the way you came to Oliver Street and then St. James Place.
16. Make a left on St. James, then turn around at Pearl Street.

17. Go right on James Street.

18. Go left on Madison Street.

19. Go left on Catherine Street.

20. Cross Bowery onto Doyers Street.

21. Walk right on Pell Street to Bowery.

22. Go left on Bowery.

23. Go left on Canal Street to one of the subway stations.

CONNECTING THE WALKS

To begin Walk 7 (The Bowery, Little Italy, and Soho), head east about six blocks on Canal Street to Chrystie Street, then walk two blocks north on Chrystie to Grand Street.

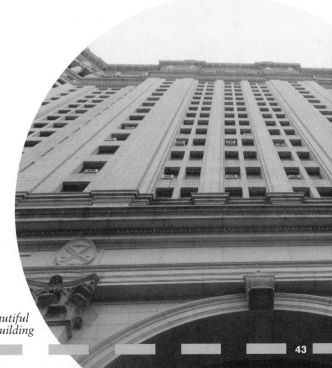

The busy, bureaucratic, yet beautiful
Municipal Building

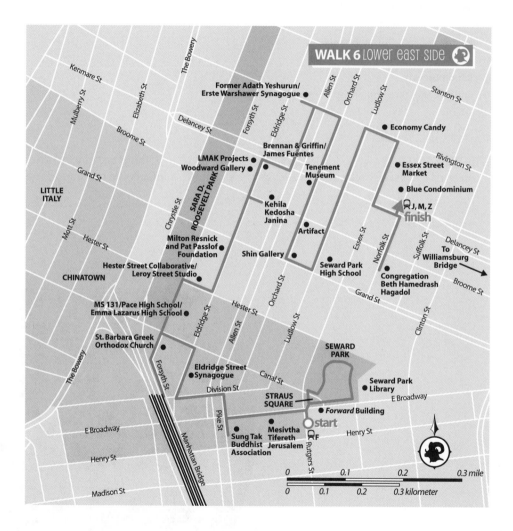

WALK 6 Lower east side

Kenmare St
The Bowery
Mulberry St
Elizabeth St
Broome St
Delancey St
Forsyth St
Eldridge St
Allen St
Orchard St
Ludlow St
Stanton St

Former Adath Yeshurun/
Erste Warshawer Synagogue

Economy Candy

Rivington St

Grand St

LITTLE
ITALY

Mott St

Hester St

Chrystie St

SARA D. ROOSEVELT PARK

Brennan & Griffin/
James Fuentes

LMAK Projects
Woodward Gallery

Tenement
Museum

Essex Street
Market

Blue Condominium

Kehila
Kedosha
Janina

J, M, Z
finish

CHINATOWN

Milton Resnick
and Pat Passlof
Foundation

Shin Gallery

Artifact

Seward Park
High School

Essex St
Norfolk St
Suffolk St

Delancey St
To
Williamsburg
Bridge

Congregation
Beth Hamedrash
Hagadol

Broome St

Hester Street Collaborative/
Leroy Street Studio

Hester St

Orchard St

Ludlow St

Grand St

Clinton St

MS 131/Pace High School/
Emma Lazarus High School

Eldridge St
Allen St

St. Barbara Greek
Orthodox Church

The Bowery

Forsyth St

Eldridge Street
Synagogue

Canal St

SEWARD
PARK

Division St

STRAUS
SQUARE

Seward Park
Library

E Broadway

Pike St

Forward Building

Manhattan Bridge

E Broadway

Sung Tak
Buddhist
Association

Mesivtha
Tifereth
Jerusalem

start

F

Rutgers St

Henry St

Henry St

Madison St

0   0.1   0.2   0.3 mile
0   0.1   0.2   0.3 kilometer

6 Lower East Side: History, Meet Hipster

BOUNDARIES: **E. Broadway, Chrystie St., Delancey St., Norfolk St.**
DISTANCE: **2.2 miles**
SUBWAY: **F to E. Broadway**

The Lower East Side has a mythic quality that is cherished by locals and tourists alike. Long known for its importance in Jewish American history, it has also been home base for generations of Latino and Chinese families and institutions. (Puerto Rican residents coined its Spanglish nickname, "Loisaida.") Lacking the polish and glamour of Midtown, the quaint historical feel of City Hall, the cultural cool of the Upper West Side, or the moneyed elegance of Fifth Avenue, the Lower East Side has long held a reputation as a gritty place where people strive, where kids run the streets, where vendors and businesspeople hustle. It's certainly more than that, of course, but it retains this essence in many ways.

The Lower East Side still shelters a mix of ethnicities, but with dollops of high style and hipster chic added to that mix. Upscale eateries, art galleries, posh or offbeat shops, and boutique hotels dwell side by side with grungy tenements and modest storefronts. And it seems like one out of five people is sipping a flavored bubble tea.

The neighborhood's major anchors include Seward Park (which my old assistant principal fondly referred to as "Sewer Park"), Sara D. Roosevelt Park, the stores of Delancey Street, and the Williamsburg Bridge, along with the many houses of worship that have sustained residents over the years.

As architectural evidence of the Lower East Side's deep Jewish roots, this walk takes you past 6 of New York City's 250 lost synagogues, which now serve non-Jewish congregations, have been repurposed for nonreligious use, or sit abandoned and in danger of being lost forever.

- **Emerge from the F station on Rutgers Street; East Broadway is half a block north. First take a look at the rustic Church of St. Teresa, housed in an old stone building that looks like it belongs in the countryside. Across the street is Captain Jacob Joseph Playground, more interesting for its name than the equipment in it. Joseph** was a World War II hero who died in battle, and the great-grandson of Rabbi Jacob Joseph, the first (and only) chief rabbi of New York City.

● Walk the half-block to East Broadway and turn right. On the north side of the street is Straus Square, a triangular plaza named for Nathan Straus, a department store mogul (Abraham & Straus, Macy's) and philanthropist. Just behind you at 173–75 East Broadway, towering above its neighbors, is the Forward Building (1912). It's pricey condos now, but for decades it served as the offices of *The Jewish Daily Forward,* the best-known Yiddish newspaper in the United States. The front entrance, the western outer wall, and other spots have FORWARD emblazoned on them. Peer up at the clock near the roof—here, the Hebrew lettering reads FORVERTS, Yiddish for "forward." Look for many opulent touches and a few surprises, such as carved heads of Karl Marx and Friedrich Engels. (Still published in print and online, *The Forward* was long associated with the socialist movement and continues to espouse progressive views today.)

● Cross East Broadway and walk into the park that's just north of Straus Square. This is Seward Park, the first permanent city playground in the US, opened in October 1903 and named for William H. Seward, the noted 19th-century statesman. It has benefited from renovations over the years, but some of its pieces are more than 100 years old. (The Jacob H. Schiff Fountain, on the west side, dates to 1895, but it was brought here in 1936 from another park.) Inside the park are play areas, sprinklers, sports fields, a white-and-blue field house, a running-dog statue, and pigeons galore. You'll often see Chinese senior citizens here working on their Tai Chi.

● Walk just east of the park to pay a visit to the Seward Park branch of the New York Public Library. It's a handsome old building (1909), heavily used, with artwork by locals festooning the walls. It's also one of 65 NYPL branches built with funding from Andrew Carnegie.

● Return to East Broadway and cross Rutgers Street heading right (west). At #145 is Mesivtha Tifereth Jerusalem, a prestigious house of learning for Orthodox Jewish men. Its main building has five stories, its annex three. Note the four arches along the ground floor of the main building. Next door to the annex is an apartment building with stores on the street level; while the building looks worn overall, it has impressive window decorations all along the third and fourth floors and roofline, including several Jewish stars. At #125, find a hybrid of Chinese and midcentury New York architecture at the Fukien Benevolent Association of America. Two grinning-lion statues flank the front door, and gilded Chinese characters are inscribed just above it. Even if you can't read the language, you can admire the style.

● Turn left at Pike Street. In the middle of the block is a large, off-white building that houses the Sung Tak Buddhist Association. Ascend the stairs and you'll see ritual items such as incense urns, statues of animals and deities, paper lanterns, and plaques. If the bright-red doors are open, peek inside to see the temple and its pieces, such as drums, firecracker strands, and bells.

The temple building (1904) was originally constructed in a hybrid Romanesque–Moorish Revival style for a prominent Jewish synagogue, B'nai Israel Kalwarie (Sons of Israel from Kalwaria, a Polish town). Better known as the Pike Street Shul, it was the birthplace of the Young Israel Modern Orthodox movement within Judaism. Out on the porch, you have views of the Manhattan Bridge, the grass dividers that partition wide Pike Street, and more.

● Return the way you came on Pike, past East Broadway, and turn left on Division Street.

● Make a right at Eldridge Street. At #12 is the Eldridge Street Synagogue, which opened in September 1887. It was the first purpose-built synagogue in the US for an Eastern European congregation. Look up, down, and all around to see the myriad decorative touches: wood carvings, faux-marble finishes, gilt stars

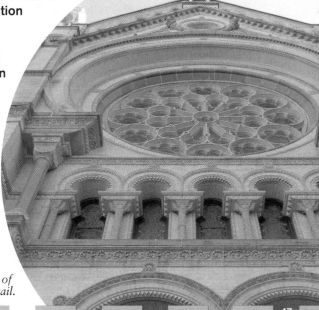

The Eldridge Street Synagogue is chock-full of astonishing architectural detail.

in heavenly domes, and such. The Moorish Revival front entrance is breathtaking, and the windows, from the small east window (2010) to the huge rose window, amply show the artistry of their creators. In addition to the congregation that still *davens* (prays) here, the building houses a museum and gift shop.

● Back out on the sidewalk, walk to the right to see another religious group's home, Pu Chao Buddhist Temple at 20 Eldridge. The doors and entrance are red and gold, and the buildings across the street are reflected in the brownish-red marble front.

● Walk north and east on Eldridge to Canal Street, and turn left.

● Just before you make a left onto Forsyth Street, note the entrance to the Manhattan Bridge, a grand archway flanked by regal columns. Cars, subway trains, bicyclists, and pedestrians all make their way over this bridge. Walk on Forsyth Street and perhaps you'll see a few itinerant vendors toiling in the shadow of the bridge during pleasant weather. On the east side of Forsyth—the only side with buildings along it— is St. Barbara Greek Orthodox Church, with its pretty three-door entrance and false dome. At this point, you may not be surprised to learn that this was also a former synagogue, Kol Israel Anshe Poland.

● Go in the other direction on Forsyth and cross Canal Street, heading north. A sprawling school complex on your right houses a middle school (Dr. Sun Yat Sen MS 131), Pace University High School (public and prestigious), and Emma Lazarus High School (also public, for English-language learners). The early-1980s building is ungainly—think a junior version of the quirky Guggenheim Museum uptown—but it has cheery paintings on the outer walls, as well as an apple statue. Sara D. Roosevelt Park is across the street and extends up to Houston Street in the East Village. It's a lovely, peaceful place, but it bears mentioning that to create it, the buildings on the west side of Forsyth Street and the east side of Chrystie Street were condemned and knocked down. Urban renewal!

● Turn right at Hester Street to see more of the school complex. At #113 is the Hester Street Collaborative/Leroy Street Studio, encompassing art, activism, and more.

● Turn left on Eldridge Street. This block is typical of the Lower East Side, full of businesses with Chinese, Spanish, and English signs, graffiti in various spots, and old buildings in varying degrees of upkeep. A plain building at #77 houses a Chinese church, but more interesting is #87: The circular multipart windows and the decorations above the top-floor windows are indicators, along with a few old signs in Hebrew, that this was a synagogue long ago. Years after the Jews left, it was a Christian church for a while. Then noted painter Milton Resnick moved in, renovated it, and used the building as his home and studio. The building now houses the Milton Resnick and Pat Passlof Foundation, an art gallery.

- Continue on Eldridge across Grand Street. Make a short detour to the right on Broome Street to #280, Kehila Kedosha Janina. An active synagogue with a museum, this is the only Romaniote (Greek Jewish) congregation in the Americas. The quaint, narrow two-story building has lovely windows and blends Moorish elements with the Judaic.

- Walk back to Eldridge Street and go right. At #133 is the Woodward Gallery, which houses modern art in a red-and-white tenement . . . that was originally a synagogue for Sephardic (Spanish–Portuguese) congregations. At 139 Eldridge is LMAK Projects, another modern-art gallery.

- Turn right onto Delancey Street to see more galleries such as #55, Brennan & Griffin, and James Fuentes next door (and if they're open, go in to visit).

- Turn left on Allen Street, called Avenue of the Immigrants here. At 133 Allen stands the white-painted Church of Grace to Fujianese, which was originally a public bathhouse—used back when many local tenement buildings lacked their own showers or baths. (Look carefully at the sign to see PUBLIC BATH in faded letters.)

- At Rivington Street, turn left. At #61 is the Lamb's Nazarene Church, but years before this was the Rivington public library. Across the street, at #60, is a peculiar building: It once housed two synagogues, first Adath Yeshurun of Jassy and later Erste Warshawer, and it was designed by Emery Roth, best known for his iconic apartment buildings along Central Park West. It's now owned by an artist who retained much of the Judaica outside but changed part of the Jewish star, removing a few metal bars of it so that it resembles a camera's lens.

You'll notice by now that the Lower East Side is one of those split-personality places: working-class folk and their a-bit-grimy buildings and stores side by side with hipster specialty shops and eateries, art galleries, and fashion. The old and the new accept each other, at times grudgingly. With that in mind, reverse direction on Rivington.

- Turn right on Orchard Street, long a haven for clothing bargains. Check out #140, The Orchard, an apartment building with its name emblazoned in golden paint. The walls of #130 are an advertisement for, and testament to, S. Beckenstein Inc. Woolens, Rayons, Silks, and Draperies. And a dangling street sign reminds everyone that on Sundays, Orchard Street is pedestrian-only for most of the day. (This was very exciting to me and my brother when we were kids and our parents brought us here—even if just to shop for clothes.)

- Now make like the romcom, carefully crossing Delancey Street along Orchard Street to the Tenement Museum, which tells the story of immigration through the real-life experiences of people who settled in the neighborhood. Besides the main museum building, you can take a tour of 97 Orchard, a tenement that was home to immigrant families from many different ethnic groups. Some rooms are carefully designed to resemble the cramped, spartan accommodations these families lived in at the turn of the century. The fact that people could live so humbly yet make their mark and (mostly) thrive is a big part of the American story. Perhaps some of the local chichi galleries are owned or frequented by descendants of the old-timers.

- Walk to 84 Orchard to see the gallery Artifact.

- Make a left at Grand Street, taking note of Shin Gallery at #322.

- Make a left at Ludlow Street. This whole block is taken up on the right by the Seward Park High School campus. This 1929 building stands on the site of the long-gone Ludlow Street Jail; the school itself had an earlier site as well. Today five smaller schools share the E-shaped campus.

- Check out stores and buildings along Ludlow (including the slightly funky Esther apartment building at #126–128) until you reach Rivington Street; then make a right. This block has one of the best candy stores in Manhattan, Economy Candy at 108 Rivington. Forget restraint—go here for candies you rarely find elsewhere, cute T-shirts, and fun collectibles. Across the street is the high-rise, so-glassy Hotel on Rivington. How do they clean all the windows? Walk to Essex Street to see the large wall mural for Schapiro's Wines, the last of the Lower East Side's kosher wine companies.

- Make a right on Essex and enter the Essex Street Market on your left. Roam. The building, which dates to 1940, was Mayor Fiorello La Guardia's effort to get food carts off the streets to relieve congestion. In recent years this outpost has become a mix of ethnic food and supply shops (Latino mostly) and hipster food stalls (artisanal meats, cheeses, and more), as well as Cuchifritos Art Gallery and a barber.

- Turn left on Delancey Street. On the left, at Norfolk Street, you can't help but gawk at the shades-of-blue-glass high-rise known as Blue Condominium. Built in 2007, it has an unconventional sculptural shape that's hard to describe—you just have to see it. A few blocks ahead in the distance is the Williamsburg Bridge to Brooklyn.

- Go one block on Norfolk Street to your right. At the corner of Norfolk and Broome Street is a very old synagogue, Congregation Beth Hamedrash Hagadol. Built in 1850 as a Baptist church, this was the first Eastern European synagogue established in New York City. The congregation was led by Rabbi Jacob Joseph, the city's chief rabbi—a post only he ever held—from 1888 to 1902 (this tour began at the playground named for his great-grandson). The building, beautiful but worn, sits unused as of this writing because of storm damage in 1997 and further storm-related damage in later years, as well as minor acts of vandalism. Its future is being debated as it grows more dilapidated. Very sad, but it deserves to be seen.

- Walk back on Norfolk Street to Delancey Street, where you can get a train at the Essex Street subway station.

POINTS OF INTEREST

Captain Jacob Joseph Playground Henry Street at Rutgers Street

Straus Square nycgovparks.org/parks/straus-square, bounded by Canal Street, Rutgers Street, and East Broadway

Forward **Building** 175 E. Broadway

Seward Park nycgovparks.org/parks/seward-park, bounded by Canal Street, Essex Street, Jefferson Street, and East Broadway

Seward Park Library nypl.org/locations/seward-park, 192 E. Broadway, 212-477-6770

Sung Tak Buddhist Association (Congregation B'nai Israel Kalwarie) 13 Pike St., 212-513-0230

Eldridge Street Synagogue and Museum eldridgestreet.org, 12 Eldridge St., 212-219-0888

St. Barbara Greek Orthodox Church stbarbaragoc.com, 27 Forsyth St., 212-226-0499

Hester Street Collaborative/Leroy Street Studio hesterstreet.org, 113 Hester St., 917-265-8591

Milton Resnick and Pat Passlof Foundation resnickpasslof.org, 87 Eldridge St., 212-226-1259

Kehila Kedosha Janina Synagogue and Museum kkjsm.org, 280 Broome St., 212-431-1619

Woodward Gallery woodwardgallery.net, 133 Eldridge St., 212-966-3411

LMAK Projects lmakprojects.com, 139 Eldridge St., 212-255-9707

Brennan & Griffin brennangriffin.com, 55 Delancey St., 212-227-0115

James Fuentes jamesfuentes.com, 55 Delancey St., 212-577-1201

Tenement Museum tenement.org, 103 Orchard St., 212-982-8420

Artifact artifactnyc.net, 84 Orchard St., 212-475-0448

Shin Gallery shin-gallery.com, 322 Grand St., 212-375-1735

Seward Park High School Campus sewardparkhs.com, 350 Grand St., 212-673-2650

Economy Candy economycandy.com, 108 Rivington St., 212-254-1531

Essex Street Market essexstreetmarket.com, 120 Essex St., 212-312-3603

Cuchifritos Gallery + Project Space artistsallianceinc.org, 120 Essex St.

route summary

1. Walk north on Rutgers Street to East Broadway, and turn right.
2. Cross Canal Street and walk into Straus Square and Seward Park.
3. Head west on East Broadway after visiting the parks and the library.
4. Walk left on Pike Street.
5. Turn around on Pike Street, cross East Broadway, and walk left on Division Street.
6. Walk right on Eldridge Street.
7. Go left on Canal Street.

8.   Stroll left on Forsyth Street for about a block; then double back on Forsyth, cross Canal Street, and continue on Forsyth to Sara D. Roosevelt Park.

9.   Walk right on Hester Street.

10. Go left on Eldridge Street.

11. Make a brief right on Broome Street, then return to Eldridge Street and turn right.

12. Walk right on Delancey Street.

13. Stroll left on Allen Street.

14. Walk left on Rivington Street, then double back and head in the opposite direction.

15. Walk right on Orchard Street.

16. Go left on Grand Street.

17. Walk left on Ludlow Street.

18. Take a right on Rivington Street.

19. Walk right on Essex Street.

20. Go left on Delancey Street.

21. Stroll right on Norfolk Street.

22. Double back to Delancey Street for the train.

CONNECTING THE WALKS

With the Williamsburg Bridge behind you, walk on Delancey to Allen Street, make a right, and cross Houston Street to arrive at the start of Walk 8 (East Village). To start the next tour, (The Bowery, Little Italy, and Soho), walk about seven blocks west on Delancey from the Essex Street station, turn left on Chrystie Street, and walk two blocks to the corner of Chrystie and Grand Street.

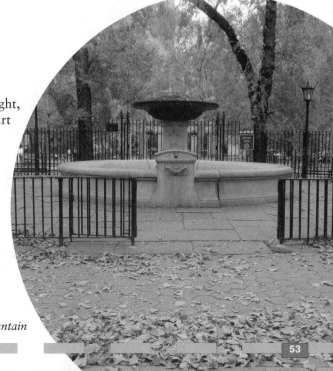

Historic Seward Park and its fountain

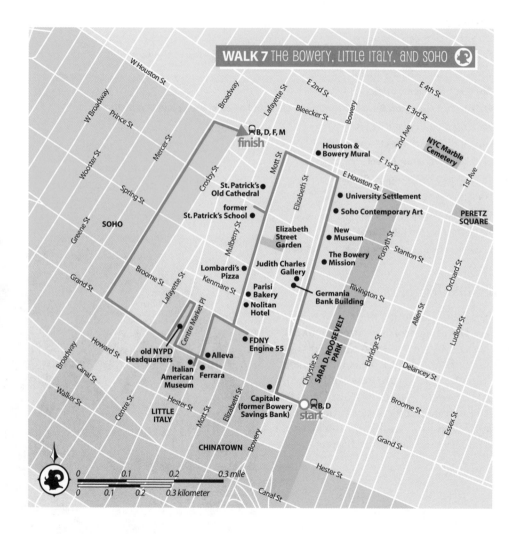

WALK 7 THE BOWERY, LITTLE ITALY, AND SOHO

finish 🚇 B, D, F, M

W Houston St

Broadway

Lafayette St

E 2nd St

Bleecker St

Bowery

E 4th St

E 3rd St

2nd Ave

NYC Marble Cemetery

Prince St

W Broadway

Mercer St

Wooster St

Greene St

Mott St

Elizabeth St

Houston & Bowery Mural

E 1st St

E Houston St

1st Ave

PERETZ SQUARE

SOHO

Spring St

Crosby St

St. Patrick's Old Cathedral

former St. Patrick's School

Mulberry St

Elizabeth Street Garden

University Settlement

Soho Contemporary Art

New Museum

Forsyth St

Stanton St

Orchard St

Broome St

Lafayette St

Grand St

Lombardi's Pizza

Judith Charles Gallery

The Bowery Mission

Parisi Bakery

Kenmare St

Nolitan Hotel

Germania Bank Building

Rivington St

Allen St

Ludlow St

Centre Market Pl

Howard St

old NYPD Headquarters

Alleva

Italian American Museum

Ferrara

FDNY Engine 55

Chrystie St

SARA D. ROOSEVELT PARK

Eldridge St

Delancey St

Broadway

Canal St

Walker St

Centre St

Hester St

Mott St

Elizabeth St

Capitale (former Bowery Savings Bank)

🚇 B, D
start

Broome St

Essex St

LITTLE ITALY

CHINATOWN

Bowery

Grand St

Hester St

Canal St

0   0.1   0.2   0.3 mile

0   0.1   0.2   0.3 kilometer

7 THE BOWERY, LITTLE ITALY, AND SOHO: FROM GRIT TO GLAMOUR

BOUNDARIES: **Grand St., Broadway, Houston St., Bowery**
DISTANCE: **3.3 miles**
SUBWAY: **B or D to Grand St.**

"The Bow'ry, the Bow'ry / They say such things / And they do strange things / On the Bow'ry! The Bow'ry . . ." That's the refrain from the famous song by Hoyt and Gaunt. As a child I saw TV commercials and heard radio ads for the Bowery Savings Bank, but I also heard about "Bowery bums," so my parents and I didn't stroll around there.

The Bowery has had quite the history, being the oldest Manhattan thoroughfare (it began life as a Native American footpath that was much lengthier). Dutch colonists dubbed it the "*bouwerij* [farm] road," and even into the 1860s it rivaled Broadway in importance. For many years it was an elegant address, but by the late 1800s it was riddled with honky-tonk entertainments and notorious flophouses. Through the early 1900s and on into the 1970s, the Bowery remained infamous as the city's Skid Row. But in the decades since (and particularly over the past 10 years), the district has been redeveloped and "rediscovered," and today it comprises a mix of chic galleries and shops, humbler wholesalers, nonprofit organizations, and residences. This walk also visits neighboring Little Italy (also see Walk 5) and Soho, a historic neighborhood that, like the Bowery, has bounced back from hard times.

● **Get off the subway and go upstairs to the sidewalk, at Grand Street and Chrystie Street. Grand Street cuts through Sara D. Roosevelt Park here, and you'll usually find a few street vendors selling newspapers or snacks. You're likely to hear Chinese and English spoken.**

● **With the park behind you, walk on Grand to the Bowery, one block away. Check out this neat little detail at 253 Grand: The street address is etched into the building, and above that is a crest that reads LB 1901. (What that means is a mystery, although** the number could allude to the year of construction.) This stretch of Grand Street has a variety of Vietnamese as well as Chinese businesses.

● Across the Bowery on the corner, check out the massive neoclassical structure (built 1893–95) with THE BOWERY SAVINGS BANK inscribed just under the clock. Its two connected buildings go back a block to Elizabeth Street; the Grand Street side has a similar sign. But the bank is no longer here; now it's Capitale, an upscale event space. Even so, the building still sports SAFE DEPOSIT VAULT signage, and you can also see ghosting where the bank's name was removed.

● Walk right (north and east) along the east side of Bowery, noting the profusion of lighting-fixture stores. At #143 is the Bowery Grand, a budget hotel that doesn't quite live up to its name. Although some of the buildings here look a bit worn, some have distinctive details. At #161 stands a seven-story commercial building from 1900, with carved-limestone pilasters and capitals, and window brackets set at an angle; #167 has Art Deco lettering up top reading CRYSTAL HOTEL. (Built during the Depression on the site of a 19th-century vaudeville theater, the Crystal was one of the Bowery's ill-famed flophouses.)

● Pause where Kenmare Street intersects on the left and widens into Delancey Street on the right. Looking right, you can see the Williamsburg Bridge in the distance. On the north side of Delancey is a beige stone building with a arched entrance: The Bowery Ballroom, a live-music venue. Directly in front of the club is the Bowery subway stop, the sole station in Manhattan with a one-word name.

● As you continue along the Bowery, notice the many restaurant-supply stores. Spring Street branches off on the left; on the corner stands a turn-of-the-century six-story building, which until very recently was covered with graffiti. The property, which is landmarked, used to be Germania Bank. The longtime owner-resident, who bought the building in the late 1960s and sold it in 2015 for a reported $55 million, apparently kept it cruddy-looking on purpose—the story goes that he balked at city orders to have the graffiti cleaned up because the city wouldn't let him do the same back in the Bowery's grittier days. Next door is the Judith Charles Gallery, a showcase for emerging artists.

● Walk farther, and on the right side past Rivington Street is The Bowery Mission. Dating to the late 1800s, this was one of the earliest mission houses for poor, homeless men. It still serves that population, and the building has some pretty features (stained-glass windows with the mission name spelled out in Old English script, mock-Tudor half-timbering). Walk a bit more to see the New Museum to the right. Bursting with cool modernity, it displays a few pieces in its windows. Look up—from this vantage point, it looks like several boxes stacked atop each other. Across the street is Bari Restaurant Equipment, established 1950. The marquee and facade resemble the grille of a vintage car.

● Continue along the Bowery past three galleries in quick succession—Sperone Westwater at #257, Soho Contemporary Art at #259, and Garis & Hahn at #263—and then come to University Settlement at the Houston Street Center. This community-services center, which operates in cooperation with the Chinatown YMCA, has a colorful mural splashed upon a wall in its yard; titled *The City as a Living Body,* it was created by high school students in collaboration with Groundswell, a public-art program. At Houston Street, another mural is painted at the northwest corner; for several years, this intersection has displayed changing murals painted by hip artists. (If you're not from these parts, now is probably a good time to mention that *Houston* is pronounced HOUSE-ton, not like the city in Texas.)

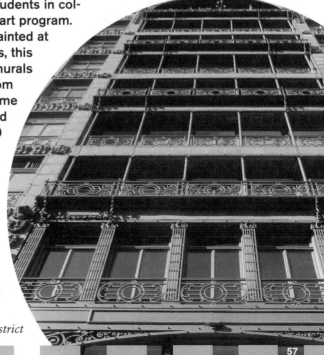

● Turn left, walk along Houston to Mott Street, and turn left again. Like other side streets in the vicinity, Mott has many boutiques and some fairly high-end retail establishments. But this block also has two notable historical sites: The Basilica of St. Patrick's Old Cathedral and the 14th Ward Industrial School. The school, at #256, was built in the 1880s, funded

One of the marvels of Soho's Cast Iron District

by an Astor family member for use by the Children's Aid Society; look for the CAS in flowery script above the engraved school name. Now the building is residential. Across the street is the cathedral, which became "old" when the Fifth Avenue building was erected in Midtown. The sanctuary was dedicated in 1815, and other sections of the building were done after, although they suffered a major fire in the 1860s. The headstones in the cemetery have quite a bit of wear. Inside, the sanctuary is a bit dark, with gracious stained-glass windows and dramatic vaulting.

● Make a right on Prince Street. Across from the church, at #32, stands a redbrick Federal-style building from 1826. A plaque here explains that the building was originally the site of the Roman Catholic Orphan Asylum—the first mission of the Sisters of Charity, founded by St. Elizabeth Ann Seton—and later St. Patrick's Old Cathedral School, the city's first Catholic school. The exterior was featured in two films by St. Patrick's alum Martin Scorsese: *Mean Streets* and *Gangs of New York.* The school closed in 2010, and the building is currently being redeveloped as condominiums.

● Go back to Mott Street and continue right (south and west). An interesting noncommercial feature of this block is the Elizabeth Street Garden, which extends back from Mott to Elizabeth Street. Among the 1,200 plantings are flowers, including lavender, daisies, and daffodils; various trees and shrubs; and vegetables and herbs. The garden also hosts such events as Tai Chi and yoga classes, poetry readings, and movie nights. (Check the website in Points of Interest for hours and an events calendar.)

● Cross Spring Street. Lombardi's Pizza, at this corner since 1905, is generally acknowledged as the first pizzeria in the United States, a fact its web address drives home. Another old-time food haunt is the Parisi Bakery, at #198. This is one of its two neighborhood shops, in business since 1903. At Kenmare Street, look across to see two modern buildings, one of them looking like it has a transistor radio plastered on it; these are the Nolitan Hotel, a play on *Nolita,* or "north of Little Italy." This portmanteau for the area (see *Tribeca* and *Soho*) was coined in the mid-1990s.

● Continue to Broome Street and make a left. The 1898 firehouse on your right at #363, Engine 55, might be one of the most likable station houses around, with its eagle bas-relief, flowing banner with the company's name, beautiful oval windows, and metalwork. Next door is Holy Trinity Ukrainian Church, even though ghosting left behind on the facade reads CHURCH OF SAN SALVATORE (that congregation left). Walk in the other direction, across Mott Street, to 375 Broome, which has several gargoyle-y faces with rather dramatic facial hair carved into window decorations, plus one near the roof that's downright spooky.

● Make a left at Mulberry Street and stroll beneath the WELCOME TO LITTLE ITALY sign that hangs across the road. Check out the many Italian eateries as you walk to Grand Street. Cross Grand to see the Italian American Museum, on your right. Then cross Mulberry and walk on Grand. To your right, Ferrara makes really fine cannoli. On the other side of the street, check out a few of the area's best (and longest-lived) Italian-food shops: DiPalo, Piemonte Ravioli, and Alleva. As a cheese fan, I was smitten by a mozzarella ball I spotted in Alleva; I took it home and it was quite tasty.

● Head back across Mulberry and make a right at Centre Market Place, a block that comes out of Baxter Street and was named for the nearby Centre Market, now long gone. On the right are townhouses in various colors. Note that street numbers run consecutively here, from 1 to 8, not even on one side and odd on the other.

● When the block ends at Broome, make a left and take a good look at the big fancy building that's also to your left. This block-long entity is 240 Centre St., which was New York City police headquarters from 1909 to 1973. In 1988, it was converted to luxury condos. (The NYPD is now based near City Hall; see Walk 5.) The dome is the loveliest part, with its clocks, columns, and cupola. This is definitely a building to admire both up close and in full. Walk around it via Broome Street and then a quick jog left on Centre Street.

● Make a right onto Grand Street again.

● At Broadway, make another right. You're now in Soho ("south of Houston"), known for its many cast iron–front buildings. (Try this cool trick: Take out a small magnet, walk up to one of these buildings, and affix. *Voilà!*) Many of these structures were erected in the 1880s and 1890s, some before, some into the early 1900s. By the 1950s, this district was nicknamed "Hell's Hundred Acres" because of its many sweatshops and factories (and the accidental fires that frequently started in them). Some historic buildings succumbed to the wrecking ball, but preservationists fought hard to save many others, and in the 1960s and 1970s artists of various stripes discovered they could set up lofts in the old industrial spaces quite cheaply. Now, of course, Soho is very expensive; in fact, it nearly rivals Madison Avenue on the Upper East Side for posh designer shops. Below I make note of my favorite buildings along this stretch of Broadway, but there are many others worth a look and a photo.

- First, at #462, see the International Culinary Center on your right, along with its Michelin-honored student restaurant, L'Ecole. The building in which they're housed dates from 1879 and takes its architectural cues from the French Renaissance. Narrow #472, an apartment building, has lovely lacelike ironwork. Impressive #478–482 (a clothing boutique) has intricate work between its pilasters and windows. The building at #486 is made of red brick but has attractive darker banding on the top floors.

- Continue along Broadway, crossing Broome Street, and gaze at #488, a feast of pillars and arches. The building at #504 is likewise an arch festival (with a Bloomingdale's!), while #508 and #510 have elegant moldings at their rooflines, both topped with rounded pediments. After you pass Spring Street, #532 has opulent Beaux Arts touches. Narrow #540 has vaguely Celtic flourishes around the windows; also note the "1867" at the roof. Next door, at #540–542, there are three caryatids to catch your eye, each slightly different, near the roof. Across the street, massive #555 reads CHARLES BROADWAY ROUSS. Charles Baltzell Rouss operated a department store here in the 1890s; a Virginia native and self-made millionaire, Rouss honored the city that gave him his fortune by changing his middle name to Broadway. Next door, at #557, is the headquarters of Scholastic, the educational publisher. The building, from 2001, only looks old. (When the last Harry Potter book, *Harry Potter and the Deathly Hallows,* came out, Scholastic—which published the series in the US—held a block-long street fair and was swamped with fans.)

- At #561, the "Little Singer Building" (nicknamed to distinguish it from the sewing machine company's now-demolished skyscraper farther downtown) has wonderful ironwork and textured terra-cotta pieces all over. Finally, don't overlook #583, the 1897 Astor Building. For some time, the New Museum of Contemporary Art was located here, but now it's residential. Perhaps best described as Beaux Arts gone wild, it has lavishly decorated bay windows sandwiched between Corinthian columns, plus terra-cotta gewgaws everywhere they'll fit: cartouches, arches, gargoyles, you name it.

- At Houston Street, turn right and walk to Lafayette Street to see the Puck Building, which once housed the printing facilities for *Puck,* a humor magazine published from

1878 to 1916 and named for the imp from *A Midsummer Night's Dream.* This redbrick Romanesque Revival building from the 1880s has two gold-leaf statues of the magazine's mascot to admire. Catch the train at the Broadway–Lafayette Street station at Houston Street.

POINTS OF INTEREST

Capitale (Old Bowery Savings Bank) capitaleny.com, 130 Bowery, 212-334-5500

The Bowery Ballroom boweryballroom.com, 6 Delancey St., 212-260-4700

Judith Charles Gallery judithcharlesgallery.com, 196 Bowery, 212-219-4095

The Bowery Mission bowery.org, 227 Bowery, 212-674-3456

New Museum newmuseum.org, 235 Bowery, 212-219-1222

Sperone Westwater speronewestwater.com, 257 Bowery, 212-999-7337

Soho Contemporary Art sohocontemporaryart.com, 259 Bowery, 646-719-1316

Garis & Hahn garisandhahn.com, 263 Bowery, 212-228-8457

University Settlement at the Houston Street Center hsc.universitysettlement.org/hsc, 273 Bowery, 212-475-5008

The Basilica of St. Patrick's Old Cathedral oldcathedral.org, 263 Mulberry St., 212-226-8075

Elizabeth Street Garden elizabethstreetgarden.org, bounded by Mott, Elizabeth, Prince, and Spring Streets

Lombardi's Pizza firstpizza.com, 32 Spring St., 212-941-7994

Parisi Bakery parisibakery.com, 198 Mott St., 212-226-6378

Nolitan Hotel nolitanhotel.com, 30 Kenmare St., 212-925-2555

FDNY Engine 55 363 Broome St.

Italian American Museum italianamericanmuseum.org, 155 Mulberry St., 212-965-9000

Ferrara ferraranyc.com, 195 Grand St., 212-226-6150

Alleva allevadairy.com, 188 Grand St., 212-226-7990

International Culinary Center/L'Ecole Restaurant lecolenyc.com, 462 Broadway, 212-219-3300

route summary

1. Walk west on Grand Street from Chrystie Street.
2. Walk right on Bowery.
3. Walk left on Houston Street.
4. Walk left on Mott Street, dipping in and out of Prince Street to the right.
5. Walk left on Broome Street, then head in the other direction across Mott Street.
6. Walk left on Mulberry Street.
7. Go left on Grand Street to Mott Street, then double back on Grand.
8. Walk right on Centre Market Place.
9. Turn left on Broome Street, then left on Centre Street.
10. Make a right on Grand.
11. Walk right on Broadway.
12. Go right at Houston Street to the subway.

CONNECTING THE WALKS

Walk 9 (Central Greenwich Village) begins at West Houston Street and Broadway, just before you turn on Houston to reach the subway. To reach the start of the West Village tour (Walk 10), walk about eight blocks west on Houston to Varick Street.

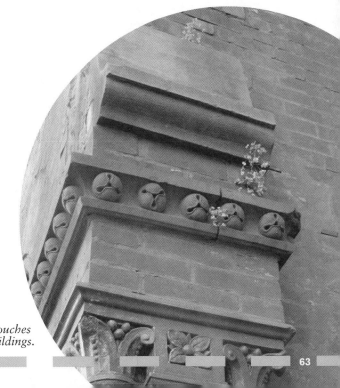

Slow your stroll to appreciate the charming touches that abound on Soho's buildings.

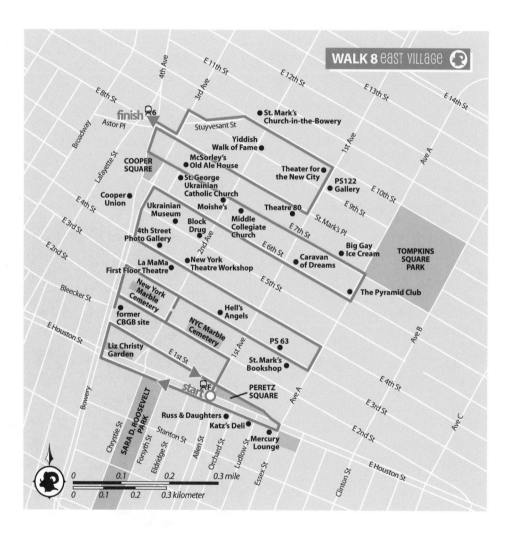

4th Ave

E 11th St

E 12th St

3rd Ave

E 13th St

E 14th St

E 8th St

Astor Pl

finish 6

Broadway

Lafayette St

Stuyvesant St

● St. Mark's
Church-in-the-Bowery

1st Ave

Ave A

**COOPER
SQUARE**

McSorley's
● Old Ale House

Yiddish
Walk of Fame ●

Cooper ●
Union

St. George
● Ukrainian
Catholic Church

E 4th St

Theater for
the New City ●

PS122
● Gallery

E 10th St

E 3rd St

Ukrainian
Museum

Moishe's
●

Theatre 80
●

E 9th St

St. Mark's Pl

4th Street
Photo Gallery
●

Block
● Drug

Middle
Collegiate
Church

2nd Ave

E 7th St

E 2nd St

La MaMa
First Floor Theatre ●

● New York
Theatre Workshop

E 6th St

Big Gay
● Ice Cream

**TOMPKINS
SQUARE
PARK**

Bleecker St

New York
Marble
Cemetery

Caravan
● of Dreams

E 5th St

● The Pyramid Club

● McSorley's Ale House

Hell's
● Angels

1st Ave

Ave B

E Houston St

● former
CBGB site

NYC Marble
Cemetery

PS 63
●

Liz Christy
Garden

E 1st St

St. Mark's
● Bookshop

start F

**PERETZ
SQUARE**

Ave A

E 4th St

Bowery

SARA D. ROOSEVELT
PARK

Russ & Daughters ●

Katz's Deli ●

Mercury
Lounge ●

E 3rd St

Ave C

Chrystie St

Forsyth St

Stanton St

Eldridge St

Allen St

Orchard St

Ludlow St

Essex St

E 2nd St

E Houston St

Clinton St

0   0.1   0.2   0.3 mile

0   0.1   0.2   0.3 kilometer

8 east village: clubs, college, culture

BOUNDARIES: **E. Houston St., Ave. A, E. 10th St., 3rd Ave.**
DISTANCE: **4.2 miles**
SUBWAY: **F train to 2nd Ave.**

The East Village is somewhat quieter, somewhat grittier, and somewhat less known than the Washington Square area, or even the West Village. But this is a neighborhood with a great deal of charm, considerable historical importance, cultural choices (and ghosts), and other C's: cinema, cemeteries, Cooper Union, and churches.

The East Village draws young and old alike with its varied offerings of music, theater, dance, ethnic meals, fashion, and knickknacks. There are sweet little parks and stirring monuments. The northern segment has two historical anchors in the Cooper Union, a highly competitive college where presidential hopeful Abraham Lincoln spoke, and St. Mark's Church-in-the-Bowery, Manhattan's oldest place of continuous religious worship.

The East Village also has legendary places that are gone but still commemorated, such as punk-rock haven CBGB, the 2nd Ave Deli (which moved), Mars Bar, the Amato Opera, and others. A visit here is nostalgic at times, forward-thinking at others.

On March 26, 2015, the block of Second Avenue just south of St. Mark's Place was rocked by a gas-line explosion and fire that killed 2 people, injured 22, and left more than 80 homeless. The blast leveled three buildings and badly damaged four others. In the true spirit of the city, area businesses, houses of worship, and nonprofits have stepped up to help the displaced.

- **Exit the subway on the First Avenue side. Just next to the station is First Park, a charming little sliver of a park and playground.**

- **Make a left onto First Avenue and then a right on East First Street. Peretz Square, a long, thin triangle of a park, is to your right. At #108 is a brick building that used to be a synagogue and a performance space and is currently pricey residences.**

Back Story: Hilly's Place

CBGB stands among the most notorious, iconic, and influential rock-and-roll venues in the United States. Along with places such as Whisky a Go Go (West Hollywood) and the Fillmore and Fillmore West (San Francisco), CBGB—which actually stood for "Country Blue Grass Blues" but rarely staged such acts—is a shorthand for live music, especially punk and new wave. The club closed in October 2006 with a concert by Patti Smith, and its building has been added to the National Register of Historic Places. The address was 315 Bowery . . . and don't you forget it.

None of this tells you much, though, about what it was like to attend a show there. I went to a number of shows at CBGB throughout the 1980s and some in the 1990s, and although it was usually fun, it was also crowded, loud, reeking of beer and sweat, and a sea of elbows. It also had remarkably disgusting bathrooms (which have been preserved and displayed at, among other places, the Metropolitan Museum of Art).

Almost every time I ventured into "CB's," the owner was at or near the door. Hilly Kristal was a gruff, disheveled guy who looked like someone's dad who wandered into the wrong place. His eyeglasses were at the tip of his nose, and he was usually involved in paperwork or talking with someone. He watched over the place like a hawk.

In July 1999, I exhibited black-and-white photographs at the adjoining CB's 313 gallery (313 Bowery) with a few other photographers, and while I was hanging up my framed prints, Hilly stood a few feet away from me, sawing away at wood planks. I'm not sure what he was working on at the time, but every once in a while he would let out a big sigh. I asked him about it and he gave an exaggerated shoulder shrug, just like my father would.

The first show I recall seeing at CBGB was The Dickies, a punk band that specialized in wacky, rapid-fire covers of mainstream rock and pop songs. Amid the proceedings, in walked actor Matt Dillon. My friend Antoinette approached him and said, "You're rich, give me some money." He handed her a dollar.

Who else did I see perform? I remember some names—the NiteCaps, Richard Hell, Token Entry, Murphy's Law—plus assorted punk bands at the Sunday-afternoon "hardcore matinees," a string of garage-rock bands, and others I just don't recall. It was always an experience, even if the ladies' room was as nasty as the men's.

● Continue along East First and merge onto East Houston Street. At Avenue A, cross the street and turn right on East Houston. At #217 is the Mercury Lounge, a well-known live-music showcase.

● Cross Ludlow Street to see the legendary Katz's Delicatessen. It has vintage signs from a few eras, serves "kosher style" food (it's complicated), and was the location for a memorable scene in *When Harry Met Sally*. Cross Orchard Street to see Russ & Daughters, a specialty-foods shop that has been in the same spot (179 E. Houston St.) since 1920. Stroll farther, and after Eldridge Street is the Sunshine Cinema at 143 E. Houston. Built in 1898 and sort of reminiscent of a synagogue, this brick structure was a Yiddish vaudeville theater and then a dumpy warehouse; now it shows indie films. Next door, at #137, is Yonah Schimmel Knish Bakery, here since 1910. (A knish is an addictive snack: a doughy pocket usually filled with mashed potato.)

● Having managed to resist all that tempting food—or not—cross Forsyth Street next to see the northern end of lengthy Sara D. Roosevelt Park. Here, it has some artsy street lamps with metal owl sculptures attached.

● Walk to the Bowery and make a right. At the right corner, across East Houston Street, is the Liz Christy Community Garden, Manhattan's first, set up in 1973.

● Pass one of the many restaurant-supply stores on Bowery and make a right onto East First Street. Avalon Bowery Place is the metal-and-glass apartment complex here. Across the street, in a nondescript brick building, is Momofuku Ko, one of five restaurants in the acclaimed Momofuku family of Asian-fusion eateries. Next to it is one of Manhattan's tiniest roads, Extra Place. Basically an alley with a sidewalk mural and graffiti, it doesn't even extend all the way to East Second Street.

● Cross Second Avenue. At #36 is one of the fabled Catholic Worker soup kitchens. A bit farther up is an 1885 brick building with alluring windows and a once-handsome entrance; this was PS 79 and is now private housing. Near the roof is a plaque that reads "1885" . . . faded glory. Walk more and be welcomed to the First Street Garden, another community garden. This one features lively wall decorations with quotes, including one by Dorothy Day (she of the Catholic Worker). As you walk to First Avenue, you pass the northern side of First Park, which you saw just after you got off the subway.

- Make a left onto First Avenue. At the corner, #29 is Gringer & Sons, an old family-run appliance business with a snazzy neon sign.

- Make a left at East Second Street. This is a mellow residential block—and very quiet at the New York City Marble Cemetery, on your right. Established in 1831, it holds the remains of some members of the Roosevelt family; President James Monroe was also interred here for a while. Note the stately turn-of-the century iron gates and signage. Across the street is the Orthodox Cathedral of the Holy Virgin Protection, a Russian Orthodox church since the 1940s. Built in 1891 as Olivet Memorial Church, this Gothic Revival limestone structure is sure to appeal to architecture fans. Its second-floor windows are the real standout here. At the corner of Second Avenue, see the redbrick building on the left, Anthology Film Archives, a major international home of experimental and avant-garde film and video. Since 1988 it's been housed here in the former Second Avenue Courthouse building.

- Turn right on Second Avenue and note the modernist Church of the Nativity, boxy and rather austere but for the bell hanging above the roof. Across from it, next to the Provenzano Lanza Funeral Home, peer through a gate to see the New York Marble Cemetery, the first nonsectarian burial place in New York open to the public. It's a year older and more hidden from view than the New York City Marble Cemetery, which you saw earlier on East Second Street.

  Though they have nearly identical names and were laid out by the same developer, these two cemeteries are completely separate entities. As a public-health precaution during a yellow fever outbreak in the early 1830s, the city outlawed burying the dead directly in the ground, so both cemeteries were constructed with underground marble burial vaults (hence "marble cemetery"). The names of those interred here at the New York Marble Cemetery are engraved on marble plaques posted on the cemetery walls, while the vaults at the New York City Marble Cemetery are more conventionally marked, with monuments or small marble squares.

- Return to East Second Street and continue in the direction (west) you'd been walking on it before. Be dazzled by the funky white-red-black-brown graffiti mural for art collective Ideal Glass, on your right. After that is Albert's Garden, a pretty little spot of green. Note the crooked tree by the left wall, its branches resembling a whip.

● Walk farther to the Bowery and stop to pay tribute to the memory of an East Village legend, remembered with a street sign: This is Joey Ramone Place, commemorating the tall, gangly singer of the Ramones, one of New York City's best-known punk bands. Don't see the memorial sign at the corner? *Look up.* The sign has been stolen several times over the past decade, and each time it's been put back, the city has had to move it higher and higher to deter souvenir seekers.

● Make a left on the Bowery. At #315, across from where Bleecker Street intersects, what's now a store for menswear designer John Varvatos used to be the pioneering punk club CBGB (see Back Story). Stop and soak up the ghosts of acts past: the Ramones, Blondie, Patti Smith, Talking Heads, the B-52s . . .

● Turn around and walk north on Bowery. At #319 pay homage to another ghost, the Amato Opera, which produced inexpensive musical performances. The building, with distinctive lettering announcing its name, sits vacant and decrepit while its current owners figure out what to do with it. At #327 is The Bowery Electric, a live-music club that sort of harks back to CBGB. At #335 is The Bowery Hotel, a hipper-than-hip boutique hotel housed in an asymmetrical brick tower.

● Turn right on East Third Street. At #8 is Renewal on the Bowery, a treatment center for substance abusers. At #30 there's an old walkup with a curious plaque and distinction: Is it truly the "SHOW ME" STATE HOUSE CIRCA 1888? (Many assume the structure is older.)

● The next block has a jumbled character, to say the least. At #55 is the Mary House, another Catholic Worker charity site. Farther down at #77 is the New York chapter of the Hell's Angels—yes, *those* Hell's Angels. Look at their colorful flags, but don't linger. And next door, at #81, is a New York Law School dorm. That's Manhattan for you: a strange mix of neighbors.

● Cross First Avenue and continue to a stately old school building. H-shaped, it houses two separate schools, Star Academy–PS 63 and the Neighborhood School. The decorations near the roof, above the entrance, would be right at home on a wedding cake. Just past the school on your right is St. Mark's Bookshop, proudly independent and always cerebral. At the corner of East Third and Avenue A is a block-length building (it goes through to East Fourth Street) that is reminiscent of apartment buildings you might see on Central Park West. Named Ageloff Towers, this 1929 co-op has pseudo-Assyrian stone carvings of animals and people above the entrance.

● Make a left on Avenue A and another left onto East Fourth Street; you'll see the other side of the Ageloff buildings. As you stroll this block, you'll pass a playground and the other side of PS 63. Farther along is another old school building, well maintained, called PS 751, the Manhattan School for Career Development.

● Cross Second Avenue for an artistic block: At #85 is an off-Broadway house, the Kraine Theater. At #79 is the New York Theatre Workshop (where the hit musical *Rent* originated), with its weathered marquee. At #74A E. Fourth is La MaMa, a premier avant-garde theatrical group; the First Floor Theatre, the very red building it's housed in, features three male busts above windows. At #67 is a storefront photography gallery with the no-frills name 4th Street Photo Gallery; it was founded by Alex Harsley, a veteran photographer who gave me two shows back in the late 1990s and early 2000s. At #66 is another La MaMa site, the Ellen Stewart Theatre (she founded the group). The building at #62, home to the Rod Rodgers Dance Company, dates to 1889; one of the more eye-catching walk-ups around, it has a chutelike fire exit, along with arches and columns.

● Make a right onto the Bowery, which becomes Cooper Square—stay to the right as the north- and southbound traffic lanes become separated by the park that gives the street its name. Across the street at 30 Cooper Square, next door to the former offices of *The Village Voice,* are the administrative offices of Cooper Union. One of a handful of US colleges and universities that charge no tuition, it specializes in art, architecture, and engineering. Its newer building is on the far corner of East Sixth Street, where you turn right. Designed by Thom Mayne and completed in 2009, it's disconcerting or amazing, depending on your inclination. The Cooper Square side seems to be folding in on itself, yet smiling; on the Sixth Street side, it looks like a piece of metal, and when the windows are open, they seem like staples sticking out of it.

● The next stretch of East Sixth Street is part of a larger section of the East Village known as Little Ukraine. Ukrainians have been living here since the 1870s; today, about a third of New York City's 80,000 Ukrainian Americans call the area home.

● Walk a bit on East Sixth and see a small street to your left, signed for both Hall Street and Taras Shevchenko Place (Shevchenko was a Ukrainian writer and political figure). Also along this street are educational facilities for younger students, such as St. George Academy, St. George's Catholic School, and the LaSalle Academy, and then, at 222 E. Sixth, the Ukrainian Museum.

● At the southwest corner of East Sixth and Second Avenue is Block Drug Stores. Dating back to 1885, this independent pharmacy is the antithesis of chain stores. Inside are a sign that reads SECOND AVENUE CHEMISTS and an old-fashioned stand-on scale. The store's neon sign glows bright red at dark. Cross Second Avenue and note the many Indian restaurants on this block. On your left, at 325 E. Sixth, is the Sixth Street Community Synagogue, a Modern Orthodox congregation. The building dates from 1848 and originally housed St. Mark's Lutheran Evangelical Church. A plaque memorializes parishioners who perished in the tragic 1904 *General Slocum* ship fire and sinking.

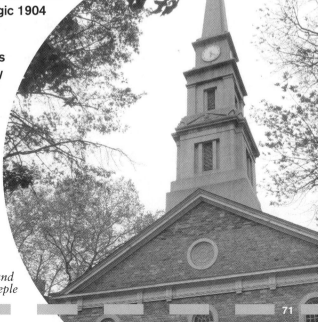

● Cross First Avenue. This next block has some thought-provoking sights, mostly on the left side. (Most of the right side is a mixed-income housing development, each of the buildings the same odd shape.) At #405 is Caravan of Dreams, a vegan restaurant here since 1991. Many of the dishes are what its website calls "live food" (read: barely cooked).

St. Mark's Church-in-the-Bowery and its dignified steeple

A bit farther down is a bittersweet story: Built in the early 1900s, 415 E. Sixth used to be an Orthodox synagogue called Anshe Meseritz. Over the years, its membership dwindled, and the building became very dilapidated. At the time of this writing, it was slated to be saved partially, but much of the building's interior will be altered and floors added, to create condos. A few doors down, you can see a few remnants of when the building at #431—now residences—was a synagogue known as the Center for the Proskurover Zion Congregation. Photographer William Wegman, famous for his endearing portraits of dogs, used to live and work here.

● Turn left onto Avenue A. The most intriguing place on this block is #101, The Pyramid Club, perhaps best known for helping launch the careers of RuPaul, Lady Bunny, and other drag divas. Over the years, The Pyramid has also hosted performances by Madonna, Nirvana, and The Red Hot Chili Peppers. The building dates to 1876; in its early days, it housed a succession of dining, drinking, and meeting halls catering to German Americans.

● Turn left onto East Seventh Street. Among the notables on this block are Big Gay Ice Cream at #125, home of irreverent-but-delicious frozen treats such as the Salty Pimp and the Bea Arthur; St. Mary's American Orthodox Greek Catholic Church at #121, with a touching Madonna painted above the main door; St. Stanislaus Catholic Church, a Polish American church with a moving 9/11 memorial plaque and a Pope John Paul II bust; and several excellent restaurants.

● The next block of East Seventh is unremarkable, but when you get to Second Avenue, take note at your left of the large Saul Birns Building, with its Art Deco intricacies (it's now an NYU site), and the longtime baked-goods fave Moishe's at 115 Second Ave. Overlook the graffiti—the sweets are delicious. Across the street is Middle Collegiate Church, a Gothic Revival masterpiece with Tiffany stained-glass windows and impressive ironwork. Burp Castle (41 E. Seventh) is a humorously retro spot for beer. Look carefully a few buildings adjacent to it for a WWII memorial plaque.

● Then you come to one of the most notorious nightlife spots in lower Manhattan: McSorley's Old Ale House, at 15 E. Seventh. It's been around since 1854, and for most of that time it served men only. It's dark and dingy and people love it; going there is a rite of passage. Across the street is the otherworldly St. George Ukrainian Catholic Church, with a magnificent dome and brilliantly colored icons trimmed in gold leaf.

- Reach Cooper Square, here also signed as Third Avenue, and cross over to Cooper Square Park. To your left, facing south, is a statue of inventor and business magnate Peter Cooper; here he sits with his cane, looking imperial. To your right, the brown building with the clock and lots of arches is the Foundation Building of Cooper Union, the college he founded. Completed in 1859, it's the school's oldest structure. Abraham Lincoln famously spoke here in 1860. Across Cooper Square on the other side of the park is the old Carl Fischer Music Publishers building. If you own any sheet music for piano, there's a good chance that they published it.

- Make a right on Cooper Square and walk to Astor Place. The small sidewalk island has a sculpture of a black cube; although its official name is *Alamo,* everyone calls it the Astor Place Cube or just The Cube. People use it as a meeting place, and nope, there's nobody living inside it, contrary to the viral-video hoax.

- With The Cube to your right, walk east on East Eighth Street past a huge apartment complex, seemingly all glass (a lot of the recent construction in Manhattan seems to be window-dominant). Cross Second Avenue and East Eighth becomes St. Mark's Place. This has traditionally been a very vibrant strip, with a tantalizing variety of shops for music, clothing, and other goodies. But some longtime residents have left, and it's harder to know the history here. Among the present and past notables are the punk-rock fashion shop Trash and Vaudeville, at 4 St. Mark's, and the Daniel LeRoy House (#20), an 1832 town house that until 2014 was home to Sounds, a much-loved music shop.

- As you continue east on St. Mark's, you'll see several quaint buildings in the block between Second and First Avenues. At #48 is a subdued but pretty church, originally First German Methodist Episcopal and now used by Church of the Village. At #62 is the even more modest Church of St. Cyril, which has one bright feature, its big central window that spans two floors. Farther down at #80 is Theatre 80 St. Mark's, another off-Broadway house with a retro-cool neon sign.

- Make a left on First Avenue to see a few more cultural highlights. On the corner to your right is PS122 Gallery, a public school–turned–performance space. Midblock on the other side, Theater for the New City is housed in the former First Avenue Retail Market, built in 1938. The theater suffered financial difficulties in the late 1990s; in exchange for removing a lien on the property, the city sold the air rights to the building, which is why you see a high-rise coming out of the back of it.

- At East 10th Street, make a left. This is a fairly low-key block with several small businesses, but take notice of buildings such as #221, with a man's face carved in stone over the door.

- When you reach the corner of Second Avenue, look at the sidewalk on your left, in front of the entrance to Chase Bank. This is the Yiddish Walk of Fame, honoring stars of the Yiddish stage. It's a vestige of the old 2nd Ave Deli, a legendary kosher restaurant that used to be where the bank is now. Once it was packed with customers clamoring for hot pastrami and kasha; sadly, though, the owner, Abe Lebewohl, was killed during a robbery in 1996, and 10 years later the restaurant relocated to Midtown. My family, friends, and I used to love this place—the food, the gruff waitstaff, the noise, the soups. Most of the Yiddish performers celebrated in the sidewalk stars are all but forgotten today, but Molly Picon and Fyvush Finkel did make it to Broadway and beyond.

- Across the avenue are a church and its yard, set at an angle. Why? Because the road used to run that way, predating the more formalized grid of streets. And a bit of it still does, sort of. This is St. Mark's Church-in-the-Bowery, New York's oldest site of continuous religious worship and the second oldest church building in Manhattan, completed in 1799. The Greek Revival steeple, from the 1820s, can be seen from quite a distance. Cross over to explore it all. The triangular sitting plaza, with trees and a small fenced patch with flags in front, is named in memory of Abe Lebewohl. Also see the statue of Peter Stuyvesant (who once owned all this land and is buried here) and the lengthy plaque on the pedestal. Other statues depict Daniel Tompkins, a state governor as well as a US vice president; the moody pair *Inspiration* and *Aspiration;* and some roaring lions.

- Proceed on East 10th Street past the church, and walk left along Stuyvesant Street, which is at odds with the other streets. (Off-grid streets are a great way to get in touch with Manhattan's past—they predate the 1811 grid system imposed on much of the island.) Pass a tiny triangle park, also dedicated to Abe Lebewohl, and admire the charming houses here. The one at #44 was built in 1795 and was owned by a Stuyvesant descendant. The group of homes at #23–35, known as the Renwick Triangle, are wonderful in their simplicity. Linger at #21, built in 1804 and known as the Stuyvesant-Fish House. This well-kept Federal-style abode was built by Petrus Stuyvesant, Peter's great-grandson, as a wedding gift for his daughter, Elizabeth, who married Nicholas Fish, an officer in the Revolutionary War. (Their son, Hamilton Fish, went on to be governor of New York, a US senator, and US secretary of state.) The tall building at #34–36 was originally the Hebrew Technical Institute, a vocational high school; now it's an NYU building.

● Bear right on East Ninth Street where it meets Stuyvesant Street. The pocket park bounded by Third Avenue, Stuyvesant, and East Ninth is actually a "sibling" of the micro-park across the triangle tip from it. Together they're called the George Hecht Viewing Gardens.

● Make a left on Third Avenue and then a right on East Eighth Street to reach the Astor Place #6 train.

POINTS OF INTEREST

Mercury Lounge mercuryloungenyc.com, 217 E. Houston St., 212-260-4700

Katz's Delicatessen katzsdelicatessen.com, 205 E. Houston St., 212-254-2246

Russ & Daughters russanddaughters.com, 179 E. Houston St., 212-475-4880

Sunshine Cinema tinyurl.com/sunshinecinema, 143 E. Houston St., 212-260-7289

Yonah Schimmel Knish Bakery knishery.com, 137 E. Houston St., 212-477-2858

Liz Christy Community Garden lizchristygarden.us, Bowery and Houston Street

Momofuku Ko momofuku.com/new-york/ko, 8 Extra Place, 212-203-8095

New York City Marble Cemetery nycmc.org, East Second Street between First and Second Avenues, 917-780-2893

Orthodox Cathedral of the Holy Virgin Protection nycathedral.org, 59 E. Second St., 212-677-4664

Anthology Film Archives anthologyfilmarchives.org, 32 Second Ave., 212-505-5181

New York Marble Cemetery marblecemetery.org, East Second Street between Second Avenue and the Bowery, 410-586-1321

The Bowery Electric theboweryelectric.com, 327 Bowery, 212-228-0228

The Bowery Hotel theboweryhotel.com, 335 Bowery, 212-505-9100

St. Mark's Bookshop stmarksbookshop.com, 136 E. Third St., 212-260-7853

Kraine Theater horsetrade.info, 85 E. Fourth St., 212-777-6088

New York Theatre Workshop nytw.org, 79 E. Fourth St., 212-780-9037

La MaMa Experimental Theatre Club lamama.org, 74A E. Fourth St., 646-430-5374

4th Street Photo Gallery tinyurl.com/4thstreetphotogallery, 67 E. Fourth St., 212-673-1021

Rod Rodgers Dance Company rodrodgersdance.org, 62 E. Fourth St., 212-674-9066

Cooper Union cooper.edu, 30 Cooper Square, 212-353-4100

Block Drug Stores blockdrugstores.com, 101 Second Ave., 212-473-1587

Sixth Street Community Synagogue sixthstreetsynagogue.org, 325 E. Sixth St., 212-473-3665

Caravan of Dreams caravanofdreams.net, 405 E. Sixth St., 212-254-1613

The Pyramid Club thepyramidclub.com, 101 Ave. A, 212-228-4888

Big Gay Ice Cream biggayicecream.com, 125 E. Seventh St., 212-533-9333

Moishe's Bake Shop moishesbakeshop.com, 115 Second Ave., 212-505-8555

Middle Collegiate Church middlechurch.org, 112 Second Ave., 212-477-0666

Burp Castle burpcastlenyc.wordpress.com, 41 E. Seventh St., 212-982-4576

McSorley's Old Ale House 15 E. Seventh St., 212-473-9148

St. George Ukrainian Catholic Church stgeorgeukrainianchurch.org, 30 E. Seventh St., 212-674-1615

Trash and Vaudeville trashandvaudeville.com, 4 St. Mark's Place, 212-982-3590

Theatre 80 St. Mark's theatre80.wordpress.com, 80 St. Mark's Place, 212-388-0388

PS122 Gallery ps122gallery.org, 150 First Ave., 212-477-5829

Theater for the New City theaterforthenewcity.net, 155 First Ave., 212-254-1109

St. Mark's Church-in-the-Bowery stmarksbowery.org, 131 E. 10th St., 212-674-6377

route summary

1. From the F stop on East Houston Street, go left onto First Avenue.
2. Walk right on East First Street.

3. Cross East Houston Street at Avenue A, and head west on Houston.

4. Go right on Bowery.

5. Walk right on East First Street.

6. Go left on First Avenue.

7. Proceed left on East Second Street.

8. Detour right on Second Avenue to the NYC Marble Cemetery, then resume walking west on East Second.

9. Go left on Bowery to the CBGB site, then turn around and head north.

10. Go right on East Third Street.

11. Go left on Avenue A.

12. Go left on East Fourth Street.

13. Go right on Bowery/Cooper Square.

14. Walk right on East Sixth Street.

15. Go left on Avenue A.

16. Travel left on East Seventh Street.

17. Cross Cooper Square to Astor Place.

18. Walk east on East Eighth Street/St. Mark's Place.

19. Go left on First Avenue.

20. Walk left on East 10th Street.

21. Make a left on Stuyvesant Street.

22. Walk right on East Ninth Street, then left on Third Avenue, then right on East Eighth Street to the train.

CONNECTING THE WALKS

From the Astor Place station, walk west a block-plus on East Eighth Street to Broadway, then south seven blocks to Houston Street for the start of the next walk (Central Greenwich Village. Or walk north about six blocks on Fourth Avenue to East 14th Street for the Union Square tour (Walk 11).

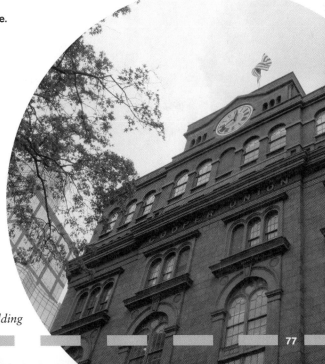

Cooper Union's iconic Foundation Building

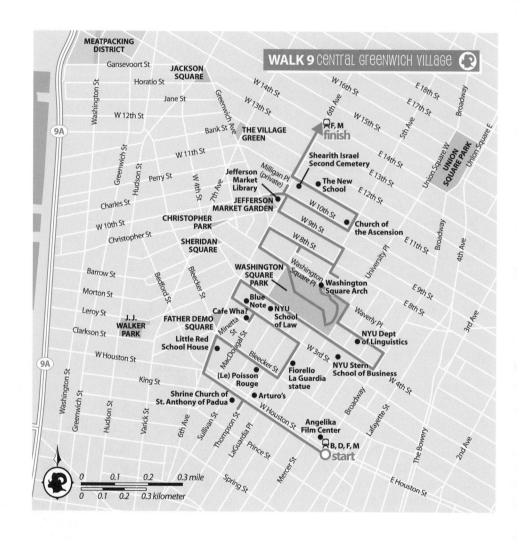

MEATPACKING DISTRICT

Gansevoort St

Horatio St

JACKSON SQUARE

Jane St

Washington St

W 12th St

W 14th St

W 16th St

E 18th St

Broadway

6th Ave

E 17th St

5th Ave

W 15th St

Union Square W

Union Square E

UNION SQUARE PARK

Bank St

W 13th St

Greenwich Ave

THE VILLAGE GREEN

9A

F, M finish

W 11th St

E 14th St

Perry St

7th Ave

Greenwich St

Hudson St

W 4th St

Milligan Pl (private)

Shearith Israel Second Cemetery

E 13th St

E 12th St

Charles St

Jefferson Market Library

The New School

JEFFERSON MARKET GARDEN

W 10th St

W 9th St

Church of the Ascension

E 11th St

University Pl

Broadway

4th Ave

W 10th St

CHRISTOPHER PARK

Christopher St

SHERIDAN SQUARE

W 8th St

Washington Square Pl

Barrow St

Bedford St

Bleecker St

WASHINGTON SQUARE PARK

Washington Square Arch

E 9th St

E 8th St

Morton St

Blue Note

Leroy St

J.J. WALKER PARK

FATHER DEMO SQUARE

Cafe Wha?

NYU School of Law

Waverly Pl

3rd Ave

Clarkson St

Minetta St

NYU Dept of Linguistics

Little Red School House

MacDougal St

W Houston St

Bleecker St

W 3rd St

NYU Stern School of Business

King St

(Le) Poisson Rouge

Fiorello La Guardia statue

W 4th St

Washington St

Greenwich St

Hudson St

Varick St

6th Ave

Sullivan St

Shrine Church of St. Anthony of Padua

Thompson St

Arturo's

LaGuardia Pl

W Houston St

Prince St

Mercer St

Broadway

Lafayette St

The Bowery

2nd Ave

9A

Angelika Film Center

B, D, F, M
start

Spring St

E Houston St

0   0.1   0.2   0.3 mile

0   0.1   0.2   0.3 kilometer

9 central Greenwich Village: Washington square affair

BOUNDARIES: **Houston St., Broadway, W. 11th St., 6th Ave.**
DISTANCE: **4 miles**
SUBWAY: **B/D/F/M to Broadway–Lafayette St., 6 to Bleecker St., or N/R to Prince St.**

When most people think of Greenwich Village, they think of Washington Square Park and the area around it. Books, movies, TV shows, and songs have long celebrated the hustle and bustle of the park and its art-all-around, life-on-stage ambience.

The other entity most closely associated with the neighborhood is New York University, spread among more than 20 schools and institutes. Named a "New Ivy" by the college-resource website Unigo, NYU is renowned for its programs in business, law, mathematics, engineering, and the visual, performing, and media arts. But it's far from the only seat of learning around here: Others include the New School, Parsons School of Design, Hebrew Union College, and Benjamin Cardozo Law School. Younger scholars attend the progressive Little Red School House, Elisabeth Irwin High School, or PS 41M. You can also educate yourself at the Jefferson Market branch of the New York Public Library.

Yet the heart of Greenwich Village offers much more than the cerebral. There are beautiful houses of worship; spots for live music and theater; and endless places to eat, drink, and shop. Architecture buffs will appreciate the myriad styles and structures represented here, particularly the jewel-like 19th-century mews houses tucked away in private alleys. For people-watching, celebrating, or chance-taking, this is a prime neighborhood for experiencing the New York life.

● **Start at Houston Street and Broadway, facing south. On the building to your right is an outdoor art piece that looks like a giant blue pegboard. This is *The Wall*, a minimalist piece created in 1973 by Forrest Myers. It marks what is generally regarded as the northern end of Soho.**

● **Walk west on Houston Street and pause at Mercer Street. On your right is the Angelika Film Center, which has been a renowned indie-movie theater since the late**

1980s. Across Mercer from it is the Coles Sports Center, part of the NYU campus. Continue walking on Houston; on the right are postwar apartment buildings with mostly NYU-related residents. At LaGuardia Place is a small park with an installation called *Time Landscape.* Farther along at #106 is Arturo's, a pizzeria where you get live jazz with your pie.

● Make a brief detour left at Thompson Street to see the Friary of St. Anthony of Padua, a stern fortress of a building. Return to Houston and continue west to the Shrine Church of St. Anthony of Padua, the oldest Italian Catholic parish in the US. Built in 1886, this Romanesque Revival church has a commanding presence. Inside, the vaulted ceiling appears like an umbrella over stained-glass windows. The side of the church has a small garden and statuary (the main entrance is on Sullivan, the next cross street).

● Proceed west on Houston to MacDougal Street, and pause. To your left, MacDougal is residential, but to your right across Houston, it's a lively strip enjoyed by tourists as well as New Yorkers who want a taste of the traditional Village café and restaurant scene.

● From Houston, make a right onto Sixth Avenue, a.k.a. Avenue of the Americas. There are cool shops and restaurants on both sides of this wide avenue, and on your right you'll pass the Little Red School House and Elisabeth Irwin High School, esteemed progressive (and private) institutions. The main entrance has a whimsical Tom Otterness sculpture called *The Lesson* (his pieces are also seen on Walk 2 and at the 14th Street A/C/E station).

● Continue along Sixth until curvy Minetta Street crops up, and walk along it briefly until it intersects Bleecker Street. Go right on Bleecker, which runs in a different direction here versus west of Sixth. At #201 is the Porto Rico Importing Co., a coffee and tea shop since 1907. At 158 Bleecker is the "multimedia art cabaret" (Le) Poisson Rouge—check out the fish motif—in the space formerly known as the Village Gate. (On the corner at Thompson Street, above the CVS sign, is an old sign from the Village Gate.) This neighborhood, and certainly Bleecker between Thompson and LaGuardia Place, has long been a stomping ground—and proving ground—for musicians (folk, rock, jazz, experimental), who pursue bookings at the small clubs on this strip, among them The Bitter End, Terra Blues, and others that have come and gone.

● When you get to LaGuardia Place, make a left. This block has a lot to offer: At #520 is a pretty building with arches and stars; #526 is the Renee and Chaim Gross Foundation, a sculpture gallery open on Thursdays and Fridays; #536 is the Center for Architecture, which has exhibits and archives. Cross the street carefully by the Citibank branch and examine the lively statue of Fiorello La Guardia, which captures (some of) the essence of this colorful, indefatigable former mayor and US congressman.

● Make a left at West Third Street. On your right is the NYU Kimmel Center for University Life, and on your left are shops. At 84 W. Third, between Thompson and Sullivan Streets is a true charmer: the decommissioned Fire Patrol 2 building (1906), with its brick-and-quoin design, bust of Mercury, and terra-cotta trim. (It's the home of CNN anchor Anderson Cooper.) At Sullivan Street on your right is Vanderbilt Hall, part of NYU Law School; it was built in 1951 in a neohistoricist style that blends well with the surrounding neighborhood. On the left is D'Agostino Hall, a residence for NYU law students. My father was the structural engineer for this building.

● At MacDougal Street, make a left. Ben's Pizzeria has anchored that corner since 1956. Caffè Reggio, farther down, has been serving coffee and pastry since 1927. Next door is Mamoun's Falafel, serving Middle Eastern fare. On the left-hand side of MacDougal, #132 has a fabulous old wrought-iron entrance. On the right side, where Minetta Lane cuts in for a block, are some iconic Village spots. Cafe Wha? is best known, its stage having been graced by the likes of Jimi Hendrix, Bob Dylan, Joan Rivers, and Richard Pryor. The Players Theatre is next door, and next to that the Comedy Cellar club and Olive Tree Café. Across

This Greenwich Village firehouse has been renovated into a residence.

Minetta Lane from Cafe Wha? is Minetta Tavern, open since 1937 and of late a pricey eatery renowned for its burgers. So many choices . . .

● Return to West Third and turn left. The club Groove is on the corner at #125, and a little more to the right is the beloved jazz spot Blue Note. Dig that piano coming out of the marquee! Also on this street, on the left, are The Village Underground (another live-music mainstay) and the Fat Black Pussycat club. West Third intersects Sixth Avenue, and if the weather is nice, there's probably a basketball game or two taking place at the West Fourth Street Courts, on the right. This storied place, also known as "The Cage," hosts some intense hoops. Film crews come here, and onlookers are reverent.

● Make a right on West Fourth Street, and, if the gates are open, amble through the Golden Swan Garden. The highlight of West Fourth here is the former Washington Square Methodist Church (#135), a stirring house of worship that is now residences. It was built in 1860 and couldn't be torn down due to landmarking.

● Past MacDougal Street/Washington Square West, West Fourth becomes Washington Square South. Among the impressive buildings in this stretch are the austere brown Hagop Kevorkian Center for Near Eastern Studies; Heyman Hall; and Judson Memorial Church (built in the 1890s and funded largely by John D. Rockefeller), its bell tower reminiscent of churches in Renaissance Italy. Then you see the brown lacelike exterior of the Catholic Center at NYU, the windows-galore look of the Kimmel Center, and the chalky red stone of the Bobst Library.

● Past Washington Square East, Washington Square South's name reverts to West Fourth Street. On your right, pass such postwar NYU buildings as the Stern Business School and the Courant Institute of Mathematical Sciences, along with the neo-Gothic Steinhardt Education Building (1930), on your left. On the corner of West Fourth and Mercer Street, Hebrew Union College is a rather plain brick structure except for the beautiful flowery menorah sculpture on its outer wall.

● When you reach Broadway, make a left. Take a long glance across the street at #704 and its opulent terra-cotta window decorations, including statues of lounging youth and caryatids. Quite a contrast with the plain red monolith that is Meyer Hall, the NYU physics building, on your left.

● Turn left onto Washington Place. The light-brown building at the corner of Mercer Street, #3–5, has exotic faces carved into the second floor. Just across Greene Street on your right is the Brown Building, home of NYU's biology and chemistry classes. But as the plaques on the building indicate, it is important also as the site of one of the most tragic events of the early 1900s: the Triangle Shirtwaist Factory Fire. Here, 146 workers, mostly young women, died on March 25, 1911.

● Make a right on Washington Square East. If you have time, go inside the Grey Art Gallery, opposite the park, to see the latest exhibitions. Make a left on Washington Square North. Here is "The Row," an elegant set of (mostly) Greek Revival town houses that were fashionable residences long ago (today, they're owned by NYU). Painter Edward Hopper lived at #3 from 1913 through 1967.

● At Fifth Avenue, turn left into Washington Square Park and behold the arch. It's one of the most photographed places in Greenwich Village, and everyone enjoys walking under and around it. George Washington is well portrayed in these statues, and the eagles seem nearly alive. To the left are a playground and a flagpole base that serves as a World War I memorial. Walk to the fountain in the center. It seems that no matter what the weather, someone is dancing, juggling, playing music, having multiple conversations with themselves, holding signs for a cause—you name it. When you tire of the action, make a left from the fountain and admire the statue of Giuseppe Garibaldi, who led the struggle for a unified Italy. Then go to the other side of the fountain to see the bust of Alexander Holley, a pioneering mechanical engineer of the 19th century.

● Follow the path to the angled left and exit the park onto Waverly Place. The building at the corner of Waverly and Washington Square West, the one with the Gothic arches and the black awning over its entrance, was home to Eleanor Roosevelt from 1945 to 1949.

● Continue to Sixth Avenue and look down the street on your left to see St. Joseph's Church, its two huge white columns gleaming in the sunlight. But go right on Sixth, then right again on West Eighth Street. West Eighth used to be an immensely lively strip of entertainment and commerce, but it has been toned down greatly (and regrettably). Still, there are some interesting things to see. Music fans can ooh and aah at Electric Lady Studios (#52), the recording studio founded by Jimi Hendrix. Stars from The Rolling Stones and Led Zeppelin to U2 and Lana Del Rey have recorded here.

● At MacDougal Street, make a right and walk half a block to tiny MacDougal Alley, a gated private street on your left. In spite of the gate, which is usually closed, you have a nice view down the alley. The buildings are beautiful, and the street is a novelty—originally it was built for horse stables. Not surprisingly, these are now pricey residences.

● Walk back to West Eighth and turn right. On your right, pass the New York Studio School of Drawing, Painting & Sculpture (#8–14), with its bold bald-eagle decoration over the entrance. The building used to house the Whitney Museum of American Art before it moved uptown. Across the street, at #5, is the Marlton House, which has a certain quaint stuffiness to it. For many years it was a dorm for the New School, but it has been remade into a boutique hotel. A plaque in the doorway explains that this was the birthplace of Galo Plaza, a president of Ecuador.

● When you reach Fifth Avenue, cross to the east side. The massive Art Deco tower in front of you is One Fifth Avenue. If you yearn to live in a high-rise, this is one to dream about. Just past it on the left is something much smaller and cozier: the one-block Washington Mews. This street is more or less a continuation of MacDougal Alley and, like that street, was originally used for stables. Now the little buildings are used by NYU. Unlike MacDougal Alley, it's open to the public during the day.

● Turn around on Fifth, walk north (away from Washington Square), and make a left onto West Ninth Street. Several buildings on this largely residential block have attractive ornamentation, such as #24 (the entrance and above it on the third and fifth floors); the town houses at #13, 15, and 17; the shimmery windows of #14; the slightly set-back windows of the Portsmouth at #38–40; and the Windsor Arms at #61, with X-shaped patterns in the brickwork. Farther on West Ninth, the PATH station has a colorful tiled mural.

● At Sixth Avenue, cross over and walk to the right to admire the busy beauty of the Jefferson Market Library. The turreted Victorian Gothic edifice was built as a courthouse and saw legal action from 1877 to 1945. But when the city threatened to demolish it, activists rallied and saved it. The interior is romantic—not your usual fusty library. But be warned: It apparently has no bathroom for public use.

- Make a left on West 10th Street. About halfway down the block on the right, you'll see another of the area's quirky alleys, Patchin Place, with an old lamp set beside the street sign. Like MacDougal Alley, this is a private street, but it affords a good view of the residences within.

- Walk back to Sixth Avenue, turn left, and on your left search out another alley, called Milligan Place. This one has a unique gate with the "street" name written in cursive, along with a crude wooden sign. Peer through the gate to see a sweet little oasis in the big city—homes with small garden plots scattered about.

- Walk back to West 10th and turn left. There are many lovely houses on the block, and the most significant is #50, the Grosvenor Private Boarding Stable. The building was renovated into a private home, and among the famous residents here were playwright Edward Albee and composer-lyricist Jerry Herman. The stately house at #18, with an entrance and parlor windows on the same level, is known as the Emma Lazarus House (it has a plaque about her). Best known for "The New Colossus," the poem on the pedestal of the Statue of Liberty, Lazarus lived here with her father and sisters. The building at #14 is nicknamed "The House of Death" because it is supposedly haunted by more than 20 ghosts. In 1987, one of America's most shocking child abuse cases—the murder of 6-year-old Lisa Steinberg—happened here.

- At Fifth Avenue, make a left. At the corner of Fifth and 10th, admire the Church of the Ascension, with its lancet windows and Gothic steeple. Then make another left, onto West 11th Street. This is another splendid block for strolling. The Larchmont at 27 W. 11th, the Charles Ives house at 70 W. 11th, and the bland modernism

Washington Square's stirring arch

of the New School building show the variety here. Of historical interest is near Sixth Avenue, on the left: a small, somewhat scraggly cemetery. This is the second cemetery of Shearith Israel synagogue; it used to be larger, but development and the street grid took their toll.

● Cross Sixth Avenue to pay homage to PS 41 on the left. One of the most prestigious public elementary schools in Manhattan, it has a slightly odd-shaped entrance area with some artwork on the wall. You can get a bus on Sixth Avenue or walk three blocks north to 14th Street for the F or M train.

POINTS OF INTEREST

Angelika Film Center angelikafilmcenter.com/nyc, 18 W. Houston St., 212-995-2570

Shrine Church of St. Anthony of Padua stanthonynyc.org, 155 Sullivan St., 212-777-2755

Arturo's 106 W. Houston St., 212-677-3820

Little Red School House & Elisabeth Irwin High School lrei.org, 272 Sixth Ave., 212-477-5316

Porto Rico Importing Co. portorico.com, 201 Bleecker St., 212-453-5908

(Le) Poisson Rouge lepoissonrouge.com, 158 Bleecker St., 212-505-FISH (3474)

Renee and Chaim Gross Foundation rcgrossfoundation.org, 526 LaGuardia Place, 212-529-4906

Center for Architecture cfa.aiany.org, 536 LaGuardia Place, 212-683-0023

Ben's Pizzeria 123 MacDougal St., 212-677-0976

Caffè Reggio caffereggio.com, 119 MacDougal St., 212-475-9557

Mamoun's Falafel mamouns.com, 119 MacDougal St., 212-674-8685

Cafe Wha? cafewha.com, 115 MacDougal St., 212-254-3706

Players Theatre theplayerstheater.com, 115 MacDougal St., 212-475-1449

Comedy Cellar comedycellar.com, 117 MacDougal St., 212-254-3480

Minetta Tavern minettatavernny.com, 113 MacDougal St., 212-475-3850

Groove clubgroovenyc.com, 128 W. Third St., 212-254-9393

Blue Note bluenote.net, 131 W. Third St., 212-475-8592

New York University nyu.edu, 70 Washington Square S., 212-998-1212

Grey Art Gallery of NYU nyu.edu/greyart, 100 Washington Square E., 212-998-6780

Washington Square Park nycgovparks.org/parks/washington-square-park, bounded by Waverly Place, University Place, West Fourth Street, and MacDougal Street

Electric Lady Studios electricladystudios.com, 52 W. Eighth St., 212-677-1366

New York Studio School of Drawing, Painting & Sculpture nyss.org, 8–14 W. Eighth St., 212-673-6466

The Marlton Hotel (Marlton House) marltonhotel.com, 5 W. Eighth St., 212-321-0100

Jefferson Market Library nypl.org/locations/jefferson-market, 425 Sixth Ave., 212-243-4334

Church of the Ascension ascensionnyc.org, Fifth Avenue and West Tenth Street, 212-254-8620

The New School newschool.edu, 68 Fifth Ave., 212-229-5108

Second Cemetery of Congregation Shearith Israel shearithisrael.org/content/eleventh-street-cemetery, 72 W. 11th St.

route summary

1. Start at Broadway and Houston Street and walk west on Houston Street.
2. Make a quick detour left on Thompson Street, then double back to Houston Street.
3. Turn right on Sixth Avenue.
4. Turn right on Minetta Street.
5. Make a quick right on Bleecker Street.
6. Walk left on LaGuardia Place.
7. Walk left on West Third Street.
8. Walk left on MacDougal Street for a block, then resume walking west on West Third.
9. Turn right on Sixth Avenue.
10. Turn right on West Fourth Street.
11. Turn left on Broadway.
12. Turn left on Washington Place.
13. Walk right on Washington Square East/University Place.

14. Walk left on Washington Square North/Waverly Place.

15. Enter Washington Square Park at Fifth Avenue.

16. Exit the park at Waverly Place and walk left (northeast).

17. Turn right on Sixth Avenue.

18. Make a right on West Eighth Street.

19. Stroll right on MacDougal Street to see MacDougal Alley, then double back to West Eighth Street.

20. Turn right on Fifth Avenue, then dip into Washington Mews, on your left.

21. Double back on Fifth Avenue, then turn left on West Ninth Street.

22. Go right on Sixth Avenue.

23. Detour left on West Tenth Street to see Patchin Place, then go back to Sixth Avenue and turn left to see Milligan Place, on your left.

24. Backtrack to West Tenth Street and head left.

25. Turn left on Fifth Avenue.

26. Go left on West 11th Street to Sixth Avenue.

27. Catch the bus on Sixth or walk three blocks north to 14th Street for the subway.

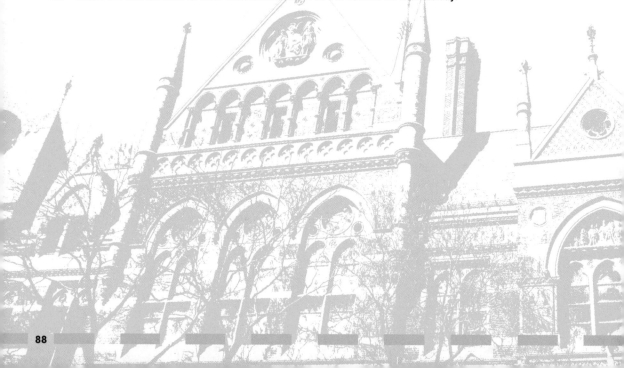

CONNECTING THE WALKS

Walk 12 (Chelsea and Madison Square Park) begins where this one ends. For the start of the Union Square tour (Walk 11), walk two blocks east on 14th Street to Union Square Park. Or walk two blocks west on 14th Street to Eighth Avenue to start Walk 13 (High Line).

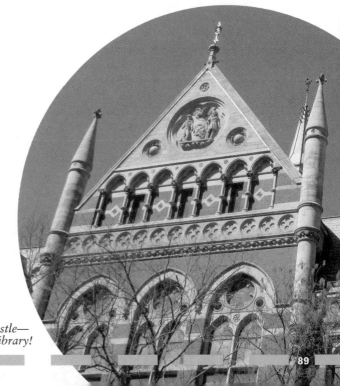

*It's not a European castle—
it's a Manhattan public library!*

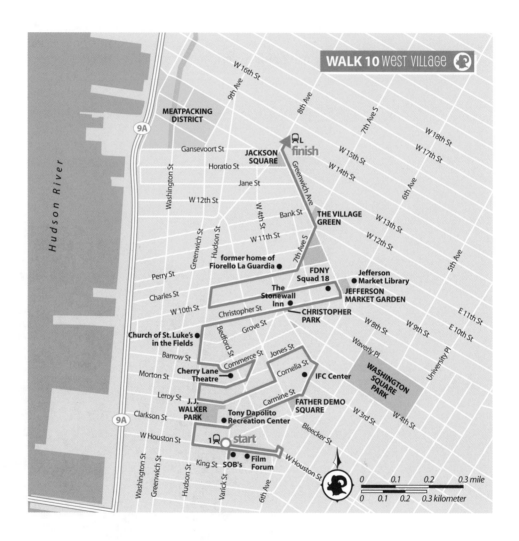

Hudson River

MEATPACKING DISTRICT

9A

W 16th St

9th Ave

8th Ave

7th Ave S

W 18th St

W 17th St

Gansevoort St

JACKSON SQUARE

L finish

W 15th St

W 14th St

Horatio St

Jane St

Washington St

W 12th St

6th Ave

Greenwich Ave

THE VILLAGE GREEN

W 13th St

W 12th St

5th Ave

W 4th St

Bank St

W 11th St

Hudson St

Greenwich St

former home of Fiorello La Guardia

7th Ave S

FDNY Squad 18

Jefferson Market Library

JEFFERSON MARKET GARDEN

Perry St

Charles St

W 10th St

The Stonewall Inn

Christopher St

CHRISTOPHER PARK

Grove St

W 8th St

W 9th St

E 11th St

E 10th St

Church of St. Luke's in the Fields

Bedford St

Waverly Pl

University Pl

Barrow St

Commerce St

Jones St

WASHINGTON SQUARE PARK

Morton St

Cherry Lane Theatre

Cornelia St

IFC Center

Leroy St

J. J. WALKER PARK

Carmine St

FATHER DEMO SQUARE

W 4th St

W 3rd St

9A

Clarkson St

Tony Dapolito Recreation Center

Bleecker St

W Houston St

1 start

Washington St

Greenwich St

Hudson St

Varick St

King St

SOB's

Film Forum

W Houston St

6th Ave

0   0.1   0.2   0.3 mile
0   0.1   0.2   0.3 kilometer

10 WEST VILLAGE: A MAZE OF STREETS AND SIGHTS

BOUNDARIES: **Houston St., Hudson St., W. 14th St., 6th Ave.**
DISTANCE: **2.2 miles**
SUBWAY: **1 to Houston St.**

Every time you walk the West Village, you'll find something new. Street patterns and naming conventions here are haphazard, rebellious; they've no doubt contributed to the neighborhood's liveliness over the years. (When the city first began imposing order on Manhattan with a grid system of numbered streets and avenues in 1811, the West Village was exempted, having been established well before the districts farther north.) Charming town houses and apartment buildings share the air with parks, public institutions, theaters and galleries, houses of worship, and shops selling everything from rare records to gourmet cheese to custom-made string instruments to literature . . . and much more.

The center of the neighborhood was ground zero for the modern American (and worldwide) gay rights movement; the Stonewall Inn and Christopher Park are testament to this. But this precinct is also home to somber war memorials, as well as the former homes of creative individuals such as Edna St. Vincent Millay and Woody Guthrie.

So get lost in the West Village—you won't regret it.

- From the subway on Varick Street, walk east on West Houston Street. There are plenty of interesting sights on this block, so just walk quickly until you hit Sixth Avenue, then turn around and make it a leisurely stroll. Start with the oddly shaped public park that separates West Houston from Bedford Street, which angles off it. There seems to be as much fence as greenery here. On the left, at #195, is Gilda's Club New York City, a cancer-support facility named after the late comic Gilda Radner. The building is quaint and cheery, with a slate roof and Tudor half-timbering. Across the street, at #196, the building looks plain, but the four bigger windows have metalwork under them, and when the sun hits them the right way they look like eyes. At #205 is the Martin Lane Gallery of Historical Americana, specializing in antique firearms, Civil War memorabilia, American Indian artifacts and jewelry, and more. At #209 is the Film Forum, a noteworthy independent-movie house. Across the street at #222 is Houston Hall, a brewpub and restaurant with a faux-old-timey lamp out front reading QUENCH THIRST on one side and FULL BELLY on the other.

● Make a left on Varick Street. On your left at #204 is SOB's, a long-lived and lively nightclub. I have to admit that even though I'd been to SOB's years ago, I never knew it was in this building with the pretty details until I created this walk. Cross the street and approach a big, serious federal building at #201. Here are offices for Homeland Security and Veterans Affairs, a post office, and more.

● Return to West Houston and make a left. Admire the redbrick school, PS M721. Designed in the Flemish Renaissance Revival style, it was the work of C. B. J. Snyder, the city's superintendent of school buildings in the late 19th and early 20th centuries.

● At Hudson Street, make a right; then turn right again onto Clarkson Street, passing James J. Walker Park on your left. Opposite the park, you see the other side of the public school on Houston; this is the main entrance, and decorated accordingly. Housed here in addition to PS M721 (a vocational school) are two alternative high schools, City As School and Independence High School. Walk up the steps of the entrance to take in the murals and other colorful art projects. On the other side of the street, see the playful Keith Haring mural at the Carmine Street Pool, one of the few diving pools left in New York City. It's part of the Tony Dapolito Recreation Center and was a location in the film *Raging Bull.*

● Make a left and walk along Seventh Avenue South. Pass the Hudson Park branch of the New York Public Library, housed in a handsome brick building from 1906. Poet Marianne Moore worked here as a library assistant in the early 1920s.

● Retreat to the previous corner, where you'll see that on the east side of the avenue, Clarkson Street curves upward and is named Carmine Street. Turn left onto Carmine. For your perusal are several shops and eateries, of varying levels of esotericism. Musicians will be agog at #42, Kelly Guitars. Across the street, at #35, is the proudly anachronistic House of Oldies, whose sign reads NO CD'S, NO TAPES, JUST RECORDS. Check out the sun-faded album covers plastered on the windows.

● At the corner of Bleecker Street, on the north side of Carmine, is Our Lady of Pompeii Church, built in the Italian Renaissance style. The bell tower is breathtaking. Go inside if you like—the main sanctuary, with its celestial frescoes and marble-and-gilt columns, seems like a direct Italian import.

- Diagonally across from the church, the triangle with benches and a trilevel fountain, often favored by resting birds, is Father Demo Square. (Father Antonio Demo served as pastor of Our Lady of Pompeii from 1900 to 1935.) People like to sit here and eat lunch or check their e-mail; I've also seen a few buskers playing here.

- Make a left on Sixth Avenue from Carmine Street and walk to the IFC Center, an indie-movie house, on your left. For many years it was known as the Waverly Theatre, and before that it was a church.

- Turn left onto West Fourth Street, passing Cornelia Street, which runs for just one block. You'll see Karavas Tavern, a Greek diner, on the corner of Cornelia and West Fourth. Across West Fourth are the Pink PussyCat Boutique, a purveyor of raunchiness for more than 40 years, and the Music Inn, a veritable garage sale of guitars, banjos, bongo drums, and what-not.

- Turn left onto Jones Street, another one-blocker, and notice the brick building with the iron balcony and medallion; this is Greenwich House Pottery. Jones dead-ends at Bleecker. Across from Jones is the famous John's of Bleecker Street—the coal-fired pizza is tasty, but as signs and the website advise, "no slices."

- Turn left on Bleecker and check out Matt Umanov Guitars at #273, Sushi Mambo at #255 (with its Japanese-style roof), and, at #254, Murray's Cheese Shop, which sells an astonishing array of specialty foods. Choose from gourmet charcuterie meats and myriad condiments in addition to cheeses.

- Turn right on Leroy Street, quietly pretty and residential. Cross Bedford Street, then Seventh Avenue South, noting that Leroy is called St. Luke's Place for one block only (Leroy picks up again at Hudson Street).

- St. Luke's Place, named for a church a few blocks away, is a collection of stately town houses. These have been the residences of some famous creative types: Marianne Moore lived at #14 and author Sherwood Anderson at #12. Jimmy Walker, the scandal-plagued mayor of New York from 1926 to 1932, lived at #6. The park across the street is named for him—you passed its Clarkson Street side earlier. A spooky element to this green acre: It was a cemetery for Trinity Church (see Walk 3) from 1812 to 1895, and some 10,000 dead remain here, in unmarked graves. The only outward reminder of the park's past is a memorial for two firemen killed on the job in the 1830s.

● Make a right onto Hudson Street, then another right on Morton Street. Another of the area's bent roads, Morton has several pretty buildings, such as #60, with lacy iron-work on its stair landing; #56 and #42, with carved stone faces flanking their entrances; and #54, with an elegant balcony.

● At Seventh Avenue South, make a left and walk to Commerce Street. Across the avenue is the Caliente Cab Co., a Mexican restaurant with a giant margarita attached to the wall.

● Turn left onto Commerce Street. Some of the houses are Federal-style and date from the 1830s.

● Make a brief detour left on Bedford Street. The house at 75½ Bedford—at 9 feet wide, Manhattan's narrowest address—has a small plaque noting that poet Edna St. Vincent Millay resided here for a year.

● Walk back to Commerce and make a left. It makes a sharp bend, just before which lies the Cherry Lane, the city's oldest continuously running off-Broadway theater. Where the street makes a right angle are two houses, at #46 and #48, that were owned by department store magnate Alexander Stewart.

● Commerce ends at Barrow Street. Make a left onto it and walk up to #72, the brick apartment building with the inner courtyard. Go in and take a look at the manicured lawn segments and colorful tile designs by the rooflines.

● Make a right on Hudson Street, but not before taking note of Barrow's cobblestoned road west of Hudson (nice to gaze at, annoying to drive on). Walk along Hudson to the Church of St. Luke in the Fields. It has a sweet little garden, and the church is pastoral and picturesque. The building dates from 1822, but most of it was rebuilt after a 1981 fire. Across the street is an elementary school, PS 3. This distinctive building was also the work of C. B. J. Snyder.

● Turn right on Christopher Street. Of particular interest is the Lucille Lortel Theatre, on your left. Ring Lardner, Samuel Beckett, Jean Genet, Wendy Wasserstein, and others are immortalized in its Playwrights' Sidewalk. The building (1926) was originally a movie house. Continue on Christopher past McNulty's (a tea-and-coffee shop, since 1895) on your left and cross Bleecker Street. In the middle of the next block is the dignified, unfussy St. John's Lutheran Church, with a charming domed cupola. This building dates to the 1820s and has served a few congregations.

● As you cross Seventh Avenue, be careful because West Fourth Street also crosses over. Christopher Street is called Stonewall Place here. Stop at the entrance to Christopher Park and cast a glance across it at Grove Street, which has pretty residences and its own micro-park. Opposite the park, at 53 Christopher St., is The Stonewall Inn, considered the birthplace of the gay rights movement. Police used to routinely raid the bar, but on June 28, 1969, the patrons rebelled and proclaimed their civil rights. New York's annual gay pride parade, held in this area in late June, commemorates the uprising. The park has statues of two gay couples, collectively called *Gay Liberation* and created by sculptor George Segal, along with a statue of Civil War general Philip Sheridan. At the eastern tip of the park, where Grove Street meets Christopher, is an unusual triangular building called the Northern Dispensary, a onetime health clinic dating to the 1830s and vacant since the 1980s. Its fate was being debated at this writing.

General Sheridan oversees his square.

● Continue along Christopher to Gay Street, on the right. It's a short, bent block lined with quaint Federal and Greek Revival town houses. (The street's name, by the way, predates the Stonewall riots by more than a century.)

● Make a left from Christopher onto Greenwich Avenue, and look over to Sixth Avenue on your right at the quirky and lovely Jefferson Market Library and park.

● Turn left on West 10th Street. On your left is the FDNY Squad 18's handsome building, whose second and third floors consist of orange brick and intricate darker orange accents. Somber plaques honor firefighters killed in 1956, 1966, and of course 2001. Cross Waverly Place, and on your left is a small corner shop, Three Lives & Company, that is the antidote to huge corporate bookstores. Past that, Seventh Avenue South crosses, creating another small, oddly shaped intersection. A short pace forward, West 10th crosses West 4th—only in New York, kids (or at least we think so). Farther along West 10th, at #233, is the NYPD's Sixth Precinct.

● Turn right on Hudson Street and notice #523, a 1880s-vintage retail–residential building that has been landmarked. Its architectural details include a dentiled roofline, a weathervane atop a cone, and terra-cotta moldings.

● Turn right again, this time onto Charles Street. The NYPD bomb squad and a police gas station are tucked into this block, along with attractive row houses that proudly display their ages on brass plates—#85 has a small plaque that reads "1868," and a few doors to the right another building's plaque reads "1897." The house at #74 has a historical sign about musician Woody Guthrie's tenure here. At #53 is Congregation Darech Emuno, established by Dutch Jews in 1838. The synagogue is housed in a renovated 1868 town home on a side of the street formerly known as Van Nest Place.

● Cross West Fourth Street and search out the curious alley on your right with a small sign, "58A." Take a peek through the fence—yet another quirky West Village address. Across the street, at #39, is the onetime home of New York City mayor Fiorello La Guardia. Continue past Seventh Avenue South to the garden patch at McCarthy Square. It mixes a patriotic war memorial with eclectic plantings and funky birdhouses.

● From the park, turn right on Seventh Avenue South. Past Perry Street on your left is the Village Vanguard, a storied jazz club. An acclaimed series of live recordings by such artists as John Coltrane, Bill Evans, Dizzy Gillespie, and Sonny Rollins originated here. At West 12th Street you'll pass a big white building on your left, covered with portholes. It's part of the former St. Vincent's Hospital complex and was originally built as the headquarters of the National Maritime Union.

● Make a left onto Greenwich Avenue, passing various shops and restaurants. Just after West 13th Street noses into Greenwich, you come to a transit-authority sub-station, tan brick with Art Deco details. The older building to the right of the substation on West 13th has whimsical clover-shaped decorations and a weathervane at the roof. To your left is Jackson Square, one of New York's oldest parks (dating from the mid-1850s), with an elegant gated entrance.

● Go right on Eighth Avenue to the 14th Street A/C/E/L train station, or relax in Jackson Square.

POINTS OF INTEREST

Martin Lane Gallery of Historical Americana historyonhand.com, 205 W. Houston St., 212-206-1004

Film Forum filmforum.org, 209 W. Houston St., 212-727-8110

Houston Hall houstonhallny.com, 222 W. Houston St., 212-675-9323

SOB's sobs.com, 204 Varick St., 212-243-4940

Kelly Guitars kellyguitars.com, 42 Carmine St., 212-691-8400

House of Oldies houseofoldies.com, 35 Carmine St., 212-243-0500

Tony Dapolito Recreation Center nycgovparks.org/facilities/recreationcenters/M103, Clarkson Street at Seventh Avenue South, 212-242-5418

Hudson Park Library nypl.org/locations/hudson-park, 66 Leroy St., 212-243-6876

Our Lady of Pompeii Church ourladyofpompeiinyc.com, 25 Carmine St., 212-989-6805

IFC Center ifccenter.com, 323 Sixth Ave., 212-924-7771

Music Inn musicinn.nyc, 169 W. Fourth St., 212-243-5715

John's of Bleecker Street johnsbrickovenpizza.com, 278 Bleecker St., 212-243-1680

Murray's Cheese Shop murrayscheese.com, 254 Bleecker St., 212-243-3289

James J. Walker Park nycgovparks.org/parks/james-j-walker-park, Hudson Street at Clarkson Street

Caliente Cab Co. calientecabco.com, 61 Seventh Ave. S., #1, 212-243-8517

Cherry Lane Theatre cherrylanetheatre.org, 38 Commerce St., 212-989-2020

Church of St. Luke in the Fields stlukeinthefields.org, 487 Hudson St., 212-924-0562

Lucille Lortel Theatre lortel.org/llt_theater, 121 Christopher St., 212-924-2817

McNulty's mcnultys.com, 109 Christopher St., 212-242-5351

St. John's Lutheran Church stjohnsnyc.org, 81 Christopher St., 212-242-5737

Christopher Park nycgovparks.org/parks/christopher-park, Christopher Street at Seventh Avenue South

The Stonewall Inn thestonewallinnyc.com, 53 Christopher St., 212-488-2705

Jefferson Market Library nypl.org/locations/jefferson-market, 425 Sixth Ave., 212-243-4334

Three Lives & Company threelives.com, 154 W. 10th St., 212-741-2069

McCarthy Square nycgovparks.org/parks/mccarthy-square, bounded by Seventh Avenue South, Charles Street, and Waverly Place

Village Vanguard villagevanguard.com, 178 Seventh Ave. S., 212-255-4037

Jackson Square nycgovparks.org/parks/jackson-square, Eighth Avenue at Greenwich Avenue

route summary

1. From Varick Street, walk east on Houston Street to Sixth Avenue, then double back.
2. Make a brief detour left on Varick Street, then continue west on Houston Street.
3. Walk right on Hudson Street.
4. Walk right on Clarkson Street.
5. Walk left on Seventh Avenue South, then return and continue east on Clarkson Street, which becomes Carmine Street.
6. Walk left on Sixth Avenue.
7. Walk left on West Fourth Street.
8. Stroll left on Jones Street.

9. Walk left on Bleecker Street.

10. Walk right on Leroy Street/St. Luke's Place.

11. Travel right on Hudson Street.

12. Walk right on Morton Street.

13. Make a left on Seventh Avenue South.

14. Walk left on Commerce Street, with a dip in and out of Bedford Street to your left.

15. Walk left on Barrow Street.

16. Walk right on Hudson Street.

17. Walk right on Christopher Street.

18. Walk left on Greenwich Avenue.

19. Travel left on West 10th Street.

20. Walk right on Hudson Street.

21. Walk right on Charles Street.

22. Head north on Seventh Avenue South

23. Walk left on Greenwich Avenue.

24. Go right onto Eighth Avenue.

CONNECTING THE WALKS

Walk 18 (High Line) begins where this one ends. To start the Chelsea tour (Walk 13), go two blocks east on West 14th Street to Sixth Avenue.

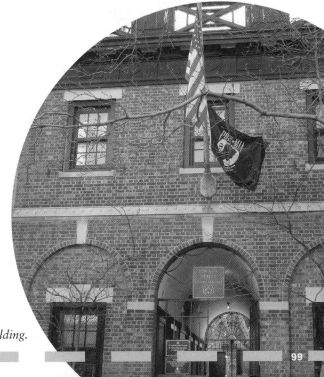

This is no ordinary Manhattan playground building.

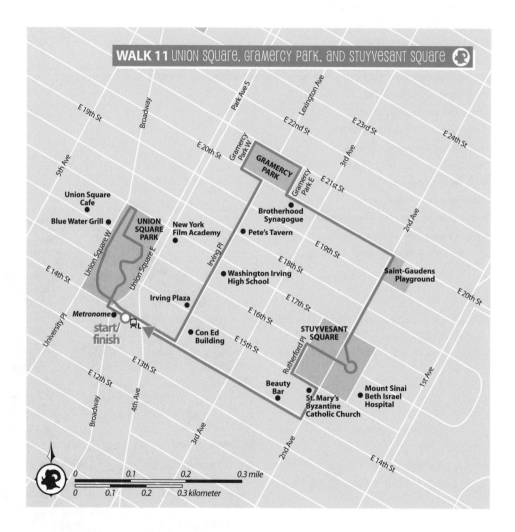

E 19th St

Broadway

Park Ave S

Lexington Ave

E 22nd St

E 23rd St

E 24th St

5th Ave

E 20th St

Gramercy Park W

GRAMERCY PARK

Gramercy Park E

3rd Ave

E 21st St

2nd Ave

Union Square Cafe

UNION SQUARE PARK

New York Film Academy

Brotherhood Synagogue

Blue Water Grill

Pete's Tavern

Union Square W

Union Square E

E 19th St

Saint-Gaudens Playground

E 14th St

Irving Pl

E 18th St

E 20th St

Washington Irving High School

Irving Plaza

E 17th St

Metronome

start/ finish

L

E 16th St

STUYVESANT SQUARE

Con Ed Building

E 15th St

Rutherford Pl

University Pl

E 13th St

Beauty Bar

E 12th St

4th Ave

Mount Sinai Beth Israel Hospital

1st Ave

St. Mary's Byzantine Catholic Church

Broadway

3rd Ave

2nd Ave

E 14th St

0   0.1   0.2   0.3 mile

0   0.1   0.2   0.3 kilometer

11 UNION SQUARE, GRAMERCY PARK, AND STUYVESANT SQUARE: TRIPLE PLAY

BOUNDARIES: **Broadway, E. 14th St., 1st Ave., Gramercy Park**
DISTANCE: **2.5 miles**
SUBWAY: **L, N, Q, R, 4, 5, or 6 to Union Square/14th St.**

Manhattan has quite a few lively public parks beyond Central Park, each with its own personality and special features. This walk brings you to three of them.

Union Square has the highest profile. It hosts a variety of activities throughout the year, is surrounded by places to eat and shop, and features a year-round farmers' market. Gramercy Park is quiet and stately; only a select few can enter its gates, but you can still peer in and appreciate its beauty. Stuyvesant Square is bordered by a hospital on the east and a school and churches on the west; it hosts live musical performances in the summer.

Within this more-or-less rectangle of east Manhattan, you'll encounter such sights as public and private schools, houses of worship, public art, historic homes, commercial establishments, and more. The Manhattan-born author, historian, and diplomat Washington Irving plays a prominent role in this neighborhood; Irving Place and Washington Irving High School are named for him, and one building bears a plaque in his memory. Such tributes are quite fitting for many reasons—for one, he popularized the nickname "Gotham" for New York City.

● **Union Square Park, where you exit the subway, has the air of a miniature Central Park, with a playground, a dog run, statues of historical figures, a spacious plaza, and a circuit of walking paths. It's surrounded on all four sides by restaurants and stores. Opposite the park, on a building on the south side of 14th Street between Broadway and Fourth Avenue, you'll see** Metronome, **a piece of public art that sort of resembles a magic wand with sparkles emanating from it in concentric circles. It also has a 15-digit counter to the left of it. Mystifying at first glance, it's actually a digital clock: The first seven digits show the time of day in 24-hour format—two digits for hours, two for minutes, two for seconds, and one for tenths of a second—and the last seven** digits show how much time is left in the day, with the previous values reversed. The center digit, between the first and last seven, represents hundredths of a second, its numbers zipping past in a blur. So if the counter reads "202126574333803," the time is 8:21 p.m. plus 26.57 seconds, and, from right to left, there are 3 hours, 38 minutes, and 33.47 seconds left in the day.

● Start exploring at the park's lower-level plaza, on the north side of 14th Street. Here, you'll often find people relaxing on the steps, eating lunch, or tending to their cell phones; occasionally, crowds gather here for a political or social rally, demonstration, or vigil. The centerpiece of this part of the park is a dignified equestrian statue of George Washington; closer to Union Square West is a fountain with decorative urns, and a bit farther up is a statue of Mohandas Gandhi, dedicated in 1986. (He looks a bit out of place amid the commercial enterprises surrounding him.) Just across the street, at 5–9 Union Square West, is the Spingler Building. This stately yellow-brick structure was completed in 1897. If you cast your eyes on the sidewalks here and there, you'll find maplike brass plaques, more than 20 in all, that explain the history of various aspects of the park.

The northern and western ends of Union Square are where you'll find the farmers' market (usually held Monday, Wednesday, Friday, and Saturday) and some street musicians. Just on the edge of the park is a sculpture of a mother and two children, which dates to 1881 and has four lion's heads at its base that used to function as drinking fountains. On Union Square West, across from the park at East 16th Street, are a few interesting older buildings. The neo-Renaissance corner building, #31, has an engraving that reads BANK OF THE METROPOLIS; the bottom floor now houses the Blue Water Grill, an upscale seafood eatery. (Around the corner, at 21 E. 16th, is another restaurant, the acclaimed Union Square Cafe.) Next door, at 33 Union Square West, the Decker Building has a vaguely Moorish look and several fancifully decorated balconies. Today it's mostly residential, but in the late 1960s and early 1970s its sixth floor was the site of the Factory, Andy Warhol's legendary studio and party pad.

● Go back inside the park and walk to Evelyn's Playground, a cheerful and quixotic place. (Even big kids like to gambol on the structures.) The Pavilion, an event space and restaurant, has a European feel to it. A big Abraham Lincoln statue watches over the festivities. Outside the park to the east is the redbrick New York Film Academy;

the Georgian Revival building (1929) started out as headquarters for the corrupt Tammany Hall political machine.

● Walk into the center of the park to admire the Independence Flagstaff. Its base displays various figures symbolizing democracy and tyranny. Stroll a bit south to see the statue of the Marquis de Lafayette; he faces outward to the sidewalk, but you can admire him from the side. Across Union Square East at East 15th Street is Zeckendorf Towers, a redbrick condo complex built in the late 1980s.

● Exit the southern end of Union Square Park and walk to your left along East 14th Street for one block, then make another left onto Irving Place. The gorgeous white limestone tower on your right, with the clocks on all four sides, is known as the Con Ed Building (after the utility). Stately in the daytime, it's sometimes lit up at night. At East 15th Street on your left is Irving Plaza, a midsize music palace in a nondescript space. I've seen a variety of rock acts here over the years, including Cheap Trick, Hot Tuna, Sonic Youth, and Children of Bodom. (If you attend a show, I recommend standing by the soundboard on the floor.)

● Walk another block, and between East 16th and East 17th Streets you'll see Washington Irving High School on the right. A quintessential big-city school building, it features a bust of Irving on the sidewalk. Go up the steps and peer inside (or just go in—why not?) to see a wondrous set of 12 murals dating to the 1920s and depicting scenes from Irving's books. In the vestibule is a plaque detailing the history of the school.

● Go outside and cross the street to gaze at the pretty row houses of

Serene Gramercy Park and its statue of Edwin Booth

East 17th Street, built in the early and mid-1800s. The one at the corner (#122) has a plaque dedicated to Mr. Irving, although there is no evidence that he actually lived here.

● Stroll to East 18th Street and you'll come upon Pete's Tavern. This corner eatery—the oldest continuously operating restaurant in the city, open since 1864—bears a street sign for O. Henry's Way (the writer was a regular here) and is full of historical and kitschy touches. "The Tavern O. Henry Made Famous" gets totally decked out at Christmastime. Across East 19th Street, check out the brick apartment building on the left corner. Designed by George Pelham, it's festooned with all kinds of kooky terra-cotta creatures.

● Walk until you're just across the street from the gated expanse known as Gramercy Park. Look to your right at the handsome redbrick residence with many black shutters at the corner of East 19th. Built in 1845, it was the home of Stuyvesant Fish, a Gilded Age industrialist, and later Benjamin Sonnenberg, a famous press agent. Now a curious white statue stands on the Gramercy Park South side.

Gramercy Park is private—keys to the gate are available only to residents of the buildings surrounding the park, along with guests of the Gramercy Park Hotel and members of several private clubs and houses of worship—but anyone can appreciate this green patch and its environs; plus, it's open to the public on Christmas Eve. Note a modern innovation on the main gate here and on the north side: flashing LED lights that warn drivers that they can't pass through. Peer into the center of the park to behold a statue of Shakespearean actor Edwin Booth, a brother of assassin John Wilkes Booth.

● Stroll to your left on Gramercy Park South, looking into the park but also at the row houses across the street, such as #17 (now serving the School of Visual Arts). Both #16, the Players (an exclusive social club founded by Edwin Booth), and #15, the National Arts Club, have lavish decoration, medallions, ironwork, a fountain, and other accoutrements. The house at #13 is more restrained, but note the quaint figure of a child over the main door.

● Take a right onto Gramercy Park West, which has a few buildings with exquisite wrought-iron entrances. Inside the park you'll see an eye-catching bird feeder on a pole. Turn right at Gramercy Park North (East 21st Street) to see more elegant houses and more park features, such as urns used as planters, informative plaques, pretty shrubbery, and more. Lexington Avenue begins at the block's center. (A plaque at 1 Lexington honors onetime resident Cyrus West Field, who oversaw the laying of the first transatlantic telegraph cable in 1858.)

- Turn right on Gramercy Park East and admire the buildings, especially #36 with its two armored knights at the entrance. The Gramercy Park House, the Queen Anne–style apartment building at the corner (#34), has a rugged, romantic quality to it.

- Make a left on East 20th Street and admire the Brotherhood Synagogue, formerly the Friends Meetinghouse, midblock on your right. It has an austere Garden of Remembrance, dedicated to Holocaust victims. Cross Third Avenue; the building at #208 has a sculpted horse head. See what's left of the old Columbus Hospital at #226–228 (at this writing, it was being renovated into housing). Farther along to the left is the city's former Police Academy, a foreboding postwar building (the academy moved to Queens in January 2015). And at #247, at the corner by Second Avenue, is the Learning Spring School, for children on the autism spectrum. The logo is pretty, and the building has a coolly metallic vibe.

- Cross Second Avenue, and to your left will be a large schoolyard, Peter's Field. There are a few public schools here; the handsomest is the castlelike, light-gray-and-cream PS 40. Going south on Second Avenue, look into the cute playground named for sculptor Augustus Saint-Gaudens. On the pavement is drawn a large face, over which kids run pell-mell.

- To your left on Second Avenue, between East 18th and East 17th Streets, is the Mount Sinai Beth Israel Hospital Center. East 17th is also named Dvorak Place, for Czech composer Antonín **Dvořák**, who lived in the area in the 1890s. You'll see a statue of him in the next park you encounter, Stuyvesant Square, bisected by Second Avenue. Walk to your left and stroll the eastern half of this park; find the **Dvořák** statue in the northeast corner. When you exit, cross Second Avenue and enter the western sector of the park. This half has a Peter Stuyvesant statue, a fountain, and gardens. Along the park's eastern edge, on Rutherford Place, are the private Friends School and St. George's Episcopal Church.

- Exit the park on Rutherford Place and walk to your left; then turn left at East 15th. St. Mary's Byzantine Catholic Church, a space-age house of worship, is on the right. The first all-glass church building in the US, it was designed in 1959 by a Franciscan monk who was also an architect. Note the dramatic icon at the entrance and the wispy silver spire holding a bell.

- Cross Second Avenue. The corner building is a school, opened in 1904 as the Hebrew Technical School for Girls. Since the late 1980s it has been a public transfer school (for off-track and older students who need to catch up on academic credits), known currently as Manhattan Comprehensive Night and Day High School; I taught here from 1989 through 1994. If you look down East 15th Street toward First Avenue, you'll see another school building past the hospital; that's the original Stuyvesant High School, and it now houses a few small schools. ("Stuy" is now on Chambers Street; see Walk 2.)

- Continue toward East 14th Street, where the New York Eye and Ear Infirmary is to your left—go right on East 14th. Walk along the block and you'll notice that the storefronts are a mixture of nationally known and local businesses. The old Italian Labor Center at #231 became a beauty salon and is now a watering hole called Beauty Bar, where you can sip a drink while sitting under a vintage hair dryer.

- Keep walking across Third Avenue. On your left is the NYU Palladium Athletic Facility; for many years, a large music club called the Palladium was on this lot. I saw several artists perform here back in the day, including Sinéad O'Connor.

- Continue walking to Fourth Avenue for the Union Square subway station.

POINTS OF INTEREST

Union Square Park nycgovparks.org/parks/union-square-park, East 14th Street at Broadway
Blue Water Grill bluewatergrillnyc.com, 31 Union Square W., 212-675-9500
Union Square Cafe unionsquarecafe.com, 21 E. 16th St., 212-243-4020
Irving Plaza irvingplaza.com, 17 Irving Place, 212-777-6800
Pete's Tavern petestavern.com, 129 E. 18th St., 212-473-7676
Gramercy Park Irving Place at East 20th Street

Brotherhood Synagogue brotherhoodsynagogue.org, 28 Gramercy Park S., 212-674-5750

Augustus Saint-Gaudens Playground nycgovparks.org/parks/augustus-st-gaudens -playground, Second Avenue between East 19th and East 20th Streets

Stuyvesant Square nycgovparks.org/parks/stuyvesant-square, Second Avenue between East 15th and East 17th Streets

St. Mary's Catholic Church of the Byzantine Rite stmarysbyzantinenyc.com, 246 E. 15th St., 212-677-0516

Beauty Bar thebeautybar.con, 231 E. 14th St., 212-539-1389

route summary

1. Tour Union Square Park, exiting onto East 14th Street and walking left.
2. Walk left on Irving Place.
3. Walk left on Gramercy Park South/East 20th Street.
4. Walk right on Gramercy Park West.
5. Walk right on Gramercy Park North/East 21st Street.
6. Walk right on Gramercy Park East.
7. Walk left on East 20th Street.
8. Walk right on Second Avenue.
9. Go into Stuyvesant Park, first east of Second Avenue and then west.
10. Go left on Rutherford Place.
11. Walk left on East 15th Street.
12. Walk right on Second Avenue.
13. Walk right on East 14th Street back to Union Square Park and the subway.

connecting the walks

To start the next walk, head three blocks west on 14th Street to Sixth Avenue. For Walk 13 (High Line), walk an additional two blocks west on 14th to Eighth Avenue.

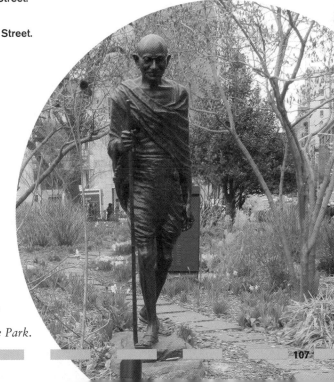

Gandhi guards a path in Union Square Park.

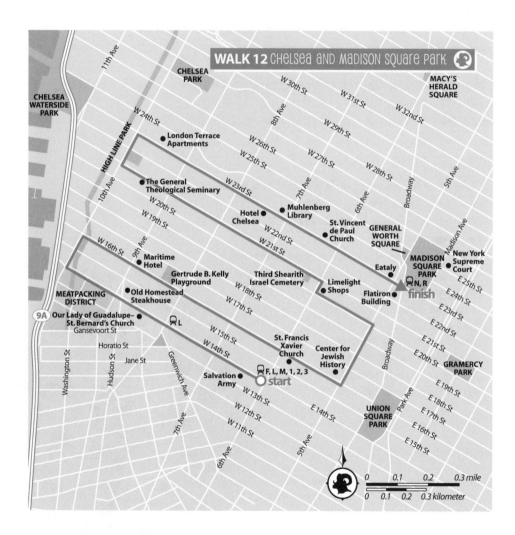

WALK 12 Chelsea and Madison Square Park

CHELSEA
WATERSIDE
PARK

CHELSEA
PARK

MACY'S
HERALD
SQUARE

11th Ave

HIGH LINE PARK

W 30th St

W 31st St

W 32nd St

8th Ave

W 29th St

W 24th St

W 26th St

W 27th St

W 28th St

● London Terrace
  Apartments

W 25th St

Broadway

5th Ave

10th Ave

● The General
  Theological Seminary

W 23rd St

7th Ave

6th Ave

W 20th St

● Muhlenberg
  Library

W 19th St

Hotel ●
Chelsea

St. Vincent
de Paul
Church

GENERAL
WORTH
SQUARE

W 22nd St

W 21st St

W 16th St

9th Ave

Maritime
● Hotel

● Eataly

Madison Ave

MADISON
SQUARE
PARK

New York
● Supreme
  Court

E 25th St

Gertrude B. Kelly
Playground

Third Shearith
Israel Cemetery

Limelight
● Shops

Flatiron ●
Building

🚉 N, R
finish

E 24th St

MEATPACKING
DISTRICT

W 18th St

E 23rd St

● Old Homestead
  Steakhouse

W 17th St

E 22nd St

9A ● Our Lady of Guadalupe–
      St. Bernard's Church
      Gansevoort St

🚉 L

W 15th St

W 14th St

Horatio St

Jane St

St. Francis
Xavier
Church

Center for
Jewish
History

E 21st St

E 20th St

GRAMERCY
PARK

Broadway

Park Ave

E 19th St

Washington St

Hudson St

Greenwich Ave

7th Ave

Salvation ●
Army

🚉 F, L, M, 1, 2, 3
○ start

W 13th St

E 18th St

E 14th St

E 17th St

UNION
SQUARE
PARK

E 16th St

W 12th St

E 15th St

6th Ave

5th Ave

W 11th St

0   0.1   0.2   0.3 mile

0   0.1   0.2   0.3 kilometer

12 Chelsea and Madison Square Park: Checking Out Chelsea

BOUNDARIES: 10th Ave., W. 14th St., 5th Ave., W. 26th St.
DISTANCE: 3.5 miles
SUBWAY: 1, 2, 3, F, M, or L to 14th St. (6th Ave.)

Chelsea is an exciting mix of old and new, residential and commercial, religious and cultural, with some iconic spots that have played significant roles in New York history (some of that history being rather sordid). From its parks to its schools, minor museums to nightclubs, this is a stimulating area to explore. Much of Chelsea has a more leisurely pace and residential feel than busy Midtown to the north and funky Greenwich Village to the south. The two main drags are 14th Street and 23rd Street, both home to a wide variety of sights; the latter has one of Manhattan's most recognizable structures, the Flatiron Building.

● Walk west on West 14th Street from Sixth Avenue. Midblock is the McBurney YMCA, located in this building since 2002 but in existence since the mid-1800s. Across the street are the New York headquarters of the Salvation Army and its Centennial Memorial Temple. This dramatic building has an arched entrance resembling thick icicles; the blog Daytonian in Manhattan calls it "Wizard of Oz Art Deco." Farther down the block at #144 is the Manhattan campus of Pratt Institute, a Brooklyn college (Pratt took over this building in 2000). At the corner by Seventh Avenue is #154, built shortly before World War I, which has many pretty terra-cotta accents of yellow and blue.

● Across Seventh Avenue, the first building on the left, 200 W. 14th, is the Jeanne d'Arc apartments, built in 1889. It features a statue of Joan of Arc above the main entrance, as well as a small balcony on the second floor, guarded by two griffins. The building at #216 houses Teamsters Local 237. It's austere in design but has the union's emblem at street level and some pleasing decorative elements on the top floor. Across the street at #229–231, two buildings from the 1840s were combined and adapted in 1902 to create Our Lady of Guadalupe Church. It served a Spanish-speaking congregation until the 2000s and is now part of the McBurney Y. The main entrance has lovely Spanish Colonial details, and the old church name is still visible, if faint.

- Both corner buildings across Eighth Avenue are elegant, weighty landmarked sites. On the left is the former New York County National Bank, from 1907, with a proud eagle standing guard atop its entrance. On the right is the former New York Savings Bank (now a CVS drugstore), from 1897. It also has an eagle, as well as a Roman-style dome and a clock topped with a sculpture of a beehive. Walk on the right side of the street and note the A/C/E station elevator; it's graced with a comical sculpture by Tom Otterness. At #328 is Our Lady of Guadalupe at St. Bernard's Church (Our Lady, whose former building you saw earlier, merged with St. Bernard's). Built in the mid-1870s, it's a darkly Gothic structure with three pointed arches over the doors. A bit farther to the right is the clumsily named but intriguing 345meatpacking, a residential and commercial building with plants growing out of linear window boxes.

- Pause at Ninth Avenue to check out a few sights. Hudson Street cuts in here at an angle, reminding us that the Chelsea neighborhood is not completely on a neat grid. Down on the right at 56 Ninth Ave., marked by a classic neon sign, is the Old Homestead Steakhouse, having held forth since 1868. There is also a seating area on the right, in a triangle formed by the intersecting streets. To the left, 675 Hudson is a triangular building from 1848 that's served various uses but still stands proud.

- Across Ninth Avenue, West 14th Street turns to cobblestones as you enter the Meatpacking District. There used to be more than 300 slaughterhouses and meat-packing plants here, but that number has dwindled greatly. In the 1970s this area had a bad rap for prostitution and drug dealing, but now it's a hipster haven with designer shops, art galleries, expensive restaurants, and popular bars. This is one neighbor-hood that has definitely surprised me with its turnaround. Continuing west, take note of all the old buildings recast into swank stores, and see the elevated High Line Park.

- Turn right on 10th Avenue and walk beside the High Line, a decommissioned freight-train line converted into a wonderful park (see the next walk). On your right between West 15th and West 16th is the NBC building—National Biscuit Company, in this case. We know the company as Nabisco, the snack empire. Now it houses the popular Chelsea Market, comprising a shopping mall, a food court, offices, and a TV studio.

- Turn right onto West 16th. A freight entrance to the Food Network studios is immediately on the right, and if the doors are up you'll see colorful murals inside. Across the street is one of the staircases up to the High Line. On the left as you near Ninth Avenue are the Fulton Houses, a public housing complex with a playground in the courtyard.

- At Ninth look to the right and see the immense former Port Authority of New York building, which now houses Google and other corporate offices. On the left is The Maritime Hotel, with its rows of porthole windows. It's a peculiar-looking building that to me resembles a game board. Originally a hotel for members of the National Maritime Union, it later served as a drug-rehab center and is now a hotel again. The porthole motif is repeated on another former NMU building next door on the left; this, too, is now a hotel, the Dream. (The union's former headquarters—also covered with porthole windows—is visited in Walk 10, East Village.)

- Farther down West 16th is part of the School of Visual Arts campus. Just across the street is Atlantic Theater Company's Stage 2 (its main stage is on West 20th Street). At 319 W. 16th there is a pretty bas-relief above the door: two robust cherubs with a cornucopia of fruit. Next door, the playground named for surgeon and philanthropist Dr. Gertrude B. Kelly goes through to 17th Street.

- Cross Eighth Avenue; this next block is pleasantly quiet and largely residential, with a particularly nice building at 253 W. 16th, Chelsea Hall. The decoration above the front entrance has three lions and a crown, giving it a British air. An especially pretty apartment building on this block is at #216, red brick with white accents and a recessed main entrance.

A small, historic cemetery in Chelsea

● Continue past Seventh Avenue to another mostly residential street. But midblock on the right is a church building that dates to the 1830s, with a motif of Renaissance Revival windows and two outer staircases. It was originally the Catholic Apostolic Church, then the French Evangelical Church. Just past it at 120 W. 16th, the cottage-like building is the former House of Industry (1878). It provided vocational training for poor women and girls and later became housing for developmentally disabled adults.

● The block after Sixth Avenue has some of the better-known institutions of this neighborhood. The Church of St. Francis Xavier, dedicated in 1882, is an imposing Roman basilica on your right. Within are five altars and much artwork; outside, arches and columns draw attention to the recessed entrance. Next door is Xavier High School, a boys' Jesuit school with pre- and post-WWII buildings. (Students can be spotted commuting to school by train, clad in tan khaki pants and emblem polo shirts.) At #17–21 are pre–Civil War buildings of the Greek Revival style; read their plaques. And #17 was a Margaret Sanger clinic. Farther down the block is the Center for Jewish History, composed of four older and two newer buildings housing five agencies: the American Jewish Historical Society, the Leo Baeck Institute, the American Sephardi Federation, the YIVO Institute for Jewish Research, and the Yeshiva University Museum.

● At Fifth Avenue cross over to the building on the left corner. B. Shackman & Co. is no longer here, selling novelties such as Kitty Cucumber Soap Crayons (I kid you not), but its nameplate lives on, as does the pretty main entrance framed by rope moldings. Turn left and walk along Fifth Avenue. In this part of town Fifth has a solid commercial presence but is far mellower than in Midtown and not nearly as posh as by Central Park.

● Turn left on West 20th Street. The Presbyterian Building, on your right at 156 Fifth Ave., dates to the 1890s and has impressive spiky dormers near the roof. Midblock on the left is the Andrew Heiskell Braille and Talking Book Library, a branch of the New York Public Library. On the right as you approach Sixth Avenue, you see a church . . . or is it something else? Make a right at Sixth to examine it more closely.

This site was built in the 1840s as the Episcopal Church of the Holy Communion. After being deconsecrated, it became Odyssey House, a drug-rehab center. In the early 1980s, nightlife impresario Peter Gatien bought it and turned it into

The Limelight, a disco and rock club. (I went there a few times to see some R&B acts and thought it was cool, with all the nooks and crannies from the original church layout.) In the 1990s, it became famous as a haunt for so-called club kids; it also became notorious for drug use and a sensational murder that inspired the movie *Party Monster.* Today it's the Limelight Shops, a collection of boutiques.

- Turn left off of Sixth Avenue onto West 21st Street, noting the golden-domed Hugh O'Neill Dry Goods Building on your left and the Beaux Arts Adams Dry Goods Building across the street on your right. Just past the O'Neill Building on your left, see the small Third Spanish–Portuguese Cemetery. This is the biggest and best preserved (and "youngest") of the very old graveyards of Shearith Israel synagogue in Manhattan (the other two are on Walks 5 and 9). Farther along to the left are old buildings now used by the School of Visual Arts.

- Cross Seventh Avenue to a largely residential block. Past Eighth Avenue in the middle of the block is PS 11, an old castlelike school building with cheery and colorful murals; a playground is next to it on the left.

- The General Theological Seminary dominates the left side of the next block. The somber red buildings that make up this Episcopalian campus occupy land once owned by poet Clement Clarke Moore ("A Visit from St. Nicholas"). The seminary has occupied this tract of land since 1827. The Chapel of the Good Shepherd has architectural elements modeled on those of buildings at Oxford University. On the right side of the block, many of the houses date to the 1850s. At 10th Avenue, look ahead to see part of the High Line.

- Turn right on 10th Avenue, passing on your left the Church of the Guardian Angel, which looks as if it were airlifted in from Italy. Built in 1930, it has a large and gorgeous rose window.

- Turn right on West 23rd Street. Taking up the entire block on your left is the massive London Terrace apartment complex, built in 1930–31. (The 4 corner buildings fronting 9th and 10th Avenues, called London Terrace Towers, are co-ops; the 10 contiguous buildings in between along West 23rd, known as London Terrace Gardens, hold rental units.) The right side of the block is lined with town houses and more apartment buildings. This block is, in fact, almost completely residential—atypical for a crosstown street.

● Cross Ninth Avenue and things become quite different and more typically Manhattan. On the left is the southern part of Penn Station South, a 1962 cooperative development built by the International Ladies' Garment Workers Union. The buildings have a streamlined look and lots of balconies. They are surrounded by a considerable amount of green space. Farther along on the left, the School of Visual Arts' SVA Theatre is kind of a concrete slab but topped with a quirky and colorful pipe-and-circles sculpture over the entrance. Just past the theater, look to the left and you'll see that the next street over, West 24th, makes an unusual curve. Across the street on the right are a few interesting smaller buildings. Stribling, a real estate firm, is located in a Greek Revival building at #340. The two buildings east of it are also that style, although their entrances vary in design. At #332 is the Leo House, a Catholic-run guesthouse that has pretty windows on the first two floors and unusual decorative motifs on the roof that are known as machicolations.

● Past Eighth Avenue, the Bow Tie Cinemas Chelsea is on the right, with an Art Deco look to the front (it was built in the late 1980s, though). Two buildings past it is the Broadway Savings Bank (1948), now an Apple Bank for Savings. The cornerstone for this marble-faced bank is still visible. After a few other pretty buildings, you reach Emunath Israel synagogue. The Jewish congregation took over the building—constructed in the 1850s as the Third Reformed Presbyterian Church—in 1920 and made adjustments, installing stained-glass windows and more. Above the main entrance is a carved Ten Commandments with two lions.

And just next door is one of the most fabled spots in the whole neighborhood: the Hotel Chelsea. It's one of those special New York places, even if it isn't as splashy as, say, the Empire State Building. Built in the mid-1880s, it's lined with rows and rows of beautiful iron balconies that would be right at home in New Orleans. There are pretty dormers at the roof, plus an eye-catching neon sign. The hotel has been the subject of movies, books, songs, and legends, and the home of artists, writers, actors, and musicians. Poet Dylan Thomas died here. Sex Pistol Sid Vicious killed his girlfriend,

Nancy Spungen, here. The building is currently undergoing an extensive renovation and is scheduled to reopen in 2016 as a boutique hotel; we hope the redo won't totally erase its shabby charm. Next to the Chelsea is the Carteret, a handsome high-rise residence built in 1926–27.

Across the street is the smaller but still-impressive Muhlenberg Branch of the New York Public Library. It dates to 1906 and is one of 65 branch libraries built with funds provided by industrialist Andrew Carnegie. The three-story limestone building is named for William Augustus Muhlenberg, rector of a neighborhood church. The tall redbrick building next door is the former McBurney Y (you saw the current site on West 14th Street at the start of this walk). Opened in 1904, this location inspired the Village People's "YMCA"; today it's condos.

● The next block of West 23rd Street is less remarkable and has a lot of commercial outlets, but a few noteworthy sites are mixed in. Take a look on the right at Chelsea Mews, at #148. This is a Gothic Revival commercial building that was converted to condos. It was built in 1910 and has appealing terra-cotta accents. Across the street farther along, see St. Vincent de Paul Church, which was finished in 1869 and was established to serve New York City's French-speaking community. The parish closed in 2013, though efforts persist to save the church from demolition.

● Cross Sixth Avenue. The building on the left corner is Masonic Hall, from 1913 (built on the site of the 1875 Masonic Hall). There is a historical plaque noting this, as well as a humbler blue and yellow flag at the entrance. Check out the Castro at 43 W. 23rd—not a tribute to Cuba's longtime ruler but Castro Convertibles

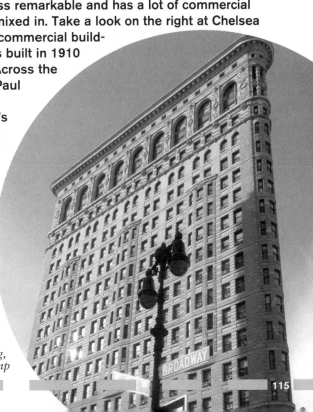

The beautiful and quirky Flatiron Building, set off by a vintage street lamp

furniture (if you're a New Yorker of a certain age, its jingle is implanted in your brain). The Girl Scouts and Touro College have offices here.

● Both corners at Fifth Avenue have distinguished buildings. On the right, the redbrick building with several dormers is the 1883 Western Union Building. It was built by Henry Hardenbergh, who also built The Plaza Hotel and The Dakota apartment building. On the left, the white building at 200 Fifth Ave. was known as the International Toy Center or the Fifth Avenue Building; it now houses the high-end Italian-foods market Eataly. It was built in 1909 and is linked to the famous Flatiron Building diagonally across from it. In front of 200 Fifth Ave., see the freestanding golden clock on the sidewalk. Then look or go across 23rd Street to the ornate, irregularly shaped Flatiron, which opened in 1903 as the Fuller Building. Architect Daniel Burnham made innovative use of the triangular plot of land. View the building from various angles; then head to the pedestrian island opposite it and then into the adjacent park, Madison Square.

Madison Square is one of my favorite parks in Manhattan—it's not overwhelming in scope and size, but it has history, it's beautiful, and it hosts a variety of fun things to do throughout the year. The park, named after James Madison, the fourth US president and chief writer and promoter of the Bill of Rights, opened in May 1847 and is rectangular in shape (with Broadway cutting through the southwest corner, creating the island). If you start at the 23rd-and-Broadway corner and walk more or less counterclockwise through the park, you'll get a good view of it all.

Wander a bit to get closer up. Among the things you will see are the William H. Seward statue; the original Shake Shack (an upscale burger joint); and the Senator Roscoe Conkling monument. Across from the southeast corner of the park stands the Metropolitan Life Insurance tower, a standout with its remarkable clock. Just outside the park at East 25th Street and Madison Avenue is the elegant Supreme Court of New York, Appellate Division: Classical design all the way, with lots of columns and statues. Toward the north end of Madison Square Park is a sweet little playground named for NYPD officer Moira Ann Smith, a 9/11 first responder who died while helping evacuate the World Trade Center. Walk a bit farther to statues of Chester A. Arthur, one of our less-illustrious presidents, and Admiral David Farragut, a Civil War hero.

When you get back to the Fifth Avenue side, across the avenue at 25th Street is General Worth Square; the general himself is buried beneath this obelisk, making his one of only two public-monument mausoleums in New York City (Grant's Tomb is the other). As you walk, you'll also see the dog run and the Eternal Light flagstaff. Look outside the park on West 24th Street: A high pedestrian bridge spans two big office buildings, part of the Toy Center complex.

● Finish at East 23rd Street and Broadway, and you can take the N or R train right outside the park.

POINTS OF INTEREST

Our Lady of Guadalupe at St. Bernard's 328 W. 14th St., 212-243-0265

Old Homestead Steakhouse theoldhomesteadsteakhouse.com, 56 Ninth Ave., 212-242-9040

High Line Park thehighline.org, 10th Avenue at West 15th Street, 212-500-6035

Chelsea Market chelseamarket.com, 75 Ninth Ave., 212-652-2110

The Maritime Hotel themaritimehotel.com, 363 W. 16th St., 212-242-4300

Dream Downtown dreamhotels.com/downtown, 355 W. 16th St., 212-229-2559

Dr. Gertrude B. Kelly Playground nycgovparks.org/parks/dr-gertrude-b-kelly-playground, bounded by West 16th Street, West 17th Street, Eighth Avenue, and Ninth Avenue

Church of St. Francis Xavier sfxavier.org, 46 W. 16th St., 212-627-2100

Center for Jewish History cjh.org, 15 W. 16th St., 212-294-8301

Limelight Shops limelightshops.com, 656 Sixth Ave., 212-255-2144

Third Cemetery of Congregation Shearith Israel shearithisrael.org/content/twenty-first -street-cemetery, 110 W. 23rd St.

The General Theological Seminary gts.edu, 440 W. 21st St., 212-243-5150

Church of the Guardian Angel guardianangelchurch-nyc.org, 193 10th Ave., 212-929-5966

London Terrace Apartments Bounded by 9th and 10th Avenues and West 23rd and 24th Streets

Leo House leohousenyc.com, 332 W. 23rd St., 212-366-0100

Hotel Chelsea *(reopens 2016)* chelseahotels.com, 222 W. 23rd St.

Muhlenberg Library nypl.org/locations/muhlenberg, 209 W. 23rd St., 212-924-1585

Eataly eataly.com, 200 Fifth Ave., 212-229-2560

Flatiron Building 175 Fifth Ave.

Madison Square Park madisonsquarepark.org, Madison Avenue at East 23rd Street, 212-538-1884

General Worth Square nycgovparks.org/parks/worth-square, Fifth Avenue at West 23rd Street

route summary

1. From Sixth Avenue, walk west on West 14th Street.
2. Walk right on 10th Avenue.
3. Turn right on West 16th Street.
4. Walk left on Fifth Avenue.
5. Turn left on West 20th Street.
6. Turn right on Sixth Avenue.
7. Walk left on West 21st Street.
8. Turn right on 10th Avenue.
9. Walk right on West 23rd Street.
10. Walk around Madison Square Park, then catch the train at the southern end of the park, at East 23rd Street and Broadway.

CONNECTING THE WALKS

To start the Lower Midtown tour (Walk 14), walk two blocks west on 23rd Street to Seventh Avenue, then five blocks north to West 28th Street.

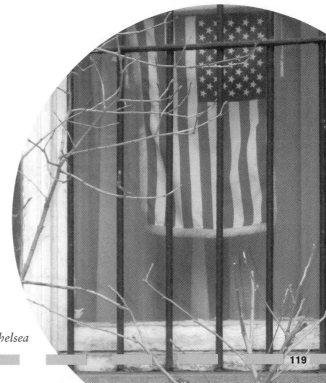

A glimpse into someone's patriotic window in Chelsea

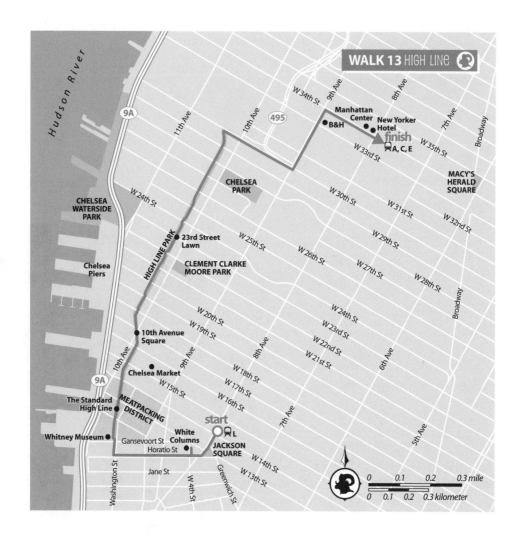

WALK 13 HIGH LINE

Hudson River

9A

11th Ave

10th Ave

495

W 34th St

9th Ave

8th Ave

7th Ave

Broadway

Manhattan
Center

New Yorker
Hotel

● B&H

W 35th St

finish
A, C, E

W 33rd St

CHELSEA
PARK

MACY'S
HERALD
SQUARE

CHELSEA
WATERSIDE
PARK

W 24th St

W 30th St

W 31st St

W 32nd St

HIGH LINE PARK

● 23rd Street
Lawn

Chelsea
Piers

CLEMENT CLARKE
MOORE PARK

W 25th St

W 26th St

W 27th St

W 28th St

W 29th St

Broadway

W 20th St

W 19th St

W 24th St

W 23rd St

W 22nd St

W 21st St

6th Ave

5th Ave

● 10th Avenue
Square

10th Ave

9th Ave

8th Ave

7th Ave

● Chelsea Market

W 18th St

W 17th St

W 16th St

W 15th St

9A

The Standard
High Line ●

MEATPACKING
DISTRICT

Whitney Museum ●

Gansevoort St

Horatio St

White
Columns
●

start
L

JACKSON
SQUARE

W 14th St

W 13th St

Washington St

Jane St

W 4th St

Greenwich St

0   0.1   0.2   0.3 mile

0   0.1   0.2   0.3 kilometer

13 HIGH LINE: an elevating experience

BOUNDARIES: **Horatio St., the High Line, W. 34th St., 8th Ave.**
DISTANCE: **2.5 miles**
SUBWAY: **A, C, E, or L to 14th St.**

Manhattan has many wonderful parks: large, medium-sized, small, and even tiny. But it has only one park located along an elevated former freight-train line. The High Line is one of the newest and certainly one of the most unusual parks of New York City, and it has become very popular in a short time.

These tracks were built by the New York Central Railroad as a freight spur in the early 1930s, but the last train rumbled along them in 1980, and it looked as if they were headed for the scrap heap. Then a community organization came together, called the Friends of the High Line, to advocate for reusing the line as a park. A large swath of this rail-trail was opened in 2009, another (up to 30th Street) in 2011, and the rest up to West 34th Street afterward. The landscape architect was James Corner of Field Operations, and Diller Scofidio + Renfro crafted the master plan. Weaving together original elements of the rail line with newer pieces, various innovations, and canny marketing have worked hand in hand to make this a prime destination in Manhattan. Buildings have begun advertising as "near the High Line"—an area that was reviled by many just a couple of decades ago.

- Exit the subway, noting the quirky sculptures by Tom Otterness in the station and on the elevator; collectively, they're called *Life Underground.* Aboveground are two elegant former banks across from each other at the intersection of West 14th Street and Eighth Avenue; you also saw these on the previous walk. With these on your right, walk on Eighth Avenue past Jackson Square (really a triangle) and make a right at Horatio Street, named for Horatio Gates, a hero of the American Revolution. There is a tiny garden where Horatio, West Fourth Street (seemingly off-grid), and Eighth Avenue create a triangle to your left.

- Make a right onto West Fourth Street and walk to the entrance of the big white building. This is White Columns, New York City's oldest alternative arts space. If it's open, check out the latest exhibit. Afterward walk back to Horatio Street and turn right, passing Corporal John A. Seravalli Playground as well as some delightful apartment buildings.

● Cross Hudson Street. The roadbed here is cobblestone, and the homes are very nice. Continue across Greenwich Street, which has some particularly quaint and well-kept older buildings.

● Make a right at Washington Street and walk one block to Gansevoort Street. This was once known as Great Kiln Street but was renamed for Revolutionary War general Peter Gansevoort (an ancestor of novelist Herman Melville).

● Cross over and take the stairs on your left up to the High Line. If you'd like to put that off and check out the new Whitney Museum of American Art, feel free. After having spent 45 years on the Upper East Side, it reopened in May 2015 at 99 Gansevoort St.

High Line Park is a slightly meandering line. Once you're on the High Line, take a good look at it—don't just stride through it. The disused freight train tracks have been meticulously augmented with plants, artworks, and much more. Sundecks have been built into some sections. As you walk the length of this park, you can partake of fascinating views throughout the neighborhoods of Chelsea and Midtown South. Certain prominent buildings, such as the Empire State, can be spotted from a distance.

When the plants are in bloom, many of them spill over the walls of the High Line, peep through the tracks and ties, and create interesting textures. The majority of plants are native to New York City. The art on display changes periodically; most of it is sculpture, and the collections have themes. By the way, no dogs or Frisbee allowed! And one complaint, if I may: There are not enough bathrooms along the route. Consider yourself warned.

What you *will* find in abundance are benches, which are cleverly designed. There are groups of benches that resemble chaise lounges, and some are even on wheels so they can be pushed around on tracks. The width of the High Line fluctuates from place to place, and in some spots you'll want to spend more time exploring because of the variety. Signs explaining the trail's history and the artwork you see abound. And you may be privy to any number of street happenings down below—a film crew at work, perhaps, or a street fair with a temporary mini–ice rink.

- The next cross street after Gansevoort is Little West 12th Street, and between it and West 13th Street is The Standard High Line—which you walk *beneath.* This hotel is seemingly all windows, and it's notorious for guests who don't close their curtains. After passing through The Standard, look out to the Hudson River to see Hoboken, New Jersey. Shortly after that on the left is the minimalist orange-brick Department of Sanitation building. At West 14th Street there is an old building with an oddly shaped crystalline crown; this houses the headquarters for fashion designer Diane von Furstenberg. Then walk under the 14th Street Passage, a brown building. A bit farther on the left is another brown building, this one shaped like a cake slice: the Liberty Inn . . . which apparently charges by the hour. Shortly after that is the Chelsea Market Passage, with exposed brick and an adaptive industrial appearance. To your right is the Chelsea Market—the High Line actually pierces the building.

- Just past West 17th Street is one of the coolest features of the High Line: 10th Avenue Square, which has stadium seating with a big window onto the street. Look to the left at the Chelsea Piers sports complex from West 17th to West 23rd Streets. Sports and events galore take place here—golf, skating, wall climbing, swimming, gymnastics, you name it.

- At West 20th, look to the left to see the 529 Arts Building. Notice the metal numbers affixed to the brick of the adjacent buildings. Then look to the right to see The General Theological Seminary (it's on Walk 12) and the High Line Hotel. Walk along to West 21st Street, and on the right you'll see the back of the Church of the Guardian Angel. A block farther are the 23rd Street Lawn and seating steps—a nice spot to rest. A faded ad on the wall to your left promotes WAREHOUSES that are U.S. BONDED. Just past this on the right, at West 23rd, are Ten23, a modern apartment building, and *Urban Rattle,* a colorful, cartoony sculpture on poles. Look to your left for a rather innovative (or strange) modern building, HL23 Residential Tower. It seems to have an uneven glass mask affixed to the front (it's really a giant truss). Next door to HL23 is High Line 519, less unusual but still decorated with oddly shaped pieces on the facade.

- In the water just north of Chelsea Piers are many wooden pilings; this is not a conceptual-art display but remnants of long-gone piers. They have a rustic beauty.

- As you continue along the High Line, look all around and note the art galleries and businesses down below, as well as the plantings on the trail. The West 26th Street

Viewing Spur is a great place to take in the cityscape. At West 29th, the High Line veers to the left, and the Radial Bench is built into the turn. Then come to the West 30th Street Cut-Out and Viewing Platform, which might make some people a bit queasy with its layout. The High Line ends at West 34th Street (just north of it is the Jacob K. Javits Convention Center), but go down to the street at West 30th Street and walk away from the river on it.

● At Ninth Avenue, turn left. From West 31st to West 33rd on your right is the back of the gigantic main US Post Office (see next walk). Spanning West 33rd to West 34th on that side is B&H, a massive electronics store. It has one of the best darkroom-photography departments still left in the city.

● Make a right at West 34th Street. On your left is the somber neoclassical building housing the West Side Jewish Center. Farther down that side of the street is the Manhattan Center; notice the ANCIENT ACCEPTED SCOTTISH RITE engraving and various carved-stone decorations. Built in 1906, this was originally the Manhattan Opera House. Now there are TV studios here as well as the Hammerstein Ballroom, a famed concert venue. At Eighth Avenue is the iconic New Yorker Hotel (completed in 1930), which exudes Art Deco style in spades. Look up—*way* up—to see the huge red neon sign. On the 34th Street side of the building, look for the brass plaque dedicated to inventor Nikola Tesla, who lived (and died) here.

● You can catch the subway at West 34th Street and Eighth Avenue.

POINTS OF INTEREST

White Columns whitecolumns.org, 320 W. 13th St. (Horatio at West Fourth), 212-924-4212

Whitney Museum of American Art whitney.org, 99 Gansevoort St., 212-570-3600

High Line Park thehighline.org, Gansevoort Street to West 34th Street west of 10th Avenue, 212-500-6035

The Standard High Line standardhotels.com/high-line, 848 Washington St., 212-645-4646

B&H bhphotovideo.com, 420 Ninth Ave., 212-444-6615

Manhattan Center mcstudios.com, 311 W. 34th St., 212-564-1072

Wyndham New Yorker Hotel newyorkerhotel.com, 481 Eighth Ave., 212-971-0101

route summary

1. Walk south on Eighth Avenue.
2. Walk right on Horatio Street.
3. Walk right on West Fourth Street.
4. Double back to Horatio Street and continue right (west).
5. Walk right on Washington Street.
6. Go up to the High Line at Gansevoort Street.
7. Follow the High Line to the end or West 30th Street. (If you're walking all the way to the end, return to West 30th to exit.)
8. Walk east on West 30th Street.
9. Walk left on Ninth Avenue.
10. Walk right on West 34th Street to Eighth Avenue.

connecting the walks

To start the next walk (Lower Midtown/Garment District), go east one block on West 34th Street to Seventh Avenue, then six blocks south to West 28th Street.

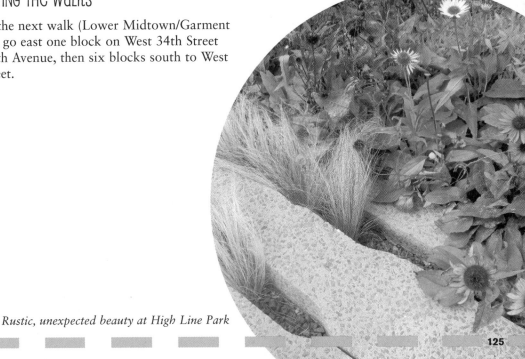

Rustic, unexpected beauty at High Line Park

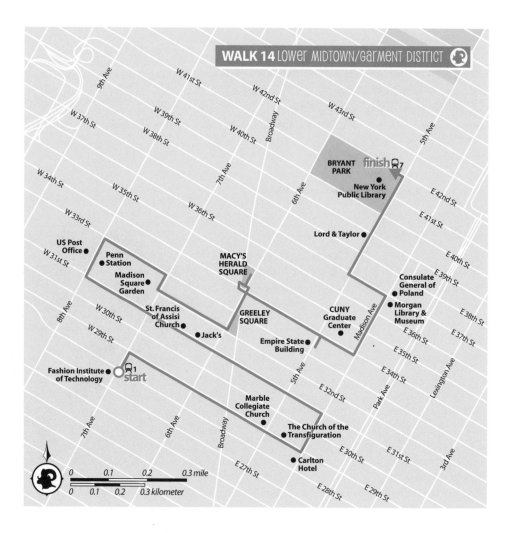

WALK 14 LOWER MIDTOWN/GARMENT DISTRICT

W 41st St
9th Ave
W 42nd St
W 39th St
W 37th St
W 38th St
Broadway
W 43rd St
W 40th St
5th Ave

BRYANT PARK   finish 7
New York Public Library

W 34th St
W 35th St
7th Ave
W 36th St
6th Ave
E 42nd St
E 41st St

Lord & Taylor

W 33rd St

US Post Office
W 31st St
Penn Station
Madison Square Garden

MACY'S HERALD SQUARE
E 40th St
E 39th St
Consulate General of Poland
Morgan Library & Museum

8th Ave
W 30th St
St. Francis of Assisi Church
Jack's
GREELEY SQUARE
CUNY Graduate Center
Madison Ave
E 38th St
E 37th St
W 29th St
Empire State Building
E 36th St
E 35th St

Fashion Institute of Technology
1 start
E 34th St
Park Ave
Lexington Ave

7th Ave
6th Ave
Broadway
Marble Collegiate Church
5th Ave
E 32nd St
E 31st St
3rd Ave

The Church of the Transfiguration
E 30th St

E 27th St
Carlton Hotel
E 28th St
E 29th St

0   0.1   0.2   0.3 mile
0   0.1   0.2   0.3 kilometer

14 LOWER MIDTOWN/GARMENT DISTRICT: SWINGIN' AROUND MIDTOWN

BOUNDARIES: **W. 27th St., 7th Ave., W. 42nd St., Madison Ave.**
DISTANCE: **2.5 miles**
SUBWAY: **1 to 28th St.**

A first-timer in midtown Manhattan is likely to be overwhelmed quickly by the mass of huge and famous sights that abound. Contrast that with the thousands of pedestrians and commuters who seem unfazed by their surroundings as they race to their jobs or meetings and the trains they're late for.

As someone who worked in and attended graduate school in Midtown, I know what it's like to be in a rush and have to dodge crowds—but I also know how much fun it is to shop in the local stores, attend events at Madison Square Garden, spend time reading and researching at the main library on Fifth Avenue, and partake of other social and cultural events. Midtown has *a lot* to offer, and even the most jaded New Yorkers know that occasionally they have to give in and enjoy the scene. From the splendid flagship Macy's to the towering Empire State Building, from Madison Square Garden sports and concerts to the quiet joys of the museums in the area, there is so much to do and see here.

This tour focuses on the area often referred to as Midtown South; 42nd Street, the Theater District, and Rockefeller Center are covered in the next three walks.

● At Seventh Avenue and West 28th Street, where you exit the subway, is the Fashion Institute of Technology (FIT), part of the State University of New York system. It offers majors in fashion, design, art, and many related courses of study. It's at the southern edge of the Garment District, where many designers and clothing companies are headquartered (hence Seventh Avenue's nickname, Fashion Avenue). You may have to dodge workers pushing around wheeled racks of clothing—just part of the scene. See FIT's Pomerantz Art and Design Center, as well as a few of the other buildings. At West 27th Street, see an abstract sculpture under the connector

BacK STory: I Love a Parade . . . From Home, THaT IS

I've been to the Macy's Thanksgiving Day Parade—a tradition that in some ways rivals turkey dinner—exactly one time, with a friend and my brother, in the early 1980s. It was so bitterly cold that day that we hung around for only a brief while before heading home on the subway. (I did, however, go to watch the balloons being inflated the evening before Thanksgiving for a few years.)

Like so many other Americans, I prefer to watch the parade on television and clips of it on YouTube. Begun in 1924, it has long featured huge balloons, floats, and hybrids thereof (variously dubbed "falloons" and "ballonicles") with likenesses of cartoon and pop-culture characters: Mickey Mouse, Yogi Bear, Superman, Popeye, SpongeBob SquarePants, Hello Kitty, Betty Boop, Dora the Explorer . . . In 2013 there was a dreidel float, because Thanksgiving and Hannukah coincided (a calendar rarity). Other highlights include marching bands, the Rockettes, and various pop singers and actors. The parade is great fun, but it's also a major marketing push for Macy's and for the TV and Broadway shows promoted by the lineup. And the parade places New York City at center stage every year, not unlike the New Year's Eve ball drop.

between FIT buildings; to me, it looks like a basketball and a sideways hoop. Also check out the Museum at FIT, the Goodman Center.

● With FIT on your left, walk north on Seventh Avenue to West 29th Street, and turn right. This block is unglamorous, full of older buildings and businesses and signs, but on your left near Sixth Avenue is an open space that has the look of a swim club dropped into the middle of the city—a fun little spot. Continue to Broadway, where buildings at three of the four corners have much charm. On your near right (southwest corner), 1201 Broadway has a lot of Art Deco decoration under the windows and as dividers. Across the street, at 1186, is the hip Ace Hotel, in a French Renaissance structure from 1904; note its rounded corner and copper mansard roof. To the left and across West 29th, the big, bold, cream-colored edifice at 1200 Broadway is highly ornate; look up to see the clock near the top. This is the former Gilsey House, a hotel from the early 1870s.

● The highlight of the next block is Marble Collegiate Church, a Dutch Reformed house of worship from the early 1850s. It's on the left, fronting Fifth Avenue, but the West 29th side has several humorous grotesques on the exterior. Go onto Fifth Avenue to take in the church, its clock tower, and more—and perhaps even go inside. Afterward, cross Fifth (which divides the West and East Sides) and walk along East 29th Street. Shortly, you come upon The Church of the Transfiguration, an Episcopal church that was consecrated in 1849. The building is pretty, but the real attraction is the garden and its features—a gazebo, the plantings, the layout, and the externals of the church (such as windows) that extend into the garden. In the 19th century, this church became famous as a spiritual haven for actors, writers, and other bohemian types who were looked down upon by polite society.

● When you reach Madison Avenue, on the right is the beautiful Carlton Hotel (#88). Alternating bands of white limestone and red brick, plus ornate black window casements and terra-cotta cartouches, make this a Beaux Arts delight. Turn left and walk north on Madison Avenue. Just past East 30th on your left is the American Academy of Dramatic Arts, the oldest acting school in the English-speaking world. The building, from 1904, was originally the Colony Club. Across the avenue, Madison Avenue Baptist Church occupies the first four stories of the Roger Williams Hotel. The Romanesque Revival church structure is in stark contrast to the rest of the building.

● Turn left on East 31st Street. On your left, Hotel Chandler, with many comely bay windows, was built in 1905 as Hotel Le Marquis. Continue to Fifth Avenue; at the corner on your left is the Textile Building, a pretty building that's a center for the home textile industry. Cross Fifth Avenue and Hotel Wolcott is on your left at 4 W. 31st. An exuberant mishmash of Beaux Arts and Neoclassicism, it has a dramatic sunburst-and-cherubs motif above the main entrance; past celebrity residents include Isadora Duncan and Doris Duke. Farther along the block on the right side is the Herald Square Hotel, with an even more ostentatious decoration (named *Winged Life*) above its entrance. It also has the word LIFE in triplicate at the second floor, "1883" in one corner, and, curiously, a bland 1960s-era sign as well. *Life* magazine called this place home from 1883 to 1936.

● Continue across Broadway on West 31st and then along the short block to Sixth Avenue. Just after you cross Sixth, look at the secondary street sign marking 31st Street; Father Mychal Judge was an FDNY chaplain and the first identified victim of 9/11.

- On the right side of the block is Jack's, one in a chain of discount stores (or, as some of us old-timers call them, "schlock stores"). Make like a dyed-in-the-wool Noo Yawker and go inside, buy something on the cheap, maybe get a snack. Then continue to 31 Penn Plaza, an understated buff building on your left. The Church of St. Francis of Assisi, Father Judge's church, will be on the right. This beautiful Catholic church was completed in 1892 and has a huge mosaic from 1928. To meet the spiritual needs of shift workers, St. Francis introduced the "Nightworkers' Mass" at midnight, plus a Mass at noon for workers on their lunch hour. Pause to consider the poignant statue at the sidewalk: A man begs, a hood over his face and his hand extended outward.

- Walk to Seventh Avenue (here co-named Joe Louis Plaza, for the legendary boxer), and across on your right is one of the sports world's most famous venues: Madison Square Garden. This is the fourth complex to be dubbed Madison Square Garden and dates to the 1960s. It sits on top of Penn Station and is home to the Knicks, Rangers, and Liberty teams. It also hosts boxing, concerts, occasional religious events, the Westminster dog show, and the circus. See more of the Garden as you walk along West 31st west of Seventh Avenue. On the left is the Capuchin Monastery of St. John the Baptist, an ascetic brown-brick box. (The actual church, on West 30th, is quite lovely.)

- At Eighth Avenue, cross over to the two-block-long neoclassical building with many pilasters on the West 31st side and many columns on the Eighth Avenue side. This is the James A. Farley Building, more commonly known as the main US Post Office. The part of the building fronting 31st and 8th was completed in 1912 (it was expanded in the 1930s).

- Walk north on Eighth Avenue alongside the post office, then make a right on West 33rd Street, passing Penn Station on your right.

- At Seventh Avenue, make a right and walk to the recessed front of Madison Square Garden. Note the big, bold marquee, the stone eagles, the flags. If an event is about to start, you'll no doubt see people wearing team attire or concert T-shirts. In addition, there are always very hurried commuters around here, going to and from the subway or Long Island Rail Road or NJ Transit trains. Opposite the Garden is the mammoth Hotel Pennsylvania, with an elegant neoclassical entrance.

● Make a left onto West 32nd Street. About halfway up the block is the other side of St. Francis of Assisi, here a pretty little courtyard. Farther up 32nd is the heart of the Koreatown neighborhood, chockablock with Korean restaurants, shops, and spas, all marked with colorful signage. Feel free to explore it on your own, but our tour continues as far as Sixth Avenue, where you cross to Greeley Square. One of those "squares" that are actually triangles, it has public seating and a statue of Horace Greeley, publisher of the long-gone newspaper *The New York Herald* (which eventually became the *Herald-Tribune*). Relax here a bit, then walk up Sixth Avenue with the park to your right.

● Before you become totally transfixed by Macy's, check out Herald Square, in front of it. (The name refers to the aforementioned *New York Herald*.) Enter the park from West 34th Street and walk between two pillars, each with a watchful owl sculpture. Continue in to see the main statue: A figure of Minerva, two at-work blacksmiths, a big clock, and more owls await you. (Minerva was the Roman goddess of wisdom, and the owl her spirit animal.) When the weather is nice, you might find musicians playing here.

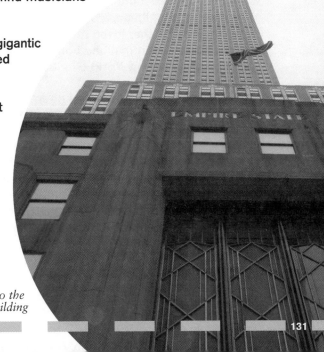

Now check out Macy's up close. This gigantic store is actually a few buildings merged into one (this is more obvious when you walk inside on the first floor). The main entrance on Sixth Avenue is best known, with MACY'S spelled out and the cubed clock in the center. But the entrance on West 34th Street just around the corner is more elaborate, with four caryatids, globe lamps, and another pretty clock.

● Now walk east on West 34th, with Macy's to your left. The stretch from Seventh Avenue to Fifth Avenue is

The massive Art Deco entrance to the Empire State Building

chock-full of big-name retail stores—sort of an open-air shopping mall. Over the years, there have been long-term anchors other than the stalwart Macy's . . . Ohrbach's, for instance, is long gone, and you kind of date yourself if you mention its name.

- When you get to Fifth Avenue, make a right and walk to the main entrance of the Empire State Building (1931). Look up, up, up, to drink in all 1,454 feet of it: the gold-embossed EMPIRE STATE logo flanked by angular griffins, the windows that create a sort of geometric pattern puzzle, the needlelike spire reaching seemingly to the heavens, King Kong running amok! On many nights, the upper section is lit in colors that commemorate a holiday or special event—red, white, and blue for Independence Day, green for St. Patrick's Day, or the colors of a local sports team when they win a championship. During the year, a few special events take place here (a race up the stairs, weddings on Valentine's Day). Touristy attractions and observation decks are located at the 86th and 102nd floors.

- Across Fifth Avenue on the other side of 34th Street, examine the beautiful building with three covered entrances that call to mind Paris Métro train stops. From 1906 to 1989, this was B. Altman, a department store more subdued than Macy's but just as respected. (My mother loved Altman's clothing and dignified air, and I still hold on to one striped T-shirt that she bought there.) The building is now used as the CUNY (City University of New York) Graduate Center and related academic offices.

- Walk along East 34th Street and notice #12, the Ditson Building, its name emblazoned above the third floor. There are other picturesque older buildings on this block as well.

- Turn left onto Madison Avenue and the back of the B. Altman building, which houses the NYPL's Science, Industry and Business Library. In contrast to its classic-department-store exterior, it's modern, sleek, and high-tech inside. Anyone can walk in and read, conduct research, or attend a lecture or workshop. Cross East 35th to admire the Episcopal Church of the Incarnation, a mottled brown edifice on your right, with its parish house next to it. The church dates to the 1860s, but after a fire it was rebuilt in the 1880s. Madison Avenue starts to get steeper at this block, but for most people it won't be a hardship. Cross East 36th to a lesser-known yet highly impressive museum of Manhattan, The Morgan Library & Museum. Manuscripts, books, prints, and drawings are exhibited and made available to serious researchers. Opposite the Morgan on East 37th Street, you'll see the Consulate General of the Republic of Poland, in a white Beaux Arts building.

● Turn left on East 37th Street. There are some handsome office buildings on this block, such as 232 Madison (with an entrance on the street) and its herald-festooned entrance. At Fifth Avenue, check out #411 (and see the side on East 37th as well), which has several attractive molded faces, many wearing hats, as well as nudes and vegetation attached to the outer walls. This 1915 building is just one of many anonymous but intriguing structures that are so common around town.

● Turn right on Fifth. On the west side at 38th Street is the tony department store Lord & Taylor. Note the baronial crests flanking the entrance, each with an interlocking *L* and *T*. Stop in and browse, or walk on to West 40th Street to behold the main New York Public Library (covered in more detail in the next walk). Go inside, hang out with the lions, sit on the steps, or make your way to the subway station at 42nd Street.

POINTS OF INTEREST

Fashion Institute of Technology fitnyc.edu, 227 W. 27th St., 212-217-7999

Marble Collegiate Church marblechurch.org, 1 W. 29th St., 212-686-2770

The Church of the Transfiguration littlechurch.org, 1 E. 29th St., 212-684-6770

Carlton Hotel carltonhotelny.com, 88 Madison Ave., 212-532-4100

Madison Avenue Baptist Church mabcnyc.org, 30 E. 30th St., 212-685-1377

Jack's 99 Cent Store jacksnyc.com, 115 W. 31st St., 212-268-9962

Church of St. Francis of Assisi stfrancisnyc.org, 135 W. 31st St., 212-736-8500

James A. Farley Building, US Post Office usps.com, 421 Eighth Ave., 212-330-3296

Madison Square Garden thegarden.com, 4 Penn Plaza, 212-465-6741

Greeley Square nycgovparks.org/parks/greeley-square-park, bounded by Broadway, Sixth Avenue, and West 32nd Street

Herald Square 34thstreet.org, bounded by Broadway, Sixth Avenue, and West 34th Street

Macy's Herald Square tinyurl.com/macysheraldsquare, 151 W. 34th St., 212-695-4400

Empire State Building esbnyc.com, 350 Fifth Ave., 212-736-3100

Science, Industry and Business Library nypl.org/locations/sibl, 188 Madison Ave., 917-275-6975

Episcopal Church of the Incarnation churchoftheincarnation.org, 209 Madison Ave., 212-689-6350

The Morgan Library & Museum themorgan.org, 225 Madison Ave., 212-685-0008

Lord & Taylor lordandtaylor.com, 424 Fifth Ave., 212-391-3344

route summary

1. From West 28th Street, walk north on Seventh Avenue.
2. Walk right on West 29th Street.
3. Walk left on Madison Avenue.
4. Walk left on East 31st Street.
5. Walk right on Eighth Ave.
6. Walk right on West 33rd Street.
7. Turn right on Seventh Ave.
8. Walk left on West 32nd Street.
9. At Sixth Avenue visit Greeley Square, then walk north.
10. Visit Herald Square and Macy's, then head east on West 34th Street.
11. See the Empire State Building to your right on Fifth Avenue, and continue onto East 34th Street.
12. Walk left on Madison Avenue.
13. Walk left on East 37th Street.
14. Walk right on Fifth Avenue to West 42nd Street.

CONNECTING THE WALKS

You can pick up the next walk (42nd Street) around its midpoint at the library (see page 140). To start the Times Square/Theater District tour (Walk 16), walk about one and a half blocks west on West 42nd to Broadway. For Rockefeller Center (Walk 17), walk one block west to Sixth Avenue and then north five blocks to West 47th Street.

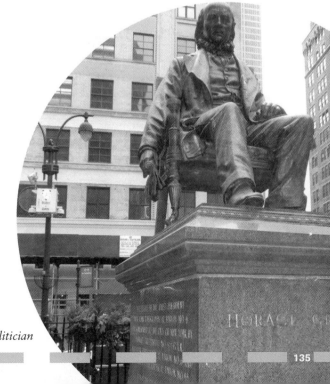

Horace Greeley, newspaperman and politician

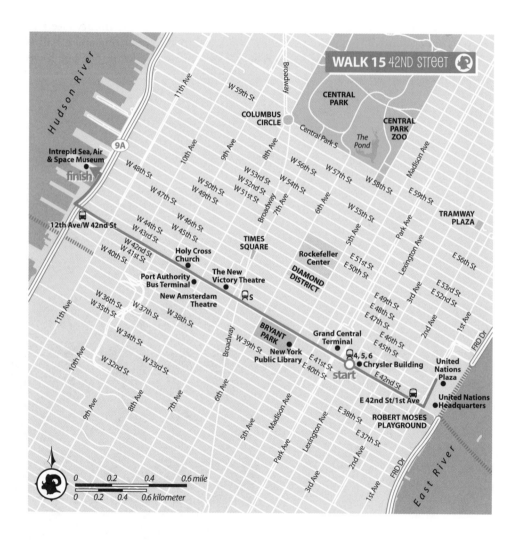

WALK 15 42ND STREET

Hudson River

11th Ave
W 59th St
Broadway

CENTRAL PARK

COLUMBUS CIRCLE

Central Park S

CENTRAL PARK ZOO

The Pond

9A

Intrepid Sea, Air & Space Museum

finish

10th Ave
9th Ave
8th Ave

W 48th St
W 53rd St
W 56th St
W 57th St
W 58th St
E 59th St

Madison Ave

W 47th St
W 50th St
W 49th St
W 52nd St
W 51st St
W 54th St
W 55th St

7th Ave
6th Ave
5th Ave

12th Ave/W 42nd St

W 44th St
W 43rd St
W 45th St
W 46th St

Broadway

TRAMWAY PLAZA

Park Ave

E 56th St

W 42nd St
W 41st St
W 40th St

Holy Cross Church

TIMES SQUARE

Rockefeller Center

E 51st St
E 50th St

Lexington Ave

E 53rd St
E 52nd St

Port Authority Bus Terminal

The New Victory Theatre

DIAMOND DISTRICT

E 49th St
E 48th St
E 47th St

3rd Ave
2nd Ave
1st Ave

New Amsterdam Theatre

S

W 36th St
W 35th St
W 37th St
W 38th St

BRYANT PARK

Grand Central Terminal

E 46th St
E 45th St

FRD Dr

11th Ave
10th Ave

W 34th St
W 32nd St
W 33rd St

Broadway
W 39th St

New York Public Library

E 41st St
E 40th St

4, 5, 6
Chrysler Building

United Nations Plaza

9th Ave
8th Ave
7th Ave
6th Ave

start

E 42nd St

E 42nd St/1st Ave

United Nations Headquarters

5th Ave
Madison Ave
Park Ave
Lexington Ave

E 38th St
E 37th St

2nd Ave

ROBERT MOSES PLAYGROUND

East River

3rd Ave
1st Ave
FRD Dr

0   0.2   0.4   0.6 mile
0   0.2   0.4   0.6 kilometer

15 42ND Street: a Street Like No Other

BOUNDARIES: **W. 40th St., 12th Ave., E. 45th St., East River**
DISTANCE: **2 miles**
SUBWAY: **4, 5, 6 to Grand Central–42nd St., then M42 bus to 1st Ave.**

No other street in Manhattan or New York City, and few other streets in the world, are as commanding or as famous as 42nd Street, from river to river. It is the very core of Manhattan: a mix of commerce, media, transportation, entertainment, and education. It's always "on." Every subway line that runs through Midtown has a stop here. It has nicknames, such as "Forty-Deuce" or just "The Deuce." A classic movie musical is named for it, the title song of which urges, "Come and meet those dancing feet / On the avenue I'm taking you to / 42nd Street."

The street holds a stunning collection of buildings and destinations along its length: the United Nations, the *Daily News* Building, Grand Central Terminal, and Bryant Park, among them. Times Square, "The Crossroads of the World," is at West 42nd and Broadway. As you saunter east to west, feel like a citizen of the world, partaking of an ever-bustling boulevard that will always fascinate. And don't assume you know it all when it comes to 42nd Street— there are always surprises, new things to experience and investigate.

● **Outside Grand Central Terminal, take the eastbound M42 bus (free transfer from the subway) to First Avenue. Walk all the way to the eastern end of the street and look out onto the East River. The small outcropping of land you see is U Thant Island (a.k.a. Belmont Island), a migratory-bird sanctuary. Past this are the larger Roosevelt Island and the borough of Queens—people tend to forget how close the water is when they're in Midtown, so savor this view. Now turn around and face west. On your left is a playground named for Robert Moses, a controversial public-works administrator and the subject of Robert Caro's biography *The Power Broker.* Among the many projects he spearheaded or had a hand in are Lincoln Center (see Walk 19), the Triborough and Verrazano-Narrows Bridges, the UN headquarters, the 1964–65 World's Fair, and Shea Stadium. Much of the play space is occupied by a ventilation structure for the Queens–Midtown Tunnel.**

● Walk back to First Avenue and make a right, walking alongside the United Nations complex on your right. The tall building is the Secretariat; the low building that seems like an air duct is the General Assembly; and the Dag Hammarskjöld Library has shimmering windows. Go until East 45th Street to admire the layout of the UN. Seeing all the nations' flags is a highlight for me, especially if a breeze is blowing.

● Turn around and walk back to 42nd Street. Many of these buildings you pass are connected to the UN. The Ronald H. Brown US Mission has a wavy-topped entrance. At 777 First Ave., the Church Center for the United Nations has a world peace–themed abstract sculpture on its bottom floor. At 43rd Street is Ralph Bunche Park, named for the diplomat and Nobel Peace Prize winner—the first person of color so honored—who brokered peace between Israel and its Arab neighbors in the late 1940s. The Isaiah Wall and the steep, dramatic steps here are often the site of political rallies. Also here is a tall silver modernist sculpture called *Peace Form One.*

● Go right on East 42nd and notice two staircases, one on each side of the street, that lead to a street above called Tudor City Place. Tudor City, a multiblock apartment complex built during the late 1920s and 1930s, is loaded with charm. Its buildings overflow with pseudo-Elizabethan details; gardens, playgrounds, and other amenities make it a very desirable place to live. Walk up to see it all. Before Tudor City was constructed, this was a rough area dominated by slums and slaughterhouses.

● As you continue along East 42nd, look over your right shoulder at the rooftop TUDOR CITY sign. On your left at #320 is Woodstock Tower, which sort of echoes the Tudor look. Next door, dwarfed by the other buildings here, is the quaint Church of the Covenant. Next door is the Hilton Manhattan East, originally the Tudor Hotel.

● Cross Second Avenue and notice the street sign designating this block Yitzhak Rabin Way. This commemorates the prime minister of Israel who was assassinated in 1995. (The Israeli Consulate General is located at 800 Second Ave., on the corner behind you.) On your right is the world headquarters of the Pfizer pharmaceutical company. On your left, with a wonderful bas-relief of city workers over the entrance, is the immense Art Deco building completed in 1930 for the *Daily News* (the newspaper's offices are now located on the West Side). The lobby has a huge globe seemingly suspended in midair with step-seats surrounding it. The ceiling is almost psychedelic, and there are clocks and other gadgets indicating the weather conditions. The Standard Time Line clock is like a prop out of a 1930s movie. This is one of my favorite buildings in all of Manhattan; in 1984, as a college student, I worked two shifts here inputting primary and election data, and I couldn't have been more excited.

● Cross Third Avenue and look up. On your left at the corner is the gracious Socony-Mobil Building, built in the 1950s. But the true gem of this block is ahead on the right, the Chrysler Building. From miles away, this is one of the most distinctive components of the Manhattan skyline, and rightly so. The famous spire emerges from a crown design. Retro-future meets Art Deco, the building is a fanciful tribute to the auto manufacturer, which was headquartered here from 1930 to the mid-1950s. The entrance is reminiscent of a sci-fi rocket ship. In the lobby, awash in marble, the walls and ceilings are richly decorated with scenes of people at work, flying planes, and much more. The elongated light fixtures call to mind organ pipes. Even the lowly letterbox is clad with a mighty eagle design. The elevator doors on the lobby level are engraved with fanlike designs. Only the lobby is open to those without business here, but even a cursory look is a real treat. Reaching 1,046 feet, the Chrysler is the fifth-tallest building in New York City, and it was briefly the tallest in the world until the Empire State eclipsed it.

● Cross Lexington Avenue, and to your left is the Chanin Building (1929), another Art Deco treasure. The lower floors seem to be clad in funky wallpaper (actually bronze) with animal and plant designs. Next door is the castlelike former Bowery Bank, now a Cipriani event space. Across the street is the ever-lively Grand Hyatt. It was built in 1920, but the spacious lobby is very modern. And next door is one of the prime landmarks of Manhattan, Grand Central Terminal (often, but erroneously, called Grand Central Station). As impressive as the exterior is, with its 50-foot-tall statue of Mercury on top and the statue of railroad magnate Cornelius Vanderbilt outside the terminal's south-facing side, the interior is just as grand. Thousands of people stream in and out of here each day, scurrying to and from commuter and subway trains, but slow down to savor the sights here. The cavernous main concourse is famous for its astronomically themed ceiling designs, an immense and gorgeous clock, the Grand Central Oyster Bar with its Guastavino-tiled vaulted ceilings, and stately Vanderbilt Hall (used for exhibitions).

● Watch the road and sidewalk traffic out here—it gets quite hectic. Cars heading up or downtown use the Park Avenue viaduct to get around Grand Central. Just north of the station, see the MetLife Building, off to your right down Vanderbilt Avenue; it looks like a gigantic pegboard. On your left, at 60 East 42nd, is the Lincoln Building, an Art Deco–Renaissance Revival hybrid. Cross Madison Avenue, and on the left is the über-glassy 300 Madison, home of PricewaterhouseCoopers. On the other side of the street, the coolly severe Emigrant Savings Bank is at #5. Other buildings on this block are worth your attention—give them a glance, but continue on to Fifth Avenue.

● One of the true cerebral and cultural joys of Manhattan comes into view on your left: the main branch of the New York Public Library. A Beaux Arts beauty, it's home to the most famous lions in New York City, Patience and Fortitude, one on each side of the main entrance on Fifth Avenue. The inside is intimidating in detail, but go on in. There are exhibitions, usually involving books, artworks, and maps, along with reading rooms and research divisions. (I worked on two of my other books here, handing request slips to librarians and waiting patiently for my research materials.) Look for the memorial plaques on the walls—quiet surprises awaiting discovery. The building is officially named in honor of Stephen A. Schwarzman, a billionaire philanthropist.

● Back on West 42nd Street, look at the nonlibrary side of the street for some worthwhile sights. The building at #11 has a "calendar" entrance, with carvings in stone to represent each month. At #33 is the SUNY College of Optometry, with delicate scrollwork above and between the fourth-floor windows. Next to it is the Grace Building, recognizable for its unusual sloping design.

● Behind the library, enter Bryant Park, which spans West 42nd to West 40th Street and is a lunchtime favorite for workers and shoppers in Midtown. Before it was a park, it was a graveyard, a reservoir, the site of the New York Crystal Palace (which burned down), and a parade ground for Civil War troops. It's named for William Cullen Bryant, the Romantic poet, journalist, and newspaper editor. As lively as the park is now, I can remember when it didn't have the finest reputation; in the 1970s especially, it was a haven for pot smokers and assorted oddballs. (Once my dad was walking here after lunch when out of nowhere some guy punched him in the nose and ran.) It took years of renovation and steady policing to upgrade the park, and today it hosts musical performances and other public events. In the winter there's ice skating; in the summer there are yoga sessions on the lawn. Search out statues of a seated Mr. Bryant with a ribbed dome above him, a seated Gertrude Stein, a bust of Johann Wolfgang von Goethe, a standing Benito Juárez (on the Sixth Avenue side), and others. See and hear (maybe even ride) the small and colorful carousel. Admire the buildings that flank the park on all sides. Choose from plentiful places to eat, semifancy as well as casual.

● Exit the park at West 42nd Street and Sixth Avenue and take note of the Bank of America Tower diagonally across the intersection; completed in 2009, it seems to have a metal exoskeleton. Across the street, adjacent to the 3 Bryant Park building, is an outdoor space with seating and changing sculpture displays.

● As you approach Broadway and Times Square, "The Crossroads of the World," the energy is palpable. Note the red-and-white Beaux Arts building on your left at Broadway and 42nd: The Knickerbocker Hotel (1906). According to legend, the martini was created here in 1912. The building was used for offices for more than 90 years but reopened as a hotel in early 2015.

● The short block bounded by Broadway and Seventh Avenue has the subway station and Times Square Tower on the left. To your right is 1 Times Square, known for "The Zipper" of news headlines, stock prices, and such. This is where the New Year's Eve ball has been dropping since 1907. Signs galore are plastered here for movies, stores, and sporting events.

● Cross Seventh Avenue to enter a block of dizzying entertainment, color, food aromas, and temptations aplenty. Among the places you will see are the New Victory Theater, an old space gussied up and sporting beautiful light fixtures; the once-decrepit, now-Disney-owned

"I'm gonna take my problem to the United Nations." —Eddie Cochran

New Amsterdam Theatre; the Lyric Theatre, which has charming early-1900s details and actually combines sections of two older theaters; the New York outpost of Madame Tussauds Wax Museum; the American Airlines Theatre, formerly the Selwyn; B.B. King's Blues Club and Grill; the Regal Cinemas, with its retro South Beach front; Ripley's Believe It or Not! museum; the too-loud arcade–restaurant Dave & Buster's (a favorite of my younger daughter); a Yankees team shop; the AMC Empire 25, a multiplex movie house in a grand former vaudeville palace; and too many eateries and gift shops to mention. Street vendors and tour-bus salespeople work the sidewalks.

Some New Yorkers gripe that Times Square has lost its grittiness, grown sanitized and hypercommercial, but I have to say I don't miss the grime and crime of the 1970s and 1980s. You should be mindful of your surroundings here as you would anywhere, but thankfully you're no longer subjected to such sights and sounds as drug dealers peddling their wares. ("Smoke, smoke" was a common refrain I used to hear around here. Ugh.)

● Cross Eighth Avenue. The left side of the block is dominated by the big brown-and-glass rectangle that is the Port Authority Bus Terminal. Built in 1950, it's the largest bus terminal in the US (it extends to West 40th Street and a full block to Ninth Avenue) and the world's busiest in traffic volume. It won't win any beauty contests, but it serves travelers and commuters and offers a wide assortment of shops, services, and places to eat—if you need it, it's here. A few 1980s-era artworks are on display, including George Segal's *Commuters* (in the main ticket area) and a statue of Jackie Gleason as bus-driving Ralph Kramden from *The Honeymooners* (outside the Eighth Avenue entrance). A bit farther along on the right is the redbrick Holy Cross Church; completed in 1870, it's the oldest building on all of 42nd Street. It's also known as "Father Duffy's Church," after an early-1900s priest (see the next walk).

● Cross Ninth Avenue, and as you do, look to the left to see the lengthy bus ramps that emerge from Port Authority and head off to the Lincoln Tunnel. On the left side of the street is a collection of off-Broadway theaters, heralded by a vertical sign that reads THEATRE ROW. Just past them runs Dyer Avenue, a short street that feeds into the Lincoln Tunnel. The right side of West 42nd has large postwar housing complexes, parking, and a few businesses.

• From here to the Hudson River, 42nd Street has much less of note than the sections you've already seen. Much of it is fairly recent residential or office buildings, but there are a few arts groups and performance spaces along the way, as well as the local police precinct and the Manhattan South Task Force. Continue past a few huge apartment complexes and parking lots. At 12th Avenue, to your left is Lucky Strike, an upscale bowling alley and restaurant, and across the street, perhaps improbably, is the Chinese consulate. The venerable Circle Line sightseeing cruises are based at Pier 83, just north of West 42nd. If you want, continue up to West 46th Street to visit the Intrepid Sea, Air & Space Museum, a splendid military- and maritime-history museum aboard a WWII-era aircraft carrier.

• When you're ready to call it a day, walk or take the M42 bus east to the Times Square or Grand Central subway station.

POINTS OF INTEREST

United Nations visit.un.org, 405 E. 42nd St., 212-963-4475

Tudor City tudorcity.com, bounded by East 40th and East 43rd Streets and First and Second Avenues, 212-949-6555

Daily News **Building** 220 E. 42nd St.

Chrysler Building tishmanspeyer.com/properties/chrysler-center, 405 Lexington Ave., 212-682-3070

Grand Central Terminal grandcentralterminal.com, 89 E. 42nd St., 212-340-2583

New York Public Library, Main Branch nypl.org/locations/schwarzman, Fifth Avenue and West 42nd Street, 917-275-6975

Bryant Park bryantpark.org, West 42nd Street and Sixth Avenue, 212-768-4242

The Knickerbocker Hotel theknickerbocker.com, 6 Times Square, 212-204-4980

Times Square timessquarenyc.org, bounded by West 42nd Street, Broadway, Seventh Avenue, and West 47th Street

Port Authority Bus Terminal tinyurl.com/portauthoritynyc, 625 Eighth Ave., 212-502-2200

Holy Cross Church 329 W. 42nd St., 212-246-4732

Lucky Strike bowlluckystrike.com, 624–660 W. 42nd St., 646-829-0170

Circle Line circleline42.com, Pier 83 (West 42nd Street and 12th Avenue), 212-563-3200

Intrepid Sea, Air & Space Museum intrepidmuseum.org, Pier 86 (West 46th Street and 12th Avenue), 212-245-0072

route summary

1.   From the Grand Central–42nd Street subway, go aboveground and take the M42 bus east to First Avenue.
2.   Walk to the East River, then head west on East 42nd Street.
3.   Turn right on First Avenue for the UN.
4.   At East 45th Street, double back to East 42nd and turn right.
5.   Continue west along 42nd to the Hudson River.
6.   Walk or take the M42 back to the subway.

CONNECTING THE WALKS

From 12th Avenue, take the M42 bus east to Times Square to start the next walk (Times Square/Theater District). On foot it's about six and a half fairly lengthy blocks.

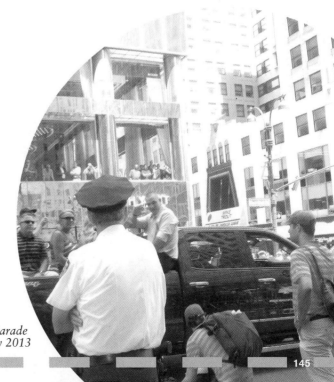

The MLB All-Star Game Parade that I attended on 42nd Street in July 2013

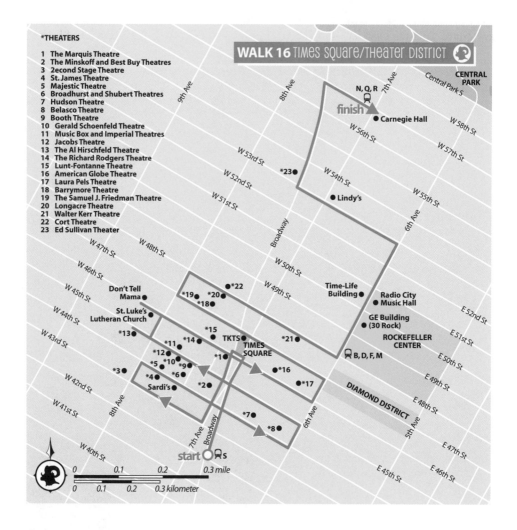

*THEATERS

1   The Marquis Theatre
2   The Minskoff and Best Buy Theatres
3   2econd Stage Theatre
4   St. James Theatre
5   Majestic Theatre
6   Broadhurst and Shubert Theatres
7   Hudson Theatre
8   Belasco Theatre
9   Booth Theatre
10 Gerald Schoenfeld Theatre
11 Music Box and Imperial Theatres
12 Jacobs Theatre
13 The Al Hirschfeld Theatre
14 The Richard Rodgers Theatre
15 Lunt-Fontanne Theatre
16 American Globe Theatre
17 Laura Pels Theatre
18 Barrymore Theatre
19 The Samuel J. Friedman Theatre
20 Longacre Theatre
21 Walter Kerr Theatre
22 Cort Theatre
23 Ed Sullivan Theater

WALK 16 TIMES SQUARE/THEATER DISTRICT

CENTRAL PARK

N, Q, R

finish

Carnegie Hall

Central Park S

9th Ave
8th Ave
7th Ave
6th Ave
5th Ave

W 58th St
W 57th St
W 56th St
W 55th St
W 54th St
W 53rd St
W 52nd St
W 51st St
W 50th St
W 49th St
W 48th St
W 47th St
W 46th St
W 45th St
W 44th St
W 43rd St
W 42nd St
W 41st St
W 40th St

E 52nd St
E 51st St
E 50th St
E 49th St
E 48th St
E 47th St
E 46th St
E 45th St

*23

Lindy's

Time-Life Building

Radio City Music Hall

GE Building (30 Rock)

ROCKEFELLER CENTER

Broadway

Don't Tell Mama

St. Luke's Lutheran Church

*19 *20 *22
     *18

*13

*15

*11 *14   TKTS
*12   TIMES SQUARE
*5 *10 *9
*4   *6   *1
*3   *2

*21

B, D, F, M

*16

*17

DIAMOND DISTRICT

Sardi's

*7

*8

8th Ave
7th Ave
Broadway
6th Ave
5th Ave

start   s

0   0.1   0.2   0.3 mile
0   0.1   0.2   0.3 kilometer

16 TIMES SQUARE/THEATER DISTRICT: WALKING THE GREAT WHITE WAY

BOUNDARIES: **6th Ave., W. 42nd St., 8th Ave., W. 57th St.**
DISTANCE: **2.7 miles**
SUBWAY: **1/2/3/7/A/C/E/N/Q/R/S to 42nd St.–Times Square**

What once was called Longacre Square was renamed for *The New York Times* in 1904, the year that the newspaper moved its offices to a spanking-new skyscraper on 42nd Street. Ever since, Times Square has been a mecca for performance and splashy advertisement, such as the huge billboard for Camel cigarettes that showed a man blowing smoke rings. That's gone, but now the Naked Cowboy strolls around strumming a guitar and wearing little more than a wide-brimmed hat. Almost all of the Broadway theaters are located here, plus innumerable stores, restaurants, and special attractions.

A considerable swath of Times Square was turned into a pedestrian-only plaza in the early 2000s. As crowded as it can get, filled with tourists and people clasping overstuffed shopping bags, Times Square is almost always a fun and energizing place to be. Through the years, it has had its special moments when people congregated for something more: Think of the end of World War II, when thousands cheered and Alfred Eisenstaedt snapped his iconic photo of a sailor kissing a nurse. Or the Super Bowl Boulevard celebration in 2014. Or more-serious occasions, such as political and antiwar protests. And of course, a huge New Year's Eve celebration has been held here each year since 1907, with the world-famous ball dropping and thousands upon thousands of revelers whooping it up while millions more watch at home.

Be mindful (of your belongings, of wayward vehicles), but enjoy watching the entertainers clad in superhero and cartoon costumes, occasional street preachers, and vendors. Only the grumpiest New Yorker wouldn't get psyched while walking around "The Crossroads of the World" these days.

● **Whichever train you alight from at 42nd Street–Times Square, follow the signs to the S—the 42nd Street Shuttle—and zero in on Tracks 3 and 4. At the tracks' western end** (where they stop), you can see the northbound 1, 2, and 3 trains go by. Look down past the metal barrier and notice an unused track: This was the connector used early in the history of the New York subways, when trains crossed between the East and West Sides. Now this separate shuttle train carries out that responsibility. Today, the subway system has only a few shuttles, and this line serves just two stations, Times Square and Grand Central.

- Walk west along Track 1. Near a staircase to the street, notice a dingy white door with an old sign above that reads KNICKERBOCKER. The building on the southwest corner of West 42nd Street and Broadway is The Knickerbocker Hotel, which originally operated from 1906 to 1921 and reopened in 2015 (it was an office building during the decades in between). This "secret" doorway was a perk for the old hotel's patrons. Several feet away is a wall sign, somewhat worn-out, that also reads KNICKERBOCKER.

- Go up to the street and find "The Zipper," the electronic news ticker encircling the 1 Times Square building. People stand still at times to read the latest dispatches and see stock quotes. Walk on the Broadway side of the building, on one of the pedestrian-only sections of Times Square. There's a sense of adventure to walking in the middle of the street in a big city, though this was a controversial move, put into place during Michael Bloomberg's tenure as mayor and disliked by many who felt it would impede vehicular traffic too much.

- On your left at West 43rd Street, the Times Square police station has its own bold blue sign, as well as an interesting wall mural. Opposite it, see the US Armed Forces Recruiting Station, serving all four branches. The nation's flag is brightly lit on the side. To the right at West 44th is the eye-poppingly huge Toys"R"Us store, with floors of toys, games, sweet treats, and what-not for kids of all ages. Among the big draws is the Ferris wheel of toy characters, which you can see through the store windows; I also like the Lego models of the Empire State Building and other local landmarks. See it all while you can—the store is set to close at the beginning of 2016. Across Times Square is the hard-to-miss Marriott Marquis hotel, big and bold.

- Past 44th Street, Broadway merges into Seventh Avenue. Walk to West 45th, which is co-named George Abbott Way in memory of a theater producer, playwright, and director who lived to be 107. Pass the Disney Store and other big-name shops. To your right, on the north side of West 46th Street, is the I. Miller Building, with the inscription THE SHOW FOLKS SHOE SHOP DEDICATED TO BEAUTY IN FOOTWEAR. *Whew.* This charming building has four statues of famous actresses of the past, clad in costumes of characters they portrayed.

● To your left, the pedestrian island, formally called Duffy Square, offers stadium-style seating that faces south; the other side of it has TKTS booths, where you can line up and purchase discounted tickets to same-day performances of Broadway and off-Broadway shows.

In front of the seating area is a statue of Father Francis P. Duffy, who presided over nearby Holy Cross Church on 42nd Street (see previous walk). Just steps away is a statue of George M. Cohan, the actor-writer-composer known for the songs "You're a Grand Old Flag," "The Yankee Doodle Boy," and, fittingly, "Give My Regards to Broadway." As you stand here, take in the gigantic ads, marquees, and buildings, and tune in to the cacophony.

● Turn around and walk south on Broadway, on the west side of Duffy Square. Past West 44th Street on your right, admire the pretty gilded front entrance of 1501 Broadway, complete with clock. Look to the left to see the cornerstone of this building, the 1926-built Paramount. It has an even more opulent entrance closer to West 43rd Street, with huge windows and a distinctive marquee, now used as the entrance to the Hard Rock Cafe.

● Turn right on West 43rd Street. See the back of the Lyric Theatre on your left. Some of the doors have quaint carvings above them, such as the word

Want to be recruited in Times Square?

MVSIC. Across the street, at #229, is the old *New York Times* building, its mansard-roofed upper floors reminiscent of a French chateau; "All the News That's Fit to Print" was published here from 1913 to 2007. Back to your left is the Hotel Carter, which opened in 1930. It has a vertical red neon sign, not to mention a history of suicides, murders, and other sordid stuff. (In 2006, 2008, and 2009, it earned the coveted distinction of "Dirtiest Hotel in America" from TripAdvisor.) A much glossier hotel at the end of this block is the Westin New York, seemingly all dark glass.

● Reach the intersection of West 43rd and Eighth Avenue. Across Eighth to the left is the Show World Center, one of the area's very few remaining adult-flick houses, and on the right is 2econd Stage Theatre. This street corner is co-named for Leon Davis, who organized hospital workers in the 1950s; their union, 1199, is in the next block of 43rd Street.

● Turn right and walk north on Eighth Avenue. West 44th Street here is co-named Rodgers & Hammerstein Row, for the musical-theater duo who wrote *South Pacific, The King and I, Oklahoma,* and *The Sound of Music.*

● Make a right on West 44th to see a few Broadway theaters, such as the St. James (from the 1920s) and the Majestic, home of *The Phantom of the Opera,* the longest-running show in Broadway history. Note the covered balconies and lamps of the Majestic—very New Orleans. Also on this block are the Helen Hayes, Broadhurst, Booth, and Shubert Theatres (the last with its striking angled title board). Rosters of hits (and misses) and scores of talented actors have graced the stages here. Also sandwiched in here is Sardi's restaurant, its walls full of caricatures of showbiz personalities. A fabled hangout for theater people and the press, Sardi's is where producer-director Brock Pemberton came up with the idea for the Tony Awards (to honor his late creative partner, Antoinette Perry).

● At Broadway, walk past the Toys"R"Us again. The Millennium Broadway Hotel, with its jazzy black-and-gray window over the entrance, is after it on the left. This stretch of West 44th has several restaurants and other hotels. The highlight of the block is the Belasco Theatre, named for theatrical impresario David Belasco. Open since 1907, it has a duplex apartment above the theater and lots of beautiful architectural detail. On the right, at #110, is the decidedly nontheatrical IRS office.

● When you reach Sixth Avenue, on the block to your right is the International Center of Photography (ICP). The building is unremarkable, but the museum has excellent photography exhibits.

● Make a left on Sixth, then a left on West 45th Street. This block is notable for its Irish pubs, such as Connolly's, The Perfect Pint, and O'Lunney's. At #120, there is an open public space with a space age–y lighting fixture suspended like a sculpture. On the right side of the street closer to Seventh Avenue is the Lyceum (1903), Broadway's oldest continuously operating theater, with six massive Corinthian columns and a wavy canopy over the entrance. At the corner is Planet Hollywood.

● Cross Broadway and Seventh Avenue to see several more theaters: the Minskoff, the Music Box (with a balcony and four columns and pilasters, plus its name written in distinctive script), the Gerald Schoenfeld (named for the late chairman of the Shubert Organization, which owns a whopping 17 Broadway theaters), the Jacobs, the Imperial, and the Golden. Most of these theaters date to the 1920s, or just before.

● Cross Eighth Avenue. This block of West 45th is co-named Runyon's Way for writer Damon Runyon, famous for his stories about people on the fringes of the Broadway scene. To the left, see The Al Hirschfeld Theatre. It was renamed in 2003 to honor the cartoonist who drew distinctive caricatures of theater, movie, and TV stars; *The New York Times* popularized his work, which he continued to do into his 90s (he died in 2003, a few months shy of his 100th birthday). His self-caricature graces the marquee.

● Go back to Eighth Avenue and turn left.

● Make a left at West 46th Street, affectionately known as Restaurant Row for its collection of eateries that cater to theater crowds. (In particular, Joe Allen restaurant is famous as a celebrity haunt.) You'll also see St. Luke's, a commanding church that dates to the early 1920s; not surprisingly for this area, it has an off-Broadway theater space as well. Farther down to the right at #343 is Don't Tell Mama, which has two cabarets, a piano bar, a restaurant, and a cute keyboard logo.

● Turn around and go back across Eighth Avenue. This block of West 46th has its share of hotels, theaters, and the Church of Scientology. The Paramount Hotel at #245 resembles a pretty theater itself. The Richard Rodgers Theatre (originally

Chanin's 46th St. Theater) dates to the 1920s and has attractive pilasters and arches. A bit farther down is the Lunt-Fontanne Theatre, built in 1910 as the Globe.

- Continue east to a block of West 46th known less for theater and eateries (although it has those) than for houses of worship and a very famous school. The Church of St. Mary the Virgin (#145), from 1895, has a dramatic set of religious statues out front—and the distinction of being the first church in the world built like a skyscraper, on a concealed iron skeleton. Across the street is a large, brown, sorta-spooky-looking school building from the early 1890s. This is the Jacqueline Kennedy Onassis High School for International Careers, but from 1948 to 1984 it was the home of the High School of the Performing Arts, immortalized in the movie *Fame* despite not actually having been used as a filming location. (In 1984, it merged with Harlem's High School of Music & Art and moved near Lincoln Center to became Fiorello H. LaGuardia High School of Music & Art and Performing Arts.) Check out the exquisite carved heads near the main door.

- At Sixth Avenue, make a left.

- At West 47th Street, look across to the east side of the avenue to the so-called Diamond District, named for all the jewelry stores located on this block. But make a left on West 47th, passing the Fox News building on the northwest corner. To the left, pass the northern end of St. Mary the Virgin Church. Cross Seventh Avenue and continue past TKTS and then the W Hotel, with its bold red *W.* After that on the left is the Hotel Edison, built in 1931; Thomas Edison himself flipped on the lights here the very first time. This Art Deco treasure also houses the Edison Ballroom, a private event space. Across the street is the Barrymore Theatre, named for one of America's acting dynasties, with BARRYMORE written in an exuberantly swoopy script on the marquee. Farther down on the right is the Samuel J. Friedman Theatre, named for a legendary Broadway press agent, and across the street from that is the Brooks Atkinson Theatre, named for the famed *New York Times* drama critic. At the corner on the left is the Copacabana nightclub. This isn't the original—it's moved a few times over the years—but it nonetheless has a rich history of entertainment, plus that Barry Manilow song to serenade it.

- Make a right on Eighth Avenue and pause at the firehouse on your right, Engine 54/Ladder 4/Battalion 9. Pay homage to the men they lost over the years, remembered on several plaques. Check out the bas-relief 9/11 memorial.

● Make a right and walk along West 48th Street. Hotels dominate this block, but closer to Broadway are the Longacre and Walter Kerr Theatres. The Longacre (as in the old name for Times Square) has French neoclassical details above the entrance level; the Walter Kerr, with its lacy balconies, used to be the Ritz.

● The intersection of 48th and Broadway could well be dubbed Candy Corner, for the Hershey's Chocolate World and M&M's World stores across from each other on your left. The M&M's store has four floors of candy, gifts, and photo ops. The block of West 48th east of Seventh Avenue used to be a musician's paradise, with several instrument stores and repair services. Sadly, hardly any are left; some relocated and others went out of business. Modest Rudy's Music Stop and Alex Musical Instruments stores are still here, but Sam Ash moved several blocks south, and the big Manny's Music is gone, although the store name is still on the sidewalk at 156 W. 48th St. Farther on the right, see the palatial Cort Theatre, modeled on the Petit Trianon at Versailles.

● Make a left on Sixth Avenue, dominated on your left by the humongous McGraw-Hill Companies building. It has a plaza where you can sit and relax, but it's not a particularly cozy corner. Publishers Simon & Schuster are across the avenue.

● Pass the wide rectangular fountain in front of the Exxon Building (1251 Sixth Ave.), and check out the sky-scraping Art Deco delight across the street from it. Long known as the GE Building (though now signed for Comcast) and more informally as "30 Rock," it's part of Rockefeller Center and home to NBC Studios. The building's recessed entrance has a brilliantly colored mosaic mural titled

The Shubert Theatre's unique angled title board

Intelligence Awakening Mankind, sort of reminiscent of church iconography. (See the next walk for more of Rockefeller Center.)

● Across West 50th Street, behold the world's largest theatrical space: Radio City Music Hall. Outside it has those iconic vertical neon signs and the bas-relief allegory *Morning, Present, Evening* on the Sixth Avenue side; highlights within include the "Mighty Wurlitzer" pipe organ, which impressed me as a little kid, and high–Art Deco interior design everywhere you look—the Grand Foyer and the sunburst proscenium of the Great Stage are simply jaw-dropping. Like many New Yorkers, I've thrilled to the Rockettes, and I've also attended concerts here (R.E.M., Pet Shop Boys, Elvis Costello, and others). The sound quality can't be beat.

● Look across Sixth Avenue to see the Time-Life Building and its bright-blue sculpture, *Cubed Curve,* and then the UBS Building between West 51st and West 52nd Streets. Walk farther on Sixth, and on the left see the Calyon Building, which features three headless Venus de Milo–inspired statues—two at 52nd Street and another at 53rd Street—collectively called *Looking Toward the Avenue.* The block of West 52nd Street heading west is co-named W. C. Handy's Place, for the African American composer known as "The Father of the Blues"; heading east, it's co-named Swing Street. (Fifty-Second Street between Fifth and Seventh Avenues was the epicenter of the New York jazz scene from the 1930s to the 1950s.) On your right, at the corner of Sixth and West 52nd, are the corporate offices of CBS.

● Make a left on West 53rd Street, with the immense New York Hilton Midtown to your right. This block has one quirky building, on your left: the 53rd Street Central Substation, which services the subway trains. The Art Deco–style building has a futuristically detailed entrance. Notice the 6½ AV street sign next to the substation, which marks the public walkway opposite it. At Seventh Avenue, on the right, is Lindy's, famous for its cheesecake and being a hangout for organized-crime heavies in decades past. Cross Seventh and walk a half-block to Broadway.

● Turn right on Broadway. To your left is the Ed Sullivan Theater. It's gone by a few other names in its history but is best known as the home base of *The Ed Sullivan Show* and, today, *The Late Show with David Letterman.* While you're not busy being starstruck, check out the vestibule with its pretty ceiling.

● West 54th Street here is co-named Big Apple Corner as well as Señor Wences Way, for the Spanish ventriloquist Ed Sullivan featured on his show many times. *S'awright!*

● Walk up to West 57th Street and turn right. Note the Art Students League of New York building, on your left at 215 W. 57th, with its vaguely exotic doors and windows. The Brooklyn Diner, across the street, is . . . vaguely authentic. Walk to the corner of 57th and 7th, and, if you're a musician, feel shock and awe: Across Seventh Avenue is Carnegie Hall. This august ochre building (1891) has long been one of the most prestigious musical venues in the world. I've not only seen a plethora of performers here—Tracy Chapman, Arlo Guthrie, Mickey Hart, and Planet Drum, among them—I've also fretted over a few annual piano exams in the studios on the upper floors.

● Catch the N, Q, or R train on Seventh Avenue and West 57th Street, just across the street from Carnegie Hall.

POINTS OF INTEREST

Times Square timessquarenyc.org, bounded by West 42nd Street, Broadway, Seventh Avenue, and West 47th Street

Duffy Square nycgovparks.org/parks/father-duffy-square/history, West 46th Street at Broadway

Sardi's sardis.com, 234 W. 44th St., 212-302-0865

International Center of Photography icp.org, 1133 Sixth Ave., 212-857-0000

Restaurant Row restaurantrownyc.com, West 46th Street between Eighth and Ninth Avenues

St. Luke's Lutheran Church & St. Luke's Theatre stlukesnyc.org/stlukestheatre.com, 308 W. 46th St., 212-246-3540 (church), 212-246-8140 (theater)

Don't Tell Mama donttellmamanyc.com, 343 W. 46th St., 212-757-0788

Church of St. Mary the Virgin stmvirgin.org, 145 W. 46th St., 212-869-5830

Diamond District diamonddistrict.org, West 47th Street between Fifth and Sixth Avenues, 212-302-5739

Hotel Edison & Edison Ballroom edisonhotelnyc.com, 228 W. 47th St., 212-840-5000

Copacabana copacabanany.com, 268 W. 47th St., 212-221-2672

Radio City Music Hall radiocity.com, 1260 Sixth Ave., 212-465-6741

Lindy's 825 Seventh Ave., 212-767-8343

Ed Sullivan Theater edsullivan.com/ed-sullivan-theater, 1697 Broadway, 212-975-4755

Carnegie Hall carnegiehall.org, 881 Seventh Ave., 212-247-7800

route summary

1. Explore the S train-track area in the Times Square–42nd Street station, then go aboveground and walk north on Broadway/Seventh Avenue.
2. At West 46th Street, cross over to Duffy Square, then go south on Broadway on its other side.
3. Walk right on West 43rd Street.
4. Walk right on Eighth Avenue.
5. Walk right on West 44th Street.
6. Walk left on Sixth Avenue.
7. Walk left on West 45th Street to The Al Hirschfeld Theatre, and turn around.
8. Walk left on Eighth Avenue.
9. Walk left on West 46th Street for Restaurant Row, then reverse direction.
10. Walk left on Sixth Avenue.
11. Walk left on West 47th Street.
12. Walk right on Eighth Avenue.
13. Walk right on West 48th Street.
14. Walk left on Sixth Avenue.
15. Walk left on West 53rd Street
16. Walk right on Broadway.
17. Walk right on West 57th Street to Seventh Avenue.

CONNECTING THE WALKS

To start the next walk (Rockefeller Center), go one block east on West 57th Street to Sixth Avenue, then turn right and walk 10 blocks to West 47th Street.

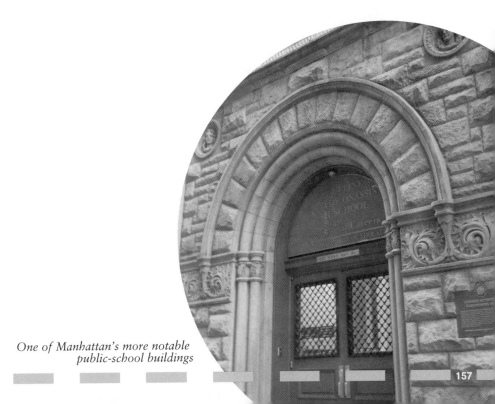

One of Manhattan's more notable public-school buildings

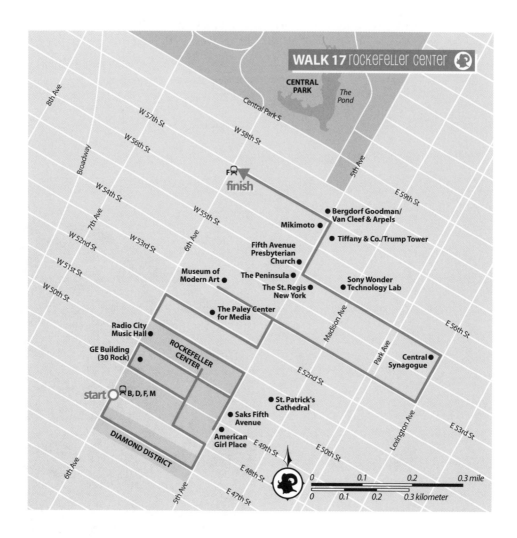

CENTRAL PARK

The Pond

Central Park S

8th Ave

W 57th St

W 56th St

W 58th St

Broadway

5th Ave

E 59th St

F finish

W 54th St

7th Ave

W 55th St

W 53rd St

6th Ave

● Bergdorf Goodman/
Van Cleef & Arpels

Mikimoto ●

W 52nd St

W 51st St

W 50th St

Fifth Avenue
Presbyterian
Church ●

● Tiffany & Co./Trump Tower

Museum of
Modern Art ●

● The Peninsula

● The St. Regis
New York

Sony Wonder
● Technology Lab

● The Paley Center
for Media

Radio City
Music Hall ●

ROCKEFELLER
CENTER

Madison Ave

Park Ave

E 56th St

GE Building
(30 Rock) ●

Central ●
Synagogue

start ○ 🚇 B, D, F, M

E 52nd St

Lexington Ave

E 53rd St

● St. Patrick's
Cathedral

● Saks Fifth
Avenue

● American
Girl Place

DIAMOND DISTRICT

E 49th St

E 50th St

6th Ave

5th Ave

E 48th St

E 47th St

0   0.1   0.2   0.3 mile

0   0.1   0.2   0.3 kilometer

17 rockefeller center: "the rock" and other midtown treasures

BOUNDARIES: **W. 47th St., 6th Ave., E. 57th St., Lexington Ave.**
DISTANCE: **2.3 miles**
SUBWAY: **B, D, F, M to Rockefeller Center/47–50th St.**

Fans of Art Deco architecture and decorative arts love midtown Manhattan because it has so many stellar specimens. In particular, the Rockefeller Center complex is eye candy for lovers of this style. But the swath of Manhattan covered in this walk has other stirring sights of artistic, spiritual, and cultural importance. St. Patrick's Cathedral touches the hearts of Roman Catholics and others. MoMA (the Museum of Modern Art) houses an unparalleled art and design collection. The Sony Building has fascinating science, technology, and media exhibitions that will thrill children and adults alike. And for shopping—or just dreaming about it—head over to Tiffany's, among other swank stores, or thrill to the Diamond District, centered on 47th Street. (Be aware that traffic, both pedestrian and vehicular, can be quite heavy in the area this walk covers.)

● **Look for the West 47th Street exit from the subway station. Upstairs, the Diamond District awaits. All along 47th Street are stores selling gemstones, pearls, rings, watches, necklaces . . . it's simply dizzying. Years ago, I was walking around here and spied Brian Setzer of the Stray Cats peering into a window, just like every other dazzled visitor. You'll hear many different languages spoken in the shops, and it may seem like half the people you see have jewelers' loupes on chains around their necks.**

● **Walk east to Fifth Avenue and turn left, looking across the avenue just past 48th Street to see the Sephora store—it used to be Charles Scribner's and Sons, one of the city's great bookstores; the old sign, flanked by cherubs, remains proudly affixed. Just around the corner, at 5 E. 48th St., is the Church of Sweden, known for its cheap and tasty lunches. (An open-faced sandwich of cheese, fish, or ham goes for about $2.50.)**

● **Turn left on West 48th Street. The Centria, a residential tower at #18, seems to be glass and nothing else. Cross the street and make a right at your entry point to Rockefeller Center.**

BacK STorY: MoMa Mia

The Museum of Modern Art is a formidable entity in the art-and-design world: It's not the New York Museum of Modern Art, it's *the* Museum of Modern Art, also known as MoMA. It began in 1929, was bankrolled by the Rockefeller family, and moved into its International-style abode on West 53rd Street in 1939. It has undergone renovations and expansions over the years and has waded into various controversies (regarding exhibits, design and construction plans, and other things), but it is known above all else for its astounding holdings. The permanent collection includes works by Picasso, van Gogh, Monet, Matisse, Cézanne, Dalí, Chagall, Kahlo, Wyeth, Warhol, Gauguin, Klee, and so many more illustrious artists.

I was a teen the first time my mom brought me here, to see Picasso's *Guernica,* which confused me. (The painting is now housed

at the Queen Sofía Museum in Spain.) I brought a dozen high school students here in late 2010, and they were fascinated—especially by the temporary exhibit of someone playing a piano from the inside and then walking with it. One of the most striking exhibits in recent years was a retrospective of performance artist Marina Abramović's work, some of it involving naked people you had to walk between. The key aspect of this was that Abramović would sit in a chair for several hours a day and not move or say anything, and people in the museum could sit across from her. My husband, daughters, and I came to watch this; at one point, she shocked everyone by putting her head in her hands, as if in anguish.

Go to MoMA to be entertained, shocked, aggravated . . . or relaxed. Its funky sculpture garden with small reflecting pools is one of the treats of a spring or summer day in the city.

● Pause to peruse the entrance to 1 Rockefeller Plaza, on your right. Each side is flanked by a massive etching of a laborer. *Industry* and *Agriculture* are their names, and they date to 1937. On your left, NBC News is in a corner building with windows that allow passersby to look in on the on-air staff. People love to congregate here, waving to the camera and holding up signs. The NBC Experience store is across West 49th Street—as is the GE (General Electric) Building, a.k.a. "30 Rock," one of the tallest buildings in Manhattan at 850 feet. The grand entrance here features three magnificent painted carvings: The middle one, a crowned and bearded sage, represents Wisdom; the male on the left, his palms facing outward, is Sound; and the female, arms outstretched, is Light. Look on the sidewalk for a circular marker that shows where the Christmas tree is installed annually.

When in residence, the tree towers above the grand ice-skating rink, open from midautumn to early April. No matter what time of year you come, the street-level perimeter of the rink is lined with flags—sometimes those of nations, sometimes the US flag and state flags. Walk alongside the flags so you can see the gem of the rink: *Prometheus,* who faces Fifth Avenue, perched on a fountain. Every detail of this great gilded statue—said to be the most-photographed monumental work in New York City—is exquisite, from the waves of his hair to his eyes to the band that encircles him (illustrated with animals and symbols) and the quote from Aeschylus etched into the wall behind him.

- Cross West 50th Street to see 50 Rockefeller Plaza. Above its entrance is *News,* a stainless-steel bas-relief created by Isamu Noguchi. Five newsmen race to get a scoop by means of different methods: pad and pencil, camera, telephone, teletype, and wire. (The former tenant here was the Associated Press.)

- Go back to West 49th Street, on the other side of the rink. There is elevator access to the Sea Grill restaurant, which borders the rink, and across from it is the side entrance of 1 Rock, with the proud and pretty *Progress* above the door. Walk with the rink to your right. Ahead on the left, at 20 Rockefeller Plaza, is Christie's, the famous auction house. Take in the triple-height entranceway. Art pieces are displayed in the windows.

- Turn right at Sixth Avenue. Here again is 30 Rock, which occupies a full block. The Sixth Avenue entrance has a lovely mosaic inside (described in the previous walk).

- Make a right at West 50th Street to ogle Radio City Music Hall. Three circular plaques grace the West 50th side: *Dance, Drama,* and *Song,* from 1932. As you walk past the neon marquee, take note of the geometric patterns running up the side of the building. Across the street is an entrance for NBC Studios, the Top of the Rock observation deck, and the Rainbow Room, a rooftop restaurant. The neon marquee here complements its Radio City sibling across the street.

- When you again reach the ice rink, on your left is 45 Rockefeller Plaza, or the International Building, with its clock and sculpted entryway mural called *The Story of Mankind.* Continue walking, and at 45 Rock's next entrance you find the bas-reliefs *Columbus Greeting a Woman* and *Boatman Unfurling a Sail* on the left and another bas-relief, *The Immigrant,* to the right. The golden carving above the door is *Swords into Plowshares,* a visual interpretation of Isaiah II:IV. At the entrance to Banana Republic, see the *St. Francis with Birds* carving. Across the street, a side entrance to 620 Fifth Ave. (a.k.a. the British Empire Building) has three etched lions called *Arms of England.*

- At Fifth Avenue, cross over and walk right to see the ever-elegant Saks Fifth Avenue. Peruse the window displays as you walk to East 49th, then cross over to American Girl Place. Many girls love American Girl dolls and their realistic clothes and accessories; the restaurant inside is popular for birthdays, so it pays to book way in advance. On the west side of Fifth, admire more of the Rockefeller Center complex. At #610, La Maison Française, are the gilded cast-bronze delight *Friendship Between America and France* and, above it, *Gallic Freedom.* Glimpse the open Promenade, which leads to the ice rink; during the holidays, it's specially decorated. On the 50th Street side of the Promenade, 620 Fifth Ave. features *Industries of the British Empire,* a high relief with nine figurines.

- Back on the east side of Fifth Avenue, at 50th Street, is St. Patrick's Cathedral, the center of Roman Catholic spirituality in New York City. Completed in 1878, this neo-Gothic masterpiece has soaring twin spires, a spectacular rose window, two massive pipe organs, and two Tiffany-designed altars, among other accoutrements. In its crypt are buried eight archbishops of New York. Cross back to the Rockefeller Center side to see 626 Fifth Ave. and the *Italia* bas-relief above its entrance. A statue of Atlas carrying the world stands in the setback entrance of 630 Fifth Ave. *Atlas* is the largest sculpture at Rockefeller Center—see how muscular he is, and how his right foot slips off the pedestal as he struggles to keep steady. And at 636 Fifth Ave., you see yet more artwork: Above the entrance are the monumental cartouche *Commerce and Industry with a Caduceus* and, just below that, the neo-Roman bas-relief *Youth Leading Industry.*

- At West 51st Street, make a left. Check out the relief etchings around the side entrance to 640 Fifth Ave., comprising such themes as communications, arts, and industry. Next door, with the flags, is the Women's National Republican Club. Across the street are another entrance to the International Building and a pretty set of heraldic symbols. Walking toward Sixth Avenue, pass on your left the FDNY Fire Zone, a hands-on fire-safety exhibit space, and then the north side of Radio City Music Hall.

- Make a right onto Sixth Avenue. At the right corner, West 52nd Street is co-named Swing Street, to commemorate the many jazz clubs that used to line the street. CBS headquarters is here, too.

- Make a right on West 52nd, passing a public space with marble seating area, trees, and a few abstract sculptures on your left, shortly before you reach The Paley Center for Media. It owns a huge collection of TV and radio recordings, and it offers exhibitions and discussions related to media and culture. The building after it has a fence with a kitschy display of lawn jockeys—this is the legendary 21 Club, a posh restaurant that started life (in a different location) as a speakeasy.

- Walk to the corner and notice the building across Fifth Avenue—this is the Manhattan flagship store for Cartier. The Renaissance Revival mansion, built in 1905 for railroad heir Morton F. Plant, is currently being renovated; until the work is completed, in 2016, Cartier is operating out of temporary digs at the General Motors Building (767 Fifth). Turn left on Fifth and catch sight of more high-end shops. On your left at West 53rd is St. Thomas, an Episcopal church in the French High Gothic Revival style. It's famous for its men's and boys' choir.

- Walk left on West 53rd Street to the middle of the block for MoMA, one of the top museums in the world (see Back Story). You need at least a few hours here to truly appreciate

Wisdom reigns over the GE Building.

the collections; happily, no admission is charged Fridays from 4 p.m. to closing. The MoMA Design Store is across the street.

● Now turn around and return to Fifth Avenue. Cross over and continue to the open space known as Paley Park (as in The Paley Center; both are named for William S. Paley, who built CBS into the huge radio and television network) on the left. As a child, I got a kick out of going to this pocket park, which is on the site of the late, lamented Stork Club.

● Continue past Madison Avenue to Park Avenue, wide and bisected by a concrete island with well-tended plantings and changing displays of sculpture. Park is the only avenue on Manhattan's East Side with such a layout. On your left, gaze up at a big building with glass in two shades of green; this is the Lever House, completed in 1952 in the International style. Many of the original glass panes have been replaced. Look to your right (south) on Park to see the MetLife Building, originally called the Pan Am Building, after the now-defunct airline. This building is also an example of the International style.

● Walk on East 53rd Street to Lexington Avenue. The southeast corner has a peculiar modernist subway station in front of a skyscraper. It's sheltered by a glass triangle—in essence, a sculpture used to access trains. Across the street from it, see the sunken plaza area, where local workers eat lunch in nice weather.

● Turn left on Lexington. The concrete-and-glass St. Peter's Church makes a statement at the corner of East 54th Street. Look to your right to see an unusual rounded skyscraper on Third Avenue, laid out with bands of windows alternating with reddish-brown granite and steel. Although formally known as 885 Third Ave., most people call it the Lipstick Building. (The Ramones sang a song about "53rd & 3rd" well before the building went up in 1986.) On your left, at East 55th Street and Lexington Avenue, see the Central Synagogue, whose building has been in continuous use longer than any other synagogue in town. Its Moorish design is based on that of a synagogue in Budapest. Built in 1872, it suffered a major fire in 1998 but was restored.

● Turn left on East 55th. Midblock is #124, with some oddball signs: ELEANOR'S BUILDING and SHE WHO MUST BE OBEYED. Both are references to the British TV show Rumpole of the Bailey and the American company that distributed it. It's a pretty building, in any case. A SUNY (State University of New York) building is past it.

- Cross Park Avenue and then Madison Avenue. On your right are the Sony Plaza Public Arcade and the Sony Wonder Technology Lab. If you have time to spare, this is a free and highly enjoyable place where you can pick and choose which tech and media exhibits you want to try. Hands-on labs involve music, video, recording techniques, and more. In the covered arcade, you may hear a musical performance. Once you pry yourself away from here, walk farther on East 55th Street to see the swank St. Regis hotel, at #2. Opened in 1904 by a member of the Astor family, it has both temporary and permanent residents. If you want to stop in for a drink, you can check out the celebrated *Old King Cole* mural by Maxfield Parrish.

- Cross Fifth Avenue and have a gander at the luxurious Peninsula hotel; built in 1905 as the Gotham Hotel, it's a Beaux Arts beauty. Across the street is Fifth Avenue Presbyterian Church, the largest Presbyterian sanctuary in Manhattan, consecrated in 1875. Duke Ellington and his orchestra recorded a live CBS broadcast here in 1966.

- Make a right on Fifth Avenue and stroll along blocks chock-full of pricey stores. Pass Henri Bendel, Harry Winston, and Prada to your left; then, on the east side, across 56th Street, see the opulent Trump Tower, with its freestanding sidewalk clock.

- Turn left on West 57th Street. Mikimoto, in the Crown Building, with a charming entrance topped by three gilded statues, is on your left, opposite Tiffany & Co. on Fifth Avenue and across 57th Street from Van Cleef & Arpels and Bergdorf Goodman. (In case you care to check them out, Chanel and Christian Dior are in the opposite direction on East 57th.)

- Pick up the subway at West 57th and Sixth Avenue.

POINTS OF INTEREST

Diamond District diamonddistrict.org, West 47th Street between Fifth and Sixth Avenues, 212-302-5739

Church of Sweden New York svenskakyrken.se/newyork, 5 E. 48th St., 212-832-8443

Rockefeller Center rockefellercenter.com, Fifth Avenue between West 48th and West 50th Streets, 212-332-6868

Radio City Music Hall radiocity.com, 1260 Sixth Ave., 212-465-6741

Saks Fifth Avenue saksfifthavenue.com, 611 Fifth Ave., 212-753-4000

American Girl Place americangirl.com/retailstore/new-york, 609 Fifth Ave., 877-247-5223

St. Patrick's Cathedral saintpatrickscathedral.org, Fifth Avenue at East 50th Street, 212-753-2261

The Paley Center for Media paleycenter.org, 25 W. 52nd St., 212-621-6600

St. Thomas Episcopal Church saintthomaschurch.org, 1 W. 53rd St., 212-757-7013

Museum of Modern Art moma.org, 11 W. 53rd St., 212-708-9400

St. Peter's Church saintpeters.org, 619 Lexington Ave., 212-935-2200

Central Synagogue centralsynagogue.org, 652 Lexington Ave., 212-838-5122

Sony Wonder Technology Lab sonywondertechlab.com, 550 Madison Ave., 212-833-8100

The Peninsula New York newyork.peninsula.com, 700 Fifth Ave., 212-956-2888

Fifth Avenue Presbyterian Church fapc.org, 7 W. 55th St., 212-247-0490

The St. Regis New York stregisnewyork.com, 2 E. 55th St., 212-753-4500

Trump Tower trumptower.com, 725 Fifth Ave., 212-832-2000

Mikimoto mikimotoamerica.com, 730 Fifth Ave., 212-457-4600

Tiffany & Co. tiffany.com, 727 Fifth Ave., 212-755-8000

Van Cleef & Arpels vancleefarpels.com, 744 Fifth Ave., 212-896-9284

Bergdorf Goodman bergdorfgoodman.com, 754 Fifth Ave., 212-753-7300

route summary

1. Walk east on West 47th Street from Sixth Avenue.
2. Walk left on Fifth Avenue.
3. Stroll left on West 48th Street.
4. Walk right on Rockefeller Plaza (pedestrian area) to the skating rink and 50 Rockefeller Plaza.
5. Go back and to the right on West 49th Street.
6. Walk right on Sixth Avenue.
7. Walk right on West 50th Street.
8. Walk right on Fifth Avenue to East 49th Street, then reverse direction on Fifth.

9.   **Walk left on West 51st Street.**

10.   **Walk right on Sixth Avenue.**

11.   **Walk right on West 52nd Street.**

12.   **Walk left on Fifth Avenue.**

13.   **Go left on West 53rd Street to MoMA, then double back past Fifth Avenue.**

14.   **Walk left on Lexington Avenue.**

15.   **Walk left on East 55th Street.**

16.   **Walk right on Fifth Ave.**

17.   **Walk left on West 57th Street to Sixth Avenue and the subway.**

CONNECTING THE WALKS

Walk two blocks north on Madison Avenue to East 59th Street and then one block west to Fifth Avenue for both Walk 22 (Central Park) and Walk 20 (Fifth Avenue).

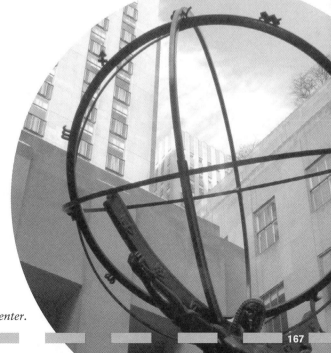

Join Atlas for a memorable day at Rockefeller Center.

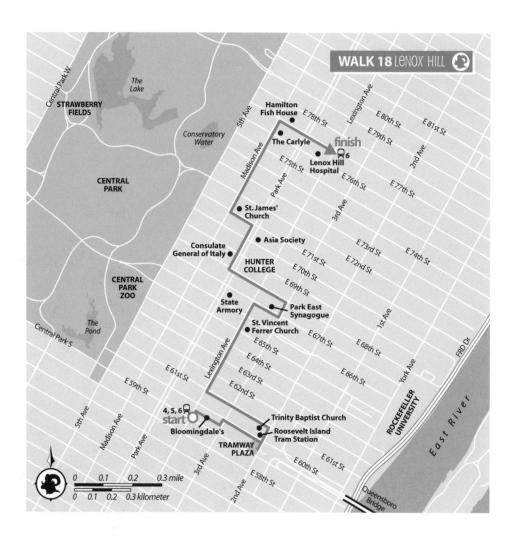

STRAWBERRY
FIELDS

The
Lake

Central Park W

Conservatory
Water

Hamilton
Fish House

E 78th St

Lexington Ave

E 80th St

E 81st St

E 79th St

5th Ave

Madison Ave

The Carlyle

finish

🚇 6

2nd Ave

CENTRAL
PARK

E 75th St

Lenox Hill
Hospital

E 76th St

E 77th St

Park Ave

St. James'
Church

3rd Ave

Consulate
General of Italy

Asia Society

E 73rd St

E 74th St

HUNTER
COLLEGE

E 71st St

E 72nd St

E 70th St

CENTRAL
PARK
ZOO

E 69th St

State
Armory

Park East
Synagogue

1st Ave

Central Park S

The
Pond

St. Vincent
Ferrer Church

E 67th St

E 68th St

E 65th St

Lexington Ave

E 64th St

E 66th St

E 61st St

E 63rd St

York Ave

FDR Dr

5th Ave

E 59th St

Madison Ave

Park Ave

E 62nd St

4, 5, 6

start 🚇

Bloomingdale's

Trinity Baptist Church

Roosevelt Island
Tram Station

ROCKEFELLER
UNIVERSITY

East River

TRAMWAY
PLAZA

E 61st St

3rd Ave

E 60th St

2nd Ave

E 58th St

Queensboro
Bridge

0   0.1   0.2   0.3 mile

0   0.1   0.2   0.3 kilometer

18 LENOX HILL: SWANKY STROLL

BOUNDARIES: **E. 59th St., Madison Ave., E. 77th St., 2nd Ave.**
DISTANCE: **1.7 miles**
SUBWAY: **4, 5, 6, N, Q, R to Lexington Ave./59th St.**

At first blush, one of the more economically intimidating sections of Manhattan would be the Upper East Side, including the section known as Lenox Hill. The neighborhood, which spans the East 60s and 70s from Fifth Avenue to Lexington Avenue, gets its name from the Lenox family, wealthy merchants and landowners who lived here in the early to mid–19th century. It has so many high-end boutiques and stores, especially along Madison Avenue—plus, of course, Bloomingdale's flagship store—that a moneyed aura is undeniable. Add to that the imposing apartment buildings on Park Avenue, and privilege seems a given here.

Lenox Hill is a place for everyone, though. Hunter College, a public institution, educates undergraduate and graduate students of many different backgrounds. Lenox Hill Hospital tends to the health needs of all, and the spiritually inclined have a variety of places to worship. This area is also within walking distance of Central Park and all its joys.

On the Upper East Side, buses run on every avenue except Park. Ever since the Second Avenue el train was discontinued in the 1940s, residents have been pleading for an underground replacement, because Lexington Avenue has the only subway service in the neighborhoods and those 4, 5, and 6 trains are very crowded. Construction on a Second Avenue subway is finally under way, with service expected to commence in 2016 at two stations.

● Exit the subway at or near Bloomingdale's, which occupies the full block between Lexington and Third Avenues, from East 59th to East 60th Street (one subway exit goes directly into the store). Take a good look at the iconic Lexington Avenue side: the name in snazzy Art Deco lettering, the two entrances with the name lit up on marquees, graceful metal grillwork, and a script *B* strategically placed in a few spots. The cornerstone reads "1930." Look up at other decorative touches and the hanging flags. Go inside and take your time strolling the first floor, which is devoted mostly to cosmetics, fragrances, jewelry, and fashion accessories.

- Exit Bloomie's on Third Avenue, noting the alternate rendering of the store name in lowercase letters; this logo dates to the 1970s. Walk left to East 60th Street, and diagonally across the intersection is one of the highest-profile sweets shops in Manhattan, Dylan's Candy Bar. This is the flagship store in a chain owned by Dylan Lauren (Ralph's entrepreneurial daughter), with a colorful and cute logo. It sells not just sweet stuff but clothing, jewelry, even candy-themed iPhone cases. Make a pit stop here, then head east on East 60th. About halfway down the block, at #225, is Serendipity 3, a kitschy restaurant most famous for its Frrrozen Hot Chocolate and the Golden Opulence Sundae, which costs $1,000, includes edible gold leaf as an ingredient, and holds a Guinness record as the world's most expensive dessert. Across the street is All Saints Episcopal Church. This pretty brown church dates to the early 1870s and, with its ribbing on the facade, resembles a chocolate cake.

- At Second Avenue, look across to see the traffic flowing onto the Queensboro Bridge—often called the 59th Street Bridge but officially renamed the Ed Koch Queensboro Bridge, for the late mayor. Simon & Garfunkel made famous reference to it in "The 59th Street Bridge Song (Feelin' Groovy)." Built in 1909, it has great architectural appeal, what with its spiky Gothic towers and vaulted, Guastavino-tile promenade under the Manhattan side (now an enclosed space housing a grocery store and an events venue). On your immediate right is the station for the Roosevelt Island Tram. The plaza has a modernist sculpture and lots of benches, as well as a bit of fenced-in greenery. Now walk left on Second Avenue to East 61st Street.

- Look across to the big, brown brick building at #1166. Constructed in 1927 and moderately Art Deco in style, this is the storage warehouse of Day & Meyer, Murray & Young Corp., a moving and storage company that specializes in artworks and touts a unique Portovault system for them.

- Now make a left onto East 61st. The second building on the left is unique even for Manhattan: an Art Deco church. Trinity Baptist Church, originally the 1929 Swedish Baptist Church, has a sort-of oval window above the decorated main doors, and above that window is a circular filled-in window that resembles a paper-cutting pattern. And the brickwork on the facade comprises at least four shades, graduating from dark to light, as if it were tie-dyed. The doors have exuberant Deco designs. The remainder of the block is largely a collection of attractive, well-maintained town houses.

- Cross Third Avenue, continue to Lexington Avenue, and make a right. For the next few blocks, Lexington is mixed-use, with stores, service businesses, and residential buildings. The redbrick building on the right corner at East 65th Street is the priory of the Church of St. Vincent Ferrer, and its affiliated school is on the street. Next to the priory on Lexington is the church, which has a dramatic main entrance featuring a sculpted crucifixion scene above the doors. This Late Gothic Revival building was finished in 1916. Go inside to see amazing paintings and other religious artwork. Much of the interior is made of limestone.

- Each side of the next block of Lexington is of interest. On the right is a stately 1906 building designed by Charles A. Platt. Across is the 7th Regiment Armory, a.k.a. the Park Avenue Armory, from 1880. Although the main entrance is on Park, there is still much to be seen here of this massive, historical site. A handful of organizations are based here now, some with military ties, others with an arts or educational emphasis.

- At East 67th Street, make a right. The Kennedy Child Study Center (#151) is housed in an elegant old building with sumptuous arched windows. Next to it is the 19th Police Precinct, a four-story Italian-style building with terra-cotta accents. After this is a gas filling station for precinct use (look carefully to find a few small, dark sculptures here), and then the Ladder 16/Engine 39 firehouse, also an elegant edifice; check out the third-floor ornamented balconies. Next door to the fire station is Park East Synagogue, a very busy Moorish Revival extravaganza from the late 1880s. It serves a Modern Orthodox congregation, and I can't think of anyone who refers to it by its official name, Zichron Ephraim. And

Intriguing statue at the Roosevelt Island Tram station

as if this weren't enough for one block, across the street are Russia's and Belarus's missions to the United Nations.

● At Third Avenue, turn left and walk to East 68th, then turn left. On your left is the Park East Day School, a big postwar building that is a bit severe for a school but does feature a remarkable statue in the front courtyard. Continue to the corner of Lexington Avenue and the train station. Look across to see the heart of the Hunter College campus, part of the larger City University of New York (CUNY) system. It was originally a teachers' college and remained a women's school until 1964. On the left is the modernist-style West Building, featuring huge windows, a plaza with seating, and another entrance to the 6 train. On the right is the gem of the campus: the castle-like Thomas Hunter Hall (1912–14).

● Proceed along East 68th, under the bridge that connects the school buildings. On the right is the Kaye Playhouse, and on the left is the Leubsdorf Art Gallery. Next to this is a charming apartment building at #116, the Milan House. It's a 1931 Art Deco confection with lots of carved stone animal figures and faces.

● When you reach Park Avenue, cross to the other side and make a right to see an impressive grouping of neo-Georgian buildings. At #680 is the Americas Society (1912), which has exhibitions; #686 is the Italian Cultural Institute, and #690 the Consulate General of Italy. All three were originally the private homes of well-heeled families. Continue along Park, which is wide and bisected by a landscaped median. Depending on the time of year, these islands have splendid flower beds, as well as changing sculpture installations. Between East 69th and East 70th Streets, take a look on the right at 709–711 Park, two reddish Queen Anne–style homes that were originally part of a larger set, from the mid-1880s. Each building is capped by a dapper black decoration. Note also the Asia Society, a museum and nonprofit organization, at #725.

● Turn left on East 71st Street. On the right, at Madison Avenue, is St. James' Church, an Episcopal congregation. Look for the gorgeous rose window and winged cherubs. Across the avenue is a Ralph Lauren store.

● Make a right on Madison. Next to St. James' parish house is the extravagant neo–French Renaissance #867, flush with statues, small columns, chimneys, dormers, and more. Continue along Madison, past pricey boutiques and fancy houses. At

East 73rd Street is Madison Avenue Presbyterian Church, opened in 1900 but with older roots—and an imposing tower. At East 74th Street is #940, the former United States Mortgage and Trust Company, now a high-end shop. The neoclassical styling and limestone carvings on the facade make it worth a look. And across the street is what used to be the Whitney Museum of American Art. In my opinion, it's an awkward modernist structure, but the exhibits were excellent. (My older daughter and I really enjoyed a psychedelic-art retrospective there in the mid-2000s.) In 2015, the Whitney moved downtown; it's a point of interest on the High Line tour (Walk 13). After East 76th Street is the ultraluxe Carlyle hotel, whose Café Carlyle is known for its jazz and pop performances. The late Bobby Short entertained here for years.

● At East 77th Street, turn right. Pretty #55 is the 1902-built Hamilton Fish House. Fish, a New York statesman, lived here with his family for just a few years, but his name remains linked to the site; the building was also featured in the film *Three Days of the Condor.* Its third-floor windows are especially graceful. At Park Avenue, all four corners feature handsome buildings. On the next block is the Eighth Church of Christ, Scientist, on the left. The redbrick building is somewhat foreboding (few windows on the facade), but they have a suave Art Deco style. Much of this block on the right is taken up by Lenox Hill Hospital, founded in 1857 and one of America's top-ranked medical centers.

● At Lexington Avenue and 77th is a stop for the 6 train.

POINTS OF INTEREST

Bloomingdale's bloomingdales.com, East 59th Street at Lexington Avenue, 212-705-2000

Dylan's Candy Bar dylanscandybar.com, 1011 Third Ave., 646-735-0078

Serendipity 3 serendipity3.com, 225 E. 60th St., 212-838-3531

All Saints Episcopal Church allsaintsnyc.org, 230 E. 60th St., 212-758-0447

Tramway Plaza (Roosevelt Island Tram) East 59th Street at Second Avenue

Trinity Baptist Church tbcny.org, 250 E. 61st St., 212-838-6844

Church of St. Vincent Ferrer csvf.org, 869 Lexington Ave., 212-744-2080

Park East Synagogue parkeastsynagogue.org, 163 E. 67th St., 212-737-6900

Hunter College hunter.cuny.edu, 695 Park Ave., 212-772-4000

Asia Society asiasociety.org, 725 Park Ave., 212-288-6400

St. James' Church stjames.org, 865 Madison Ave., 212-774-4200

Madison Avenue Presbyterian Church mapc.com, 921 Madison Ave., 212-288-8920

The Carlyle rosewoodhotels.com/carlyle, 35 E. 76th St., 212-744-1600

Lenox Hill Hospital lenoxhillhospital.org, 100 E. 77th St., 212-434-2000

route summary

1. See Bloomingdale's on Lexington Avenue, then walk through the first floor to Third Avenue and go left.

2. Walk right on East 60th Street.

3. Walk left on Second Avenue.

4. Walk left on East 61st Street.

5. Walk right on Lexington Avenue.

6. Walk right on East 67th Street.

7. Walk left on Third Avenue.

8. Walk left on East 68th Street.

9. Walk right on Park Avenue.

10. Walk left on East 71st Street.

11. Walk right on Madison Avenue.

12. Walk right on East 77th Street to Lexington Avenue.

CONNECTING THE WALKS

Walk nine blocks north on Lexington Avenue to East 86th Street for Walk 23 (Yorkville).

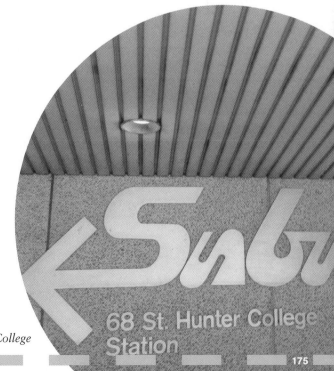

A pop-art subway sign near Hunter College

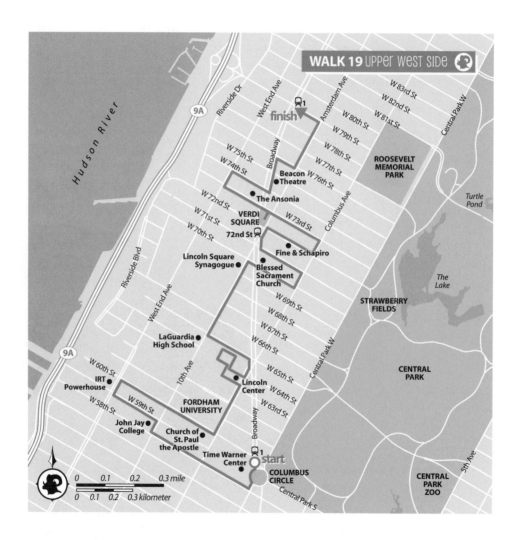

WALK 19 UPPER WEST SIDE

Hudson River

9A

Riverside Dr

West End Ave

finish

Amsterdam Ave

W 83rd St
W 82nd St
W 81st St
W 80th St
W 79th St
W 78th St
W 77th St

Central Park W

ROOSEVELT
MEMORIAL
PARK

W 75th St
W 74th St

Broadway

Beacon
Theatre

W 76th St

Turtle
Pond

The Ansonia

W 72nd St

W 73rd St

Columbus Ave

VERDI
SQUARE

W 71st St

W 70th St

72nd St

Fine & Schapiro

The
Lake

Riverside Blvd

Lincoln Square
Synagogue

Blessed
Sacrament
Church

STRAWBERRY
FIELDS

W 69th St
W 68th St
W 67th St
W 66th St

West End Ave

LaGuardia
High School

Central Park W

CENTRAL
PARK

9A

W 60th St

IRT
Powerhouse

W 65th St

10th Ave

Lincoln
Center

W 64th St

W 63rd St

W 59th St

FORDHAM
UNIVERSITY

W 58th St

John Jay
College

Church of
St. Paul
the Apostle

Broadway

Time Warner
Center

start

COLUMBUS
CIRCLE

Central Park S

CENTRAL
PARK
ZOO

5th Ave

0   0.1   0.2   0.3 mile

0   0.1   0.2   0.3 kilometer

19 Upper West Side: a West Side Story . . . or several

BOUNDARIES: **8th Ave./Central Park W., W. 58th St., West End Ave./11th Ave., W. 79th St.**
DISTANCE: **2.5 miles**
SUBWAY: **A, B, C, D, 1 to Columbus Circle**

The Upper West Side is an exciting part of Manhattan. Home to the Lincoln Center for the Performing Arts, it's also a heavily residential area with many examples of beautiful architecture. Parts of it have been immortalized in pop culture: *Seinfeld, Will & Grace,* and *How I Met Your Mother* are just a few of the TV shows whose characters have lived here or that have featured exterior shots of the neighborhood; it's also been a location in such movies as *You've Got Mail, Heartburn,* and *Die Hard with a Vengeance.*

In the early 1900s, the section in the West 60s had a heavily African American population and was known as San Juan Hill (possibly a reference to black veterans of the Spanish-American War who settled here); later, this area provided the setting for *West Side Story.* Starting in the early 1960s, waves of urban renewal took place throughout the Upper West Side, including the demolition of the tenements of San Juan Hill to build Lincoln Center. Before more-widespread gentrification began in the 1980s, the Upper West Side had been down at the heels for a while, and it's still perceived as slightly edgier than its counterpart across town, the Upper East Side. But prices for genteel older apartment complexes and town houses, as well as newer developments, have helped make this a much tonier address than it used to be.

This walk focuses on the West 60s and 70s, the southern segment of this sizable neighborhood. Lincoln Center, the anchor of this part of Manhattan, is one of America's premier performing-arts complexes (with ballet, classical and jazz music, opera, and more), and a destination in itself. Its architecture and layout, with a central fountain and prized artworks, are iconic. In the summer, you can see outdoor music and dance performances here.

The Upper West Side is also known for its educational facilities—John Jay College, Fordham University, LaGuardia High School of Music & Art and Performing Arts, among others—and its religious institutions (Christian and Jewish in particular), museums and libraries, and proximity to both Central and Riverside Parks. But there are lesser-known gems to discover here, too.

- Start at the Time Warner Center, situated between West 58th and West 60th Streets opposite Central Park. There are several high-end stores here, such as Williams-Sonoma and Swarovski, as well as more-modest ones (Whole Foods and Jamba Juice are in a lower level). A few artworks are placed about the complex. The three venues of Jazz at Lincoln Center are found here, as are CNN Studios. It is a shiny, busy place, but for some of us old-timers, it's bittersweet because we remember the building that used to stand here: the New York Coliseum, a convention and exhibition center (1956–2000).

- Exit the Time Warner Center at Columbus Circle and go right on Eighth Avenue, then make a right onto West 58th Street. You pass residential high-rises, buildings of Mount Sinai Roosevelt Hospital, and assorted stores and businesses.

- At 10th Avenue, notice a modern building on the corner with three arches at the entrance. The engraved stone on the lawn commemorates "James Henry Roosevelt, a true son of New York, the generous founder of this hospital." (He was a distant relative of Theodore Roosevelt and FDR.) Cross the street to see John Jay College of Criminal Justice, part of the CUNY (City University of New York) system. The main building here was built in 1903 as Haaren Hall of DeWitt Clinton High School, which moved north to the Bronx a long time ago. This building—especially its big stone eagle—is by far the campus's most attractive. Proceed right on 10th.

- Make a left at West 59th Street, passing more John Jay buildings. Farther down the block on the right side, at #555, is the Element condo complex, a 35-story glass tower. At 11th Avenue/West End Avenue, look across at the Interborough Rapid Transit (IRT) Powerhouse and its big smokestack. The IRT operated New York City's original subway system; this grand Renaissance Revival building generated its electrical power, and today it produces steam for the city's underground heating and cooling system. From here, you see the West Side Highway and, beyond it, the Hudson River and New Jersey.

- Turn right on West End Avenue, then right again on West 60th. At #248 is the Manhattan Movement and Art Center, in a thought-provoking modern facility. A little farther down to the right is the Gertrude Ederle Recreation Center, a former public bathhouse renovated for modern fitness. Across the street is the Lander College for

Women, part of the Yeshiva University system of schools. Just to the right of Lander is Hudson Honors Middle School and PS 191, with a playground on the 10th Avenue side. Continue across Amsterdam Avenue (Ninth Avenue south of West 59th). On your right is the Professional Children's School, for kids who perform. On the left side of the street is part of Fordham University's Manhattan campus; the main campus is up in the Bronx.

● At Columbus Avenue, make a quick jog around the corner to see the Church of St. Paul the Apostle. This building, on the northern edge of the Hell's Kitchen neighborhood, was dedicated in 1885 and is the mother church for the Paulist Fathers of the US. The most interesting element of this Catholic church is the blue-with-white bas-relief above the main entrance. It also has John La Farge–designed stained-glass windows, which you're welcome to go inside to see.

● Go in the other direction on Columbus Avenue and cross West 60th Street to see more of Fordham University's Lincoln Center campus, which includes the business and law schools. The grassy plaza by the avenue features some statues and sculptures; some are of a religious nature, reflecting the university's Jesuit roots, while others are abstracts.

● When you cross West 62nd, Lincoln Center is to your left. One of the many urban renewal projects led by city planner Robert Moses, it was begun in 1959 and officially opened in 1962, but work continued on various venues through the end of the decade. The first building you pass is the David H. Koch Theater (formerly the New York State Theater), where the New York City Ballet has performed since 1964. From this side it

The Dublin House's quirky bar sign

179

looks austere and forbidding, but the stage door is near the 62nd Street corner, and after performances you'll see dancers and musicians exiting. From the age of 4, I went to ballets here—among the dancers I saw perform were George Balanchine, one of the NYCB's founders; Mikhail Baryshnikov; Edward Villella; Suzanne Farrell; and Jacques d'Amboise. For several years, choreographer Jerome Robbins would sit several seats away from my mom and me, but only to see the first dance of the program. Our lucky Row J seats!

● Walk up to the plaza of Lincoln Center to take in the full scene. No other place in New York City looks quite like this. With your back to Columbus Avenue, the Metropolitan Opera House—probably the complex's most distinctive building, with its huge arches—is straight ahead; Avery Fisher Hall, home of the New York Philharmonic, is to the right. Behind the Koch Theater is Damrosch Park, where outdoor performances, the circus, and crafts fairs are held. On the other side of the opera house are the New York Public Library for the Performing Arts, the Vivian Beaumont Theater, a shallow reflecting pool, and the Illumination Lawn.

● Leave Lincoln Center in front of the plaza, on Columbus Avenue. Look across to Dante Park, a triangle with a Dante statue and a freestanding clock set into an asymmetrical post. Then walk left on Columbus to West 65th and turn left. To your right are more Lincoln Center buildings, such as the Rose Building (home of the School for American Ballet), the Walter Reade Theater (a screening venue for the Film Society of Lincoln Center), The Juilliard School, and Alice Tully Hall (home stage of The Chamber Music Society of Lincoln Center).

● At Amsterdam Avenue, across on your left is Fiorello H. LaGuardia High School of Music & Art and Performing Arts, a public but very prestigious and highly competitive school. Built in the early 1980s, the school has a modern but less severe look than the Martin Luther King Jr. Educational Campus across Amsterdam on your right. This 1970s building was originally just Martin Luther King Jr. High School, but like several other large high schools in New York City, it has been carved up into smaller schools with the goal of improving student achievement. Six schools are now housed in the building, which is transparent on the Amsterdam side, with brown-tinted windows. A lengthy staircase leads up to the plaza area, the most remarkable element of which is a cubic statue of weathered steel displaying quotes from Dr. King.

- Walk to your right on Amsterdam. Pass the local library branch, Riverside, which is big and modern. At the corner is the Engine 40/Ladder 35 firehouse. It has several plaques dedicated to the memory of fallen firefighters, plus a few firefighter figurines. Notice that the crouching figure has a badge that reads "343," to signify the number of firefighters who died on 9/11, and, similarly, the police-officer figure has a "23."

- Just past West 68th Street on your left is a dark gray building with undulating panels, flanked by two other gray sections. This is the Lincoln Square Synagogue, a well-known Modern Orthodox congregation. Right next to it is the West End Synagogue, a Reconstructionist congregation housed in a former public library building (note the book-deposit slot to the left of the main entrance). At West 69th Street on your left, see the Lincoln Square Synagogue's former building, an unusual white sanctuary in the round. At West 70th is Sherman Square, a tiny triangle of a park created by the angled crossing of Amsterdam and Broadway.

- Cross Broadway carefully and walk on West 70th. At #147 is the Blessed Sacrament School, a stately Gothic building accented with religious statuary. And at #135 is The Pythian, a former Knights of Pythias site with flamboyant Egyptian Revival decorative touches; now it's luxury condos. As you walk to the end of the block, admire the variety of town houses and apartment buildings. The Stratford Arms (#117), student housing for the American Musical and Dramatic Academy, has a distinctive entrance with a plumed-cap decoration.

- Turn left on Columbus Avenue. In the 1980s it seemed like Columbus had more curbside seating for eating than any other major street in Manhattan.

- Turn left on West 71st Street. Midblock is the cozy brownstone of Grace & St. Paul's Lutheran Church, built in 1890. Its name reflects the merging of two congregations (one came in from Harlem). Farther down the block on the other side is the Roman Catholic Church of the Blessed Sacrament, a far more lavish edifice in the French Gothic style. The triangle above the main entrance has astonishing detail; the number of finely crafted figures of people is amazing; the rose window is like a fantastical flower. Inside are breathtaking stained-glass windows. On the right at Broadway is the opulent Dorilton, its entrance topped with two darling cherubs who clutch a *D* in a herald. Completed in 1902, these are posh apartments, albeit on a now-noisy corner. *The New York Times* once described the Dorilton's over-the-top Beaux Arts design, replete with quoins, brackets, and terra-cotta frippery, as "the architectural equivalent of a fist fight."

● Cross Broadway halfway and walk right on the center island to the 72nd Street subway station. The first entrance you come to dates to 1904, part of the original subway system. This quaint cottage was deemed too small for current traffic, so a newer entrance to the north was added in 2002. Go into the newer control house; the roof calls to mind some major European train stations.

● Exit the newer building and, with it to your left, cross Amsterdam on West 72nd Street. West 72nd is a wide, two-way street with notable shopping and restaurants. To your right, notice the Art Deco design of the Citibank, with two turretlike outer sections. On the left, Tip Top Shoes has been on the strip, and family-owned, since 1940. The building at #137 looks like a medieval castle in miniature. Fine & Schapiro, a kosher delicatessen at #138, has been serving sandwiches and such since 1927.

● Turn left at Columbus Avenue, then left again on West 73rd Street. This quiet residential block is lined with lovely apartment buildings. The tall, narrow structure at #126 is particularly pretty, white stone with lots of carved detail, and #160 has a figure above the main doors of a seated musician blowing into pipes.

● Cross Amsterdam Avenue and turn left into Verdi Square. This small park features an interesting pseudoplanetary design on the pavement, along with a life-size statue of opera composer Giuseppe Verdi surrounded by four of his famous characters; changing sculpture exhibitions add visual variety. Verdi Square is very pleasant now, but in the 1960s and '70s, it was dubbed "Needle Park" because heroin addicts would congregate here. In 2006, Verdi Square began hosting an annual Festival of the Arts in September. Across West 73rd Street from the park is the august Apple Bank building (1928), which originally housed the Central Savings Bank.

● Continue on West 73rd across Broadway. The magnificent Beaux Arts apartment building on your right is the Ansonia, originally a residential hotel. Finished in 1904, it once upon a time had a lobby fountain with seals! Famous former tenants included Babe Ruth, Isaac Bashevis Singer, Igor Stravinsky, and Enrico Caruso. From 1977 to 1980, the swingers' club Plato's Retreat was located in the basement; before that, it was the Continental Baths, a gay bathhouse that showcased the singing talents of a young Bette Midler. One building in on the left is the sedate Rutgers Presbyterian Church. Walk farther, and to the right see one of the most bizarrely decorated Upper West Side buildings: the Level Club, at #253. Erected in 1927, its facade decked out with myriad Freemasonry symbols, the building hit bad times in the 1960s and became a low-income SRO (single-room occupancy) residence. But in the early 1980s, it was cleaned up and converted to upscale condos.

● Make a right on West End Avenue.

● Turn right on West 74th Street. At #245 are the Alfie Arms apartments; we're not sure what the name's all about, but it adds a light touch to an otherwise dignified residential block. At the corner on the right you can see more of The Ansonia—the street-level windows here are particularly ornate.

● Cross Broadway and walk left to see the Beacon Theatre. Built for movies and vaudeville in 1929, it has become well known in recent decades for concerts and other productions, even the occasional religious revival. For several years, the Allman Brothers Band played multiple concert runs here. I saw the British band UB40 and a few other shows here. The ticket kiosk out front is precious, the lobby gilded and gaudy.

● Continue north on Broadway, then make a right onto West 76th Street. To your right on Amsterdam Avenue are two remarkable buildings at the corners. The modern, glassy site is the Jewish Community Center Manhattan (2001). It offers a wide variety of religious, cultural, educational, and physical-fitness activities and has an exhibition space on the first floor. Across the avenue, in a reddish-brown brick, stucco, and terra-cotta building, is the Riverside Memorial Chapel, a funeral home built in 1925.

● Turn left on Amsterdam Avenue. Much of the block at West 77th Street to your right is occupied by the whimsical, Western-themed Tecumseh Playground; beyond it is PS 87, the William T. (Tecumseh) Sherman School. Across West 79th Street to your left, gaze at The Lucerne Hotel, with its banded entrance columns. Before it was a hotel, it served for a few years as a dormitory for Barnard College, located farther uptown.

● Walk west on West 79th Street, with The Lucerne to your right. Up the block is the Dublin House, around since the 1920s and probably the only bar in NYC to have a neon harp protruding from it. Cross to the center island on Broadway for a view of the upcoming corners: To the left is The Apthorp, an immense and beautiful apartment building that spans a complete block and has an interior courtyard. On the right is the First Baptist Church, a lively jumble of architectural styles dating to 1894.

● The 1 subway stop is at West 79th and Broadway.

POINTS OF INTEREST

Time Warner Center theshopsatcolumbuscircle.com, 10 Columbus Circle, 212-823-6300

John Jay College of Criminal Justice www.jjay.cuny.edu, 899 10th Ave., 212-663-7867

Fordham University–Lincoln Center Campus tinyurl.com/fordhamlincolncenter, West 60th to West 62nd Street between Columbus and Amsterdam Avenues, 212-636-6000

Church of St. Paul the Apostle stpaultheapostle.org, 405 W. 59th St., 212-265-3495

Lincoln Center for the Performing Arts lincolncenter.org, Columbus Avenue between West 62nd and West 65th Streets, 212-875-5456

LaGuardia High School laguardiahs.org, 100 Amsterdam Ave., 212-496-0700

Lincoln Square Synagogue lss.org, 180 Amsterdam Ave., 212-874-6100

West End Synagogue westendsynagogue.org, 190 Amsterdam Ave., 212-579-0777

Church of the Blessed Sacrament 152 W. 71st St., 212-877-3111

The Dorilton 171 W. 71st St.

Fine & Schapiro fineandschapiro.com, 138 W. 72nd St., 212-877-2721

Verdi Square nycgovparks.org/parks/verdi-square, bounded by Broadway, Amsterdam Avenue, West 72nd Street, and West 73rd Street

The Ansonia ansoniarealty.com, 2019 Broadway, 212-877-9800

Beacon Theatre beacontheatre.com, 2124 Broadway, 212-465-6500

Jewish Community Center Manhattan jccmanhattan.org, 334 Amsterdam Ave., 646-505-4444

The Lucerne Hotel thelucernehotel.com, 201 W. 79th St., 212-875-1000

Dublin House dublinhousenyc.com, 225 W. 79th St., 212-874-9528

First Baptist Church firstnyc.org, 265 W. 79th St., 212-724-5600

OF CRIMINAL JUSTICE

route summary

1. From the Time Warner Center, walk right on Eighth Avenue.
2. Walk right on West 58th Street.
3. Stroll right on 10th Avenue.
4. Walk left on West 59th Street.
5. Walk right on 11th Avenue/West End Avenue.
6. Walk right on West 60th Street.
7. Go left on Columbus Avenue.
8. Walk into Lincoln Center, exiting onto Columbus.
9. Walk left on West 65th Street.
10. Stroll right on Amsterdam Avenue.
11. Walk through Sherman Square and across Broadway onto West 70th Street.
12. Walk left on Columbus Avenue.
13. Walk left on West 71st Street.
14. Go right on the median between Broadway and Amsterdam.
15. Walk east on West 72nd Street.
16. Walk left on Columbus.
17. Walk left on West 73rd Street.
18. Walk right on West End Ave.
19. Walk right on West 74th Street.
20. Go left on Broadway.
21. Walk right on West 76th Street.
22. Walk left on Amsterdam.
23. Walk left on West 79th Street; catch the 1 train at Broadway.

connecting the walks

Walk 20 blocks south on Broadway to West 59th Street and Columbus Circle for Walk 21 (Central Park West). (Because Broadway curves eastward, the trip isn't quite as long as it seems.)

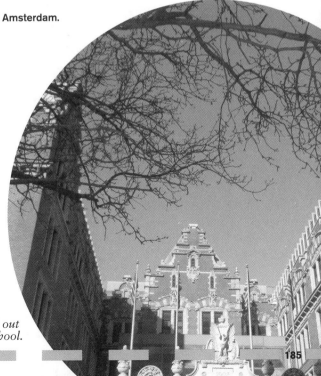

This John Jay College building started out as a high school.

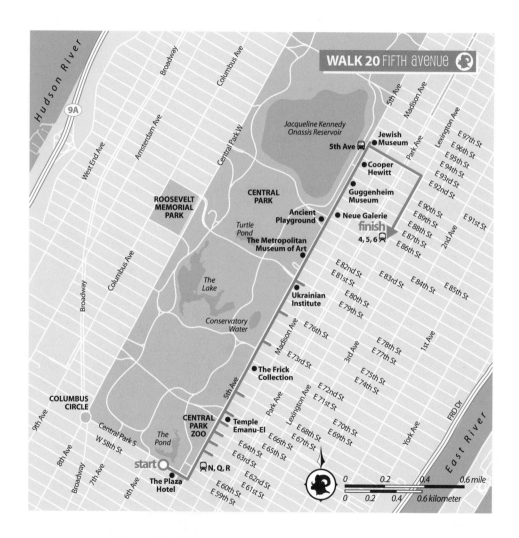

WALK 20 FIFTH AVENUE

Hudson River

9A

Broadway

Columbus Ave

Central Park W

Amsterdam Ave

West End Ave

Jacqueline Kennedy
Onassis Reservoir

5th Ave

Jewish
Museum

Cooper
Hewitt

Guggenheim
Museum

Neue Galerie

finish

4, 5, 6

Park Ave

5th Ave

Madison Ave

Lexington Ave

E 97th St
E 96th St
E 95th St
E 94th St
E 93rd St
E 92nd St

E 90th St
E 89th St
E 88th St
E 87th St
E 86th St

E 91st St

2nd Ave

ROOSEVELT
MEMORIAL
PARK

CENTRAL
PARK

Turtle
Pond

Ancient
Playground

The Metropolitan
Museum of Art

The
Lake

Conservatory
Water

Columbus Ave

Broadway

E 82nd St
E 81st St

E 80th St
E 79th St

Ukrainian
Institute

E 83rd St

E 84th St

E 85th St

Madison Ave

E 76th St

3rd Ave

E 78th St
E 77th St

1st Ave

E 73rd St

The Frick
Collection

Park Ave

Lexington Ave

E 72nd St
E 71st St

E 75th St
E 74th St

COLUMBUS
CIRCLE

9th Ave

Central Park S

W 58th St

The
Pond

CENTRAL
PARK
ZOO

Temple
Emanu-El

E 70th St
E 69th St

E 68th St
E 67th St

E 66th St
E 65th St

E 64th St
E 63rd St

York Ave

FDR Dr

8th Ave

Broadway

7th Ave

6th Ave

start

N, Q, R

The Plaza
Hotel

E 62nd St
E 61st St

E 60th St
E 59th St

East River

0   0.2   0.4   0.6 mile

0   0.2   0.4   0.6 kilometer

20 FIFTH AVENUE: MUSEUM MILE AND THE GOLD COAST

BOUNDARIES: **Central Park S., 5th Ave., E. 92nd St., Madison Ave.**
DISTANCE: **2.5 miles**
SUBWAY: **N, Q, or R to 5th Ave./59th St.**

The Big Apple loves its big parades, and several of these lengthy displays flow along Fifth Avenue, on Central Park's eastern border. Among them are annual parades celebrating St. Patrick's Day (Irish heritage), Greek Independence, Puerto Rican Day, Israel, Steuben Day (German heritage), Columbus Day (Italian heritage), and Pulaski Day (Polish heritage).

But Fifth Avenue is extraordinary for many other reasons. From East 82nd Street to East 110th Street is Museum Mile, an astonishing collection of first-class museums. The Metropolitan Museum of Art is the best known, but the others—such as the Guggenheim, Cooper Hewitt, Jewish Museum, Museum of the City of New York, and El Museo del Barrio—are excellent, too. (One evening a year, usually in June, these museums throw a block party, the Museum Mile Festival.)

Much of this part of Manhattan, just east of Central Park, is known as the Gold Coast, due to the large number of grand, stately town houses and institutional buildings dating to the late 19th and early 20th centuries. Many wealthy New Yorkers put down stakes here, and today their homes continue to be very pricey residences; in recent decades, many of these gorgeous sites have also been repurposed as foreign consulates and nonprofit foundations.

In addition, Fifth Avenue has numerous high-profile houses of worship, including Temple Emanu-El and an assortment of churches. The consulates and foundations on or just off the avenue, with their different flags and crests, complement the ethnic parades. Posh hotels dot Fifth by Central Park, and elegant apartments rise high all along the avenue. And there are features of Central Park, such as monuments and gates, that are best viewed from Fifth.

This walk travels along Fifth Avenue, with short back-and-forth movements onto the side streets.

- Exit the subway and start your walk just west of Fifth Avenue on Central Park South (that is, West 59th Street beside the park). Look over the fence into Central Park to see The Pond, a boot-shaped body of water. Turn around and gaze at The Plaza Hotel, or venture on over for a closer look. It's an iconic building, with its gabled roof and corner turrets. (When I was in college, my senior ball was held here. Ah, memories.) Celebrities and the super-rich have stayed and sashayed here, but even regular folks out for a stroll can waltz in, buy a little something in one of the shops, and use the restrooms. Also take a look at the Grand Army Plaza statues, including the goddess Pomona and a gilded General William Tecumseh Sherman. Across Fifth at East 59th is The Sherry-Netherland, another of Fifth Avenue's famed luxury hotels; the tower above the 24th floor contains apartments.

- Now walk along Fifth Avenue, on the park side. The Strand Bookstore has a kiosk here with a good selection of books. Across the avenue at East 60th Street is The Pierre, yet another dignified hotel, with stone urns arrayed on its facade.

- Cross over at East 62nd Street and notice the Knickerbocker Club at the corner. Walk onto East 62nd for a closer look at "The Knick," as this exclusive men's club is called, as well as a curious building at #5 with a series of ovals punctuating its face. This is the Fifth Avenue Synagogue, and it also features a menorah statue out front. Now focus on #11, an opulent Beaux Arts building originally known as the Edith Fabbri House. Now an Episcopal retreat, it has a pipe organ inside.

- Walk back to Fifth Avenue and make a right. Go right on East 63rd Street. At #11 is the somber Edmond J. Safra Synagogue, built in the early 2000s.

- Return to Fifth Avenue and walk to your right. Cross to the park side at East 64th and check out The Arsenal. This castlelike building from the late 1840s has served as a military facility, a police station, and an early version of the American Museum of Natural History; for many years now, it has been the main offices of the NYC Department of Parks and Recreation. The doorway, with its eagle-and-cannonballs motif, is stirring.

- Stroll back across Fifth on East 64th. The French Renaissance Revival building at #3, originally in the Astor family, is now the Consulate General of India. Check out the round windows near the roofline, called *oculi* because they resemble eyes.

- Walk back to Fifth Avenue, then detour to East 65th to see a few interesting buildings. At #12 is the Pakistani consulate, in a narrow white marble town house; #15 was the Van Alen House, built by a wealthy man who married an Astor, but since 1945 it has housed the Kosciuszko Foundation, which promotes educational and cultural exchange between the US and Poland. (The Classical Revival house was modeled on the childhood home of the late Queen Mother of England.) At #19 is a tall, slim redbrick apartment building with graceful arches on the ground floor and the name MARY LOUISE PLUMBRIDGE inscribed above them.

- Go back to Fifth Avenue, and to the right behold the fantastic Temple Emanu-El, the world's largest synagogue. It has Moorish and Renaissance Revival flair; the entrance and window coverings are so intricate they look like lace. You may be able to go inside and be wowed by the stained-glass windows and other accoutrements. At other times, its museum is open; check the website for hours.

- Turn onto East 66th St. and find #3, which has a plaque dedicated to President Ulysses S. Grant, as well as jazzy Art Deco doors. At #5, you'll find opulent wooden doors and a plaque about the Lotos Club, the posh literary society within. Its illustrious members, past and present, range from Mark Twain and Andrew Carnegie to Stephen Sondheim and Angela Lansbury.

- Back at Fifth Avenue, continue right. At #854 is the Serbian Mission to the United Nations, housed in a building with an oculus-decorated copper roof. At East 67th, cross to the park to examine the World War I memorial—a statue depicting the 107th Infantry, seemingly in action, with several "doughboys" on the move.

- Recross Fifth and turn right on East 68th to see the Indonesian consulate at #5. Originally the John J. Emery House, built by an English-born real estate magnate, it has bay windows and a dentiled roofline.

- Walk back onto Fifth, heading right (north). Between East 70th and East 71st Streets is The Frick Collection, an art museum housed in famous industrialist and philanthropist Henry Frick's mansion. (Pay what you wish on Sundays from 11 a.m. to 1 p.m.; otherwise, it's kind of pricey.) The collection is focused on the Old Masters

(Renaissance through 18th century) and 18th-century French decorative arts. The garden is tranquil, and the gates are fussy-pretty with all their details.

- Across Fifth from the Frick is the Richard Morris Hunt Memorial. Resembling a miniature stage, it has as its centerpiece a bust of Hunt—a leading architect of the late 19th century, among whose achievements are the pedestal of the Statue of Liberty, Biltmore House in North Carolina, and the Metropolitan Museum of Art (which you'll see a bit later). The bust was sculpted by Daniel Chester French, who also created the famous statue of Abraham Lincoln at his Washington, D.C., memorial.

- Cross carefully at East 72nd Street—crosstown traffic is heavy here. Turn right on East 73rd Street to see #11, where the Pulitzers (as in the prize) lived. The mansion was built in 1900–1903 by famed architect Stanford White, who modeled it on the Palazzo Pesaro in Venice. At #22 is the Cameroon Mission to the UN, its pretty balcony bearing the African nation's flag.

- Back on Fifth, continuing north, pass the French consulate at #934, originally the Charles E. Mitchell House. The European Union flag also flies here. (Mitchell was a famous but controversial banker who played a key role in the Stock Market Crash of 1929.) Continue along Fifth, then turn right at East 76th. At #9 is the Lebanese consulate, with a beautiful bay window. Then admire #11½, one of a handful of fractional Manhattan addresses. The white limestone mansion has a charming doorway, its extended entrance flanked by Corinthian columns. Turn around to see #16, red brick with quoins and dormer windows—currently the residence of the Italian consul general, it's the onetime home of designer Calvin Klein.

- Get back onto Fifth and then swing right onto East 77th to see the Mongolian Mission to the UN at #6. Its entrance is flanked by scrolls topped with Doric columns. And at #12 is the mansion that until recently was Brandeis House, an alumni club of Brandeis University; before that, it was the home of Reginald Vanderbilt, great-grandson of Cornelius and father of Gloria. Farther down the block to your left is The Mark, a luxury hotel.

- Walk back to Fifth and go right. At the corner of East 78th Street is the NYU Institute of Fine Arts. Take a brief look at 3 East 78th—the entrance is surrounded by fanciful animal statues. Photo-worthy! Kids will love it.

● Back on Fifth, at #972 is the Cultural Services of the French Embassy, a division of the main embassy in Washington. Designed by Stanford White, this beauty has two dozen (count 'em) pilasters. Make a quick right to see the mansion at 2 East 79th, which is now the Ukrainian Institute of America. Built in 1897–99, this cultural center is French Gothic in style and has oodles of detail at and above the entrance. The center hosts art exhibits, poetry readings, musical performances, kids' programs, and more.

● Walking along Fifth again, you reach a more modern building at #985 that may not fascinate but has a curious sculpture set in its small front garden. (Birdhouses? Abstracts?) Walk farther, and at #991 is the American Irish Historical Society, in a handsome brick-and-limestone Beaux Arts mansion with a bowed facade. The society hosts cultural events and has a library and archives (available by appointment).

● At East 81st Street, cross to the park side and there it is—one of the true cultural treasures of Manhattan: The Metropolitan Museum of Art, as grand as any palace. Walk by it slowly and take in as much of the architectural detail as you can. The main entrance, with all those steps, affords one of the best sites for people-watching around. Enter now or, even better, return another time for a dedicated visit.

● After the museum, carefully cross East 84th Street leading into the park. Next up on the left is the Ancient Playground, one of the coolest play-grounds in the city—even if you don't have kids with you, you have to check this out. Note the pyramid-like climbing structures (an homage to The Met's exhibit on the Temple of Dendur in Egypt), the bronze gates with animals, and much more. I enjoyed this place as a kid, and so have my own girls. Across from

Temple Emanu-El's breathtaking exterior

the park, at 1040 Fifth Avenue, is the apartment building where Jacqueline Kennedy Onassis lived from 1964 until her death in 1994. Next to it, at the corner of Fifth and East 86th Street, is Neue Galerie, a renowned collection of German and Austrian art in a Beaux Arts building.

● Walk two more blocks on Fifth, and you'll come upon one of the more bizarre buildings in Manhattan. Is it a depiction of a tornado? A spinning water-park ride? No, it's the Guggenheim Museum, filled with modern and contemporary art: Impressionist, Cubist, Expressionist, Pop, you name it. The building, controversial when built and polarizing even today, was designed by Frank Lloyd Wright. It's fun to walk inside of, following a ramp along its contours.

● A block up on your right, at 1083 Fifth Ave., find art in a more conventional setting— a turn-of-the-century mansion—at the National Academy Museum. Around the corner on 89th Street is its School of Fine Arts. Next door to the museum on Fifth is The Episcopal Church of the Heavenly Rest, a neo-Gothic–meets–Art Deco building from 1929. The congregation was established in 1865 by a group of Civil War veterans.

● Just inside Central Park at East 90th Street, check out two memorials: Straight ahead on the wall is an understated tribute to John Purroy Mitchel, a former mayor of New York City (see Walk 28 for another Mitchel memorial); to your left, along East Drive, is a bronze statue of Fred Lebow, who founded the New York Road Runners Club and the New York City Marathon.

● On the buildings side of Fifth, from East 90th to East 91st, is the Cooper Hewitt, Smithsonian Design Museum. Its collections, comprising examples of historic and contemporary design (such as jewelry, textiles, tableware, furniture, and wallpaper), reside in Andrew Carnegie's former mansion.

● Cross East 91st and behold on the corner a massive Italian Renaissance–style limestone mansion, the former Otto and Addie Kahn house. It has a grand covered entrance and now composes part of the Convent of the Sacred Heart school. Sufficiently dazzled, cross to the park side of Fifth and consider the memorial to W. T. Stead, a British journalist who perished on the *Titanic.*

● Walk along the park and cross to your right at East 92nd Street. The French chateau-ish building on the northeast corner is the Jewish Museum, originally the Felix M.

Warburg mansion. (Warburg was a German American banker and philanthropist; in 1944, his widow donated the mansion to the Jewish Theological Seminary for use as a museum.) The museum's collections, consisting of historical/religious artifacts and modern/contemporary art, are the largest of any Jewish museum outside of Israel. Much of the interior retains the home's decorative touches.

● Catch a Fifth Avenue bus back to the N/Q/R subway, or walk six blocks south on Fifth Avenue to East 86th Street, then three blocks east to Lexington Avenue for the 4/5/6 train.

POINTS OF INTEREST

The Plaza Hotel theplazany.com, 768 Fifth Ave., 212-759-3000

The Arsenal tinyurl.com/arsenalcentralpark, East 64th Street and Fifth Avenue, 212-408-0100

Kosciuszko Foundation thekf.org, 15 E. 65th St., 212-734-2130

Temple Emanu-El emanuelnyc.org, 1 E. 65th St., 212-744-1400

The Frick Collection frick.org, 1 E. 70th St., 212-288-0700

Ukrainian Institute of America ukrainianinstitute.org, 2 E. 79th St., 212-288-8660

American Irish Historical Society aihs.org, 991 Fifth Ave., 212-288-2263

Metropolitan Museum of Art metmuseum.org, 1000 Fifth Ave., 212-535-7710

Ancient Playground tinyurl.com/ancientplayground, East 84th Street and Fifth Avenue

Neue Galerie New York neuegalerie.org, 1048 Fifth Ave., 212-628-6200

Guggenheim Museum guggenheim.org, 1071 Fifth Ave., 212-423-3500

National Academy Museum nationalacademy.org, 1083 Fifth Ave., 212-369-4880

The Episcopal Church of the Heavenly Rest heavenlyrest.org, 2 East 90th St., 212-289-3400

Cooper Hewitt, Smithsonian Design Museum cooperhewitt.org, 2 E. 91st St., 212-849-8400

Jewish Museum thejewishmuseum.org, 1109 Fifth Ave., 212-423-3200

route summary

1. From the Fifth Avenue station, walk briefly on Central Park South.
2. Turn left on Fifth and head north.
3. Walk in and out of East 62nd Street, then resume going north on Fifth.
4. Walk in and out of East 63rd Street, then backtrack to Fifth and go right.
5. Walk in and out of East 64th Street, then cross Fifth to see The Arsenal at Central Park.
6. Walk in and out of East 65th Street, then resume going north on Fifth.
7. Walk in and out of East 66th Street, then continue on Fifth.
8. Cross East 67th Street to see the WWI memorial at Central Park.
8. Recross Fifth, walk in and out of East 68th Street, and backtrack to Fifth.
9. Walk in and out of East 73rd Street and continue up Fifth.
11. Walk in and out of East 76th Street, then return to Fifth.
12. Walk in and out of East 77th Street, then head north again on Fifth.
13. Walk in and out of East 79th Street, then backtrack to Fifth.
14. Get the bus at Fifth Avenue and 92nd Street, or walk to Lexington Avenue and East 86th for the subway.

CONNECTING THE WALKS

For the next two walks (Central Park West and Central Park), take the bus back to Fifth Avenue and Central Park South; for the following walk, also walk west on Central Park South/59th Street about three long blocks to Columbus Circle. For Walk 23 (Yorkville), walk six blocks south on Fifth Avenue to East 86th Street, then three blocks east to Lexington Avenue.

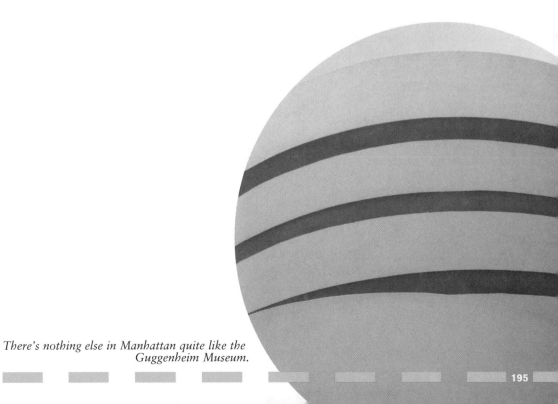

There's nothing else in Manhattan quite like the Guggenheim Museum.

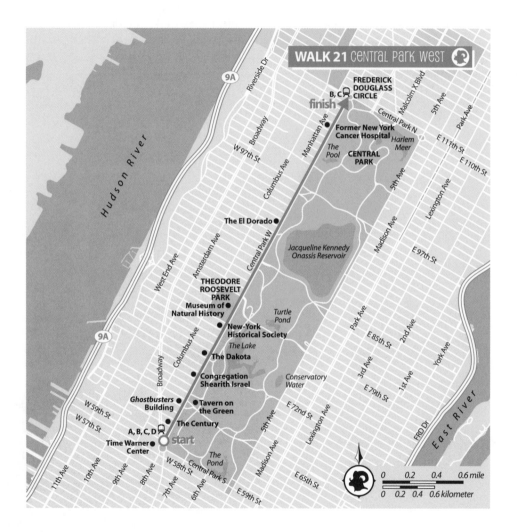

WALK 21 central park west

FREDERICK
DOUGLASS
CIRCLE

B, C

finish

Former New York
Cancer Hospital

The
Pool

CENTRAL
PARK

Harlem
Meer

The El Dorado

Jacqueline Kennedy
Onassis Reservoir

THEODORE
ROOSEVELT
PARK

Museum of
Natural History

Turtle
Pond

New-York
Historical Society

The Lake

The Dakota

Congregation
Shearith Israel

Conservatory
Water

Ghostbusters
Building

Tavern on
the Green

The Century

A, B, C, D

Time Warner
Center

start

The
Pond

Hudson River

Riverside Dr

Broadway

W 97th St

Manhattan Ave

Central Park N

Columbus Ave

Central Park W

West End Ave

Amsterdam Ave

Columbus Ave

Broadway

W 59th St

W 57th St

W 58th St

Central Park S

11th Ave

10th Ave

9th Ave

8th Ave

7th Ave

6th Ave

W 59th St

Malcolm X Blvd

5th Ave

Park Ave

E 111th St

E 110th St

5th Ave

Lexington Ave

Madison Ave

E 97th St

Park Ave

3rd Ave

2nd Ave

1st Ave

York Ave

E 85th St

E 79th St

E 72nd St

E 65th St

E 59th St

Lexington Ave

Madison Ave

5th Ave

FRD Dr

East River

0   0.2   0.4   0.6 mile
0 0.2 0.4 0.6 kilometer

21 CENTRAL PARK WEST:
TAKE A WALK ON THE WEST SIDE

BOUNDARIES: **Central Park W. (8th Ave.) from W. 59th St. to W. 110th St.**
DISTANCE: **2.4 miles**
SUBWAY: **A, B, C, D, or 1 to Columbus Circle**

To walk along Central Park West is to be dazzled by some of the most extraordinary apartment buildings in Manhattan and the United States. Fans, students, and practitioners of architecture will find much to appreciate and study. Among the most celebrated are The Dakota and The San Remo, but there are many other splendid structures. Some occupy a whole block; others are more modest in size. Walking this straight line brings together fine and decorative arts on your left, nature and playtime on your right (the western side of Central Park).

In addition to residences, you'll see the beloved American Museum of Natural History and the New-York Historical Society, impressive churches, and the synagogue of the oldest congregation in the Americas. You will also notice that the start and end of this tour take place at park circles featuring meaningful monuments.

Although this West Side tour bears similarities to the Fifth Avenue walk, which borders the east side of Central Park, it has a very different feel and tempo—mellower and more residential. Let yourself be bowled over by this easy-to-follow route, but be mindful when crossing the roads that travel through Central Park, which are indicated.

● The large Columbus Circle subway station can be confusing, but it was renovated in recent years and has a few distinctive features. One is a circular hole on the upper plaza area, which affords you a view of the tracks below (many people probably use it to find out if they should race downstairs for their train). There are several exits; once at street level, look around at all the high-rise buildings, many of which are of recent vintage. Contrast these with the low-rise delights and greenery of Central Park. Stop in the Time Warner Center, opposite the southwest corner of the park between West 58th and West 60th Streets. It's full of high-end shops and contains

Back Story: New-York Historical Society

For one week in late July 2012, I was part of a group of educators who met at the New-York Historical Society for a workshop on the American Revolution period and the early republic. But we were able to investigate other eras of American history, especially pertaining to New York City history and culture, and were allowed into the Historical Society's restricted research archives and protected vaults, which house the Gilder Lehrman Collection, an astounding assortment of American historical artifacts and documents. Sandra Trenholm, its curator and director, showed us a rare print of the Emancipation Proclamation, General Ulysses S. Grant's razor from his Civil War days, and several rare old books and maps. We also got to see the special temperature-control equipment and fire-prevention materials, high-tech and humbling indeed.

The New-York Historical Society is the oldest museum in NYC, founded in November 1804. Its Central Park West building was constructed during the first decade of the 1900s and underwent a major renovation completed in 2011. Over the years, I've seen several fascinating exhibits here, on topics such as the history of beer in New York City (richer than you might think), the Stork Club, and the Grateful Dead and Deadhead culture. A harsh, haunting exhibit on the history of lynching in the US packed an immense emotional wallop. (One of my high school students who saw the exhibit told me he cried afterward at home.)

Too many people overlook the New-York Historical Society because the American Museum of Natural History across the street is so familiar and famous. But the Historical Society has wonderful exhibits and holdings, of art and artifacts, including lots of Tiffany glass items.

A couple of years ago, my daughters, their friend, and I were approaching the museum when a group of young adults came up to us. They said they had just bought tickets to the Historical Society but were in a rush and couldn't use them—would we like them? Oh yes, we would (and did)! Thank you, nice tourists, wherever you are.

two big, voluptuous statues—*Adam* and *Eve,* if you please—by Fernando Botero. Jazz at Lincoln Center is based here, too.

● Outdoors, go into the minipark in the middle of Columbus Circle, dominated by the dramatic statue of Christopher Columbus. The pedestal has a panel portraying Columbus's landing in the New World and inscriptions in English and Italian. Carefully cross to Central Park—traffic whips around here in various patterns. The golden-topped monument at the park entrance is the USS *Maine* National Monument. Among its historical plaques, the one with depictions of armor is memorable, as is the one with two men flanking a seated buck.

● Start walking with the park on your right. You can use the first crosswalk to go to the elevated silver sculpture of the globe, which bears more than a passing resemblance to the Unisphere in Queens (an enduring symbol of the 1964 World's Fair). The building beside it is now Trump International Hotel and Tower, but old-timers still call it the Gulf and Western Building.

● I recommend staying on the park side of Central Park West for this walk so you can look into the park and also see the apartment buildings opposite it. But at times you may want to cross over for a better look at a building. As you walk along, note the many charming light posts of varying styles. Benches are placed intermittently for your resting pleasure.

● Between West 62nd and 63rd Streets, 25 Central Park W. is The Century, a twin-towered Art Deco apartment building featuring contrasting horizontal bands of tan and brown, plus vertical dark-brown bands. At West 63rd Street, look down the block on the right (north) side to see the weighty YMCA building. The Ethical Culture School and the New York Society for Ethical Culture (offering "non-theistic services in a congregational setting") are side by side on Central Park West. If you look down West 64th, you catch a view of Lincoln Center.

● At 50 Central Park W., The Prasada, a French Second Empire–style apartment building from 1907, has a wonderful four-columned entrance and ornamentation galore. Across the street at West 65th is Holy Trinity Lutheran Church, which has an appealing rose window. Art Deco aficionados and movie buffs will appreciate #55, also known as the *Ghostbusters* Building—look up to the roof for the templelike spires. As you cross West 66th Street, look into Central Park for an outside view of the legendary Tavern on the Green restaurant, which was renovated and reopened in April 2014. Walk a bit more to see #65. This is a more subdued building, but the entrance is attractive and there are eye-catching touches at the upper floors: faces, urns, cherubs, and more. At West 68th is the stately First Church of Christ, Scientist . . . formerly the Second Church of Christ, Scientist. (The First Church's congregation merged with the Second Church's in 2004.)

● Walk two more blocks, and at West 70th is Congregation Shearith Israel, more commonly known as the Spanish and Portuguese Synagogue. This building is about 120 years old, but the congregation is the oldest Jewish prayer group in the Americas, dating to the 1650s, and many ritual items from its earlier sites are inside this synagogue.

● Stroll up two blocks to West 72nd. On the northwest corner is the always-impressive Dakota, New York's first luxury apartment house, dating to the 1880s. The gables, dormers, spandrels, and other delicacies at the roof are worth savoring. John Lennon and Yoko Ono, along with Lauren Bacall, were among The Dakota's best-known residents, and the film thriller *Rosemary's Baby* used exterior shots of the building.

● At 135 Central Park W. is The Langham, a turn-of-the-century apartment building in the French Second Empire style. Look into the park from here to see The Lake. Just across West 74th Street, at #145, is The San Remo, designed by Emery Roth. Its twin towers, topped with cupolas, are an integral part of the Central Park West skyline. Approach The Kenilworth at #151, brimming with Beaux Arts delights, especially the mansard roof and the window details at floors five and nine. Then step over to the corner of West 76th to see the Fourth Universalist Society, whose church building resembles Oxford University buildings. On the next block is one of my favorite museums of all, the New-York Historical Society. The building has stately columns and an exterior statue of Abraham Lincoln. Around the corner on West 77th is the other entrance, which has a statue of Frederick Douglass.

● Some entrances to Central Park have special names: See the Naturalists Gate plaque on the pillar at West 77th St. Nearby is a bust of Alexander von Humboldt, who was a German naturalist.

● Fittingly, just a short walk up Central Park West is the amazing American Museum of Natural History, a temple of science and nature. (My personal favorite is the gems-and-minerals section, but the dinosaurs seem to get top billing.) Even if you don't venture in now, examine the castlelike building. The outside is full of engravings and statues. The Hayden Planetarium/Rose Center for Earth and Space, on the north side of the museum, is more modern and full of light. I dare you to find a schoolkid—or adult—who doesn't enjoy an excursion here. The museum plot along West 81st Street is filled by Theodore Roosevelt Park. Across 81st, at #211, is The Beresford, also designed by Emery Roth. Like The San Remo, it features twin towers, only these are topped with octagonal structures.

● Stroll farther on Central Park West and look at #225, The Alden, another Emery Roth building. The entrance features a pretty stone face, and a bit above it are two angels unfurling a banner. The penthouse is cool, too, so look up. (Roth lived here until his death in 1948.) As you cross West 83rd, look down the block to see a classically adorned synagogue with a three-part entrance, Rodeph Shalom. (The inside is like a theater.) The block between West 84th and West 85th has an apartment building that Art Deco and terra-cotta fans will enjoy, as well as three town houses, harmonious as a trio even though they're different. Each has a charming roof. Across the street at Central Park are the Mariner's Gate and a playground with a nautical theme. Be careful—roads go in and out of the park here and at West 86th. Walk more and admire #262, known as The White House. This a less ornate and more subtle luxury apartment building than many others around here.

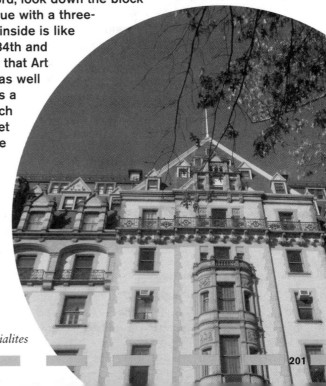

● At West 89th Street, see #285, The St. Urban, which has a regal double

The Dakota, home to celebs and socialites

entrance and attractive vertical lines of highlighted bay windows. On the northwest corner is the private Dwight School. A bit farther up, at #300, is a fine Art Deco building: The El Dorado, yet another Emery Roth creation with twin towers. Note the intricate metalwork panels over the entrance.

● The West 91st–West 92nd block has two stately buildings, the traditional redbrick Brookford and the Art Deco Ardsley, both designed by (you guessed it) Emery Roth. The first three floors of The Ardsley are especially attractive, with pale-colored bands and embellishments. On the next block, #325 is only seven stories but has lovely Renaissance Revival details, including pediments, Ionic columns, and balustrades that frame the four center windows. By West 93rd Street, inside the park is the cute Wild West Playground, and #336 across the street is an Art Deco delight whose fluted buff-stone entrance contrasts with the red brick used elsewhere.

● The building at 350 Central Park W. takes up the whole block: A weighty structure, it has attractive terra-cotta work around the second-floor windows. Cross carefully at West 96th, where a road enters the park, and admire the former First Church of Christ, Scientist, with its steeple and bold columns. (It served another congregation from 2004 to 2014 and is slated to become condominiums.) Within the park is the cheery, round Rudin Family Playground.

● At West 97th Street is one of my favorite unsung apartment buildings: #370, a large Tudor-style structure that wraps around onto the side street. It was designed by the Fred F. French Company, which also created Tudor City in Midtown East (see Walk 12, 42nd Street). I love the rugged main doors and half-timber detailing.

● As you continue north, the whiz-bang apartment buildings disappear for a bit, but there are still various interesting things to see, including the playground in the park at West 100th Street, which has a funky climbing igloo in it. Central Park is more rustic up here, and the languid body of water named The Pool can be seen. Look down and you realize that Central Park West is at a higher elevation here than the park itself.

● At the northwest corner of West 101st is The Central Park View, an apartment building at #415. Its various cast-stone elements contrast handsomely with its red brick. At West 102nd is the lavishly styled #418, The Braender. It mixes French Renaissance, Spanish, and Baroque elements and has a bold main entrance with a courtyard. The wide building at #425 looks quite similar to #415 a few blocks south, and it has a pretty half-sunburst near the roofline (a detail that you see a lot on buildings in the Lower East Side and the East Village). On the northwest corner of West 104th, #444 has lovely Moorish details on the two floors above the main entrance, as well as the penthouse.

● Between West 105th and 106th Streets is something very special. This regal block of castlelike redbrick buildings was originally New York Cancer Hospital, built in the 1880s and now a condo complex known simply as 455 Central Park West. (The hospital moved to the East Side in 1955 and is now Memorial Sloan-Kettering Cancer Center.) The Central Park West side has rounded turrets, gorgeous windows, and an outdoor arcade with arches. On the park side are the Strangers Gate, a steep staircase going up, and rock outcroppings. One of the last classy older apartment buildings along Central Park West, now a hotel, is at #465: Astor on the Park. Its seven prewar floors are, alas, marred by a bland modern addition on top.

● At West 110th Street, you come to Frederick Douglass Circle, a memorial to the great African American writer and speaker completed in 2010. The modern apartment complex on the southwest and northwest corners is bland but interesting for being set at angles to the circle. From here you can catch the B or C trains at the Cathedral Parkway/110th Street station.

POINTS OF INTEREST

Columbus Circle tinyurl.com/columbuscirclenyc, West 59th Street and Central Park West

Time Warner Center theshopsatcolumbuscircle.com, 10 Columbus Circle, 212-823-6300

New York Society for Ethical Culture nysec.org, 2 W. 64th St., 212-874-5210

Holy Trinity Lutheran Church holytrinitynyc.org, 3 W. 65th St., 212-877-6815

Ghostbusters **Building** 55 Central Park W.

Tavern on the Green tavernonthegreen.com, West 67th Street and Central Park West, 212-877-8684

First Church of Christ, Scientist firstchristiansciencechurchnyc.com, 10 W. 68th St., 212-877-6100

Congregation Shearith Israel shearithisrael.org, 2 W. 70th St., 212-873-0300

The Dakota 1 W. 72nd St.

The San Remo 145 Central Park W.

Fourth Universalist Society 4thu.org, 160 Central Park W., 212-595-1658

New-York Historical Society nyhistory.org, 170 Central Park W., 212-873-3400

American Museum of Natural History amnh.org, Central Park West and West 79th Street, 212-769-5100

The Beresford 211 Central Park W.

The El Dorado 300 Central Park W.

455 Central Park West Central Park West between West 105th and 106th Streets

Frederick Douglass Circle tinyurl.com/frederickdouglassmemorial, Central Park West and Central Park North

route summary

1. Begin at Columbus Circle.
2. Walk north along Central Park West.
3. End at the Cathedral Parkway/110th Street station.

CONNECTING THE WALKS

Walk four blocks west on West 110th Street/Cathedral Parkway to Broadway to start Walk 24 (Morningside Heights). Walk six blocks east on West 110th Street/Cathedral Parkway to Lexington Avenue for Walk 25 (Lower Harlem). Or walk six blocks north on Frederick Douglass Boulevard (the continuation of Central Park West) for Walk 26 (Central Harlem).

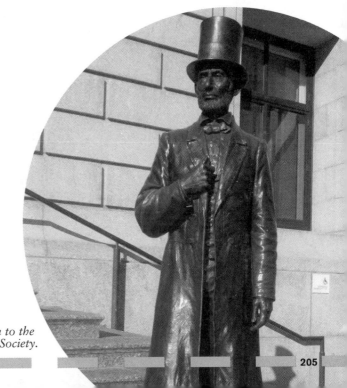

Mr. Lincoln welcomes you to the New-York Historical Society.

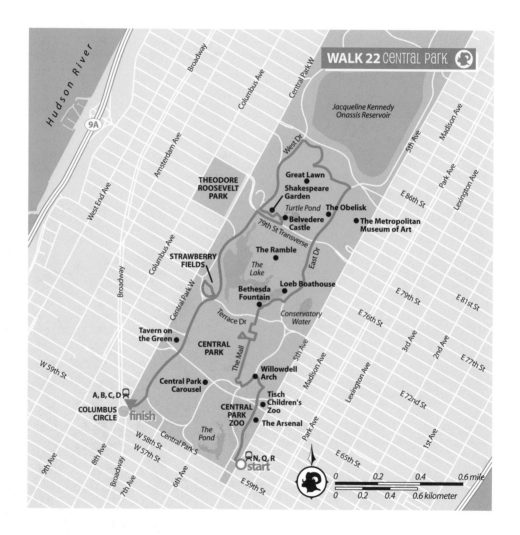

Hudson River

9A

Broadway

Columbus Ave

Central Park W

Jacqueline Kennedy
Onassis Reservoir

5th Ave

Madison Ave

Park Ave

Lexington Ave

Amsterdam Ave

West End Ave

West Dr

E 86th St

THEODORE
ROOSEVELT
PARK

Great Lawn

Shakespeare
Garden

Turtle Pond

The Obelisk

Belvedere
Castle

The Metropolitan
Museum of Art

79th St Transverse

Columbus Ave

The Ramble

East Dr

STRAWBERRY
FIELDS

The
Lake

Loeb Boathouse

E 79th St

E 81st St

Broadway

Central Park W

Bethesda
Fountain

Conservatory
Water

E 76th St

3rd Ave

2nd Ave

E 77th St

Terrace Dr

Tavern on
the Green

CENTRAL
PARK

The Mall

5th Ave

Madison Ave

Lexington Ave

E 72nd St

W 59th St

Central Park
Carousel

Willowdell
Arch

A, B, C, D

COLUMBUS
CIRCLE

finish

CENTRAL
PARK
ZOO

Tisch
Children's
Zoo

The Arsenal

Park Ave

1st Ave

9th Ave

8th Ave

Broadway

7th Ave

6th Ave

W 58th St

W 57th St

Central Park S

The
Pond

N, Q, R

start

E 65th St

E 59th St

0   0.2   0.4   0.6 mile

0   0.2   0.4   0.6 kilometer

22 Central Park: Manhattan's Backyard

BOUNDARIES: **5th Ave., W. 59th St. (Central Park S.), Central Park W., mid-80s in the park**
DISTANCE: **3.9 miles**
SUBWAY: **N/Q/R to 5th Ave./59th St. or F to 57th St.**

Few places in New York City are as enjoyable as Central Park. Fifty-one streets long, three avenues wide, it is the playground for anyone and everyone: wealthy and poor, young and old, native and guest, human and animal and plant. With its simple, direct name and its hearty embrace of nature, it offers so much in the way of activity or plain old rest and relaxation. From the simple joys of strolling and sitting upon wooden benches or craggy rocks to a wide variety of group and individual sports, from highly touted cultural events to historic exploration, from posh eating to casual snacking—Central Park is enormous fun. Birds, fish, small mammals (cute and not so cute) abound, as do trees and plants.

The park is the locus of such annual events as the New York City Marathon, which ends here; it hosts occasional major concerts and other public gatherings; and day in and day out, it houses a zoo, a reservoir, a charming carousel, two outdoor ice-skating rinks, an outdoor pool (open in season), many quaint bridges, and statues and memorials.

No matter what time of year, Central Park is in use. I've seen crowds here on the hottest, sunniest days as well as just hours after a snowstorm. On weekdays, people stop in to eat lunch; on weekends, people engage in all types of sports. Kite flying? Sure. Indulgent birthday parties and picnics? Absolutely.

This tour takes you through about two-thirds of the park, except for the northernmost section.

● **If you arrive at the Fifth Avenue/59th Street station, note the tiled mosaics of animals and other nature on the walls, reflecting a primary theme of Central Park. Out of the station, this intersection forms the southeastern entrance to the park. But before you head in, check out Grand Army Plaza across from the park. Here stands a dramatic golden statue of General William T. Sherman astride his horse. He faces a luxurious fountain with a statue of Pomona, the Roman goddess of fruit trees and gardens.**

Back Story: My Own Private Central Park

I am very partial to Central Park for way too many reasons. In September 1981, I was one of thousands who attended the legendary Simon and Garfunkel concert. In 2007, my old friend Cindy and I went to the Bon Jovi concert, part of the festivities the week New York hosted baseball's All-Star Game. In the final year of the now-discontinued Dr Pepper–sponsored concerts before they moved to Pier 84 on the west side of Midtown, I saw Steven Stills perform. I've gone to a Dave Brubeck show at Rumsey Playfield and Shakespeare plays such as *Julius Caesar* and *The Tempest* at the Delacorte Theater. Then there are the occasional unusual art exhibits that make the park into an open-air gallery, such as Christo's *The Gates* (2005), an installation of more than 7,000 saffron-colored fabric panels.

I also have fond memories of visiting Central Park with students I taught. When I worked at Manhattan Comprehensive Night High School, we took some Sunday trips to the park, ice-skating at both Wollman and Lasker Rinks. And my family has enjoyed many wonderful excursions here, especially because my husband works for the NYC Department of Parks and Recreation and his office is in the historic Arsenal building.

Across the street from her on one side are the famed Plaza Hotel and, on the other, the FAO Schwarz toy store.

- Walk into the park and get on the pedestrian path—you'll see a sign for it. This is Wien Walk, named for philanthropist Lawrence A. Wien. Vendors and street artists/portraitists may be vying for your attention here. (Avoid East Drive, which gets vehicular traffic.) Pass trees with labels identifying them, such as ginkgo. Shortly you'll pass on your left a small brick building with a pretty dome. Next, there is a handy self-service eatery called the Dancing Crane Café, which has restrooms. You also pass a gift shop up on your right, as well as some fanciful animal statues, such as the "dancing goat" (it balances on one hoof). Next on your right is a turreted brick building, The Arsenal. For more than 90 years, the NYC Department of Parks and Recreation has been headquartered here. Built in the 1840s, it originally stored munitions for New York

State; it was also briefly a police precinct in the late 1850s. The fourth floor usually has art or photography exhibits. At the front of The Arsenal, facing Fifth Avenue, are the main entrance and a set of stairs that lead to the street.

- Come back to the walk, and next up is the beloved Central Park Zoo. It's not huge on the level of the Bronx Zoo, but it is entertaining. If you want, pay the admission ($12 adults, $7 kids, $9 seniors) and visit. Watch sea lions and penguins get fed. Rare and beautiful bird species reside here, among them parrots, toucans, and the regal Victoria-crowned pigeon. The snow leopard and the cuddly red pandas are favorites with visitors. (Sadly, Gus the polar bear, who got so much attention for his endless lap swimming, died in 2013.) Look for the large eagle statues and other stone creatures as well.

- Shortly you'll be at the Delacorte Clock, above a passageway with four arches and festooned with animals that play musical instruments. (I particularly like the kangaroo that plays French horn, its baby also tooting a noisemaker.) The best time to be here is on the hour, when the animals rotate in a circle to a harmonious tune.

- Keep walking and you'll pass under one of the many lovely pedestrian bridges, so classic in appeal. To your right is Tisch Children's Zoo, which has a delightful entrance with frolicking animals and kids playing pan pipes. Walk a bit more and you'll see the Billy Johnson Playground, one of 20 playgrounds in the park. This one has a rustic wooden entrance. If you look across the playground, you'll see the back of a statue; that's the 107th Infantry Memorial on Fifth Avenue (you see it better on Walk 20). Also look up on some rocks to see a wood-beamed gazebo. Scale the rock to it if you're so inclined, or just snap a photo.

- At a Y-shaped fork in the path, go left onto Wallach Walk, marked by a drinking fountain and named for Ira D. Wallach, a businessman and philanthropist. Walk farther, and up on a rock you will see a cheery statue of a dog, Balto. His tongue lolls, and you wish you could pitch a stick to him. Continue to your left past Balto, and walk under a redbrick overpass, the Willowdell Arch.

- Make a left onto East Drive, then make a right on the footpath and approach a group of statues. The first is of William Shakespeare, in a contemplative pose. On the ground are many stones engraved with donors' names. Circle to the left of Shakespeare to see Christopher Columbus and his flag.

- Continue around the circle and go left onto the path named The Mall. A floor design with compass points announces The Mall and Literary Walk. The first two writers you will encounter are Sir Walter Scott and Robert Burns. You also pass a statue of an Indian hunting with his dog. As you stroll along The Mall, admire the canopy of trees, the many plants, the people, and the handsome old-fashioned lampposts. Keep walking to see Fitz-Greene Halleck, now obscure but a popular poet and satirist in the 1820s and '30s. There are also marble urns to see, as well as the vaulted Naumburg Bandshell, where concerts are held. A set of stairs leads behind it, and opposite the band shell is a brooding bust of Beethoven; behind him flies a flag for missing-in-action military. Also look for the Victor Herbert bust and the seemingly in-action statue of birds and a goat, *Eagles and Prey*.

- Continue straight on The Mall and arrive at Bethesda Terrace, the open plaza area in front of the Bethesda Fountain. This is one of the grandest and best-known features of Central Park. Take in the two large staircases, the many carved stone effects such as fences, and a sign for Olmsted and Vaux Way (a tribute to the two primary designers of the park). Walk downstairs through the Lower Passage, its exquisite walls and ceiling covered in colored tiles. Then walk toward the fountain, with its wonderful statue of a winged angel. There's lots to see here, so don't rush. Sometimes you'll see temporary art pieces on display (one past installation featured carved-ice versions of statues in the park).

- Go to the end of the walkway to get up close to The Lake. Make a right on the pedestrian path that hugs The Lake; soon you'll see the Loeb Boathouse on your left. Beyond the boathouse is The Ramble, the "wild garden" of Central Park (and we mean "wild" in more ways than one—it's long had a reputation for public trysting).

- Walk to your left along East Drive again, and you'll pass the 79th Street Transverse, one of a few such cut-across roads in the park. Soon you will come across a dramatic statue of man on a horse, swords crossed in the air—this is the 14th-century Polish king Jagiello. Onward along East Drive, you'll see another quaint bridge and then, to your right, the back of The Metropolitan Museum of Art (see Walk 20). To your left stands The Obelisk, an Egyptian relic more than 3,500 years old. It is commonly called Cleopatra's Needle but actually predates her, and it was originally paired with a structure of similar age now located in London. Go up and examine it; plaques offer translations of the hieroglyphics. Glimpse the crab claws at the base. Also note the view of The Met while you're here: quite different from the view along Fifth Avenue.

● Walk farther along East Drive, passing a statue of Alexander Hamilton. About a block up, a pedestrian path meets East Drive at nearly a right angle; turn left and follow it to a huge field with baseball diamonds—the Great Lawn. Maybe you'll catch some sports action, or just think about the large concerts that have been here: rock (Bon Jovi), country (Garth Brooks), classical (the New York Philharmonic), and pop (Diana Ross), to name a few. Walk right on the path between ball fields to see the police precinct for Central Park and then the Arthur Ross Pinetum, a lovely grove of pine trees.

● When you reach West Drive, go left (south). Pass on your left an outdoor theater: the Delacorte, home of the popular Shakespeare in the Park, held each summer. After that, you will see a dainty, more modest structure on your left, the Swedish Cottage Marionette Theatre. To your right in the distance, outside the park, is the American Museum of Natural History (which you see up close on the previous walk). Take the pedestrian path to the Swedish Cottage and then past it, carefully ascending the steps to the Shakespeare Garden, featuring plants mentioned in the works of the Bard. A path behind the garden leads to Belvedere Castle, a fanciful structure located at the highest point in the park. From here you have great views of the Turtle Pond, the Delacorte Theater, and the Great Lawn.

● Retrace your steps to West Drive and turn left. Pass a picturesque waterway, narrow at first, then opening wider. This is another side of The Lake, which you saw earlier. You will also pass the Oak Bridge and the Ladies Pavilion, and shortly on your right is Strawberry Fields. Watch on your left for the back of a standing statue (Daniel Webster), and take the path opposite it (on your right) into Strawberry Fields. Its IMAGINE mosaic is an artistic tribute to John Lennon, who lived just outside the park in the Dakota. On his birthday and on the anniversary of his death, as well as other occasions, people gather here to place flowers and artwork, light candles, play music and sing, and meditate. The benches around here, as in some other spots in Central Park, have dedication plaques, some of which memorialize people who died in the terror attacks of September 11, 2001.

● Walk back to see the statue of Daniel Webster, the esteemed politician and writer of the early 1800s. West Drive merges here with Terrace Drive—stay left to get back onto

West Drive. You'll pass the 7th Regiment Memorial, a monument to the Civil War, then the bust of Italian statesman Giuseppe Mazzini on your right and the peaceful Sheep Meadow to your left. Soon after, the ever-popular eatery Tavern on the Green will be on your right. The path just north of it is John V. Lindsay Drive, named for the mayor of New York City from 1966 to 1973. A path to your left leads to the carousel ($3 per ride), housed in a circus-y brick building. It's definitely worth a detour if you love riding carousels: The horses are big and beautiful, and the music is happy and upbeat.

● From West Drive as you approach the southern end of the park, a few different paths will take you to the park's southwest entrance, at Columbus Circle. From there you can get the A, B, C, D, or 1 train.

POINTS OF INTEREST

Central Park centralparknyc.org, bounded by Fifth Avenue, Central Park South/West 59th Street, Central Park West, and Central Park North/West 110th Street, 212-310-6600

Central Park Zoo centralparkzoo.com, West 64th Street and Fifth Avenue, 212-439-6500

Tavern on the Green tavernonthegreen.com, West 67th Street and Central Park West, 212-877-8684

ROUTE SUMMARY

1. Exit the subway and explore the Grand Army Plaza just south of Central Park.

2. Enter Central Park at the southeast entrance (Fifth Avenue and West 59th Street) and get on Wien Walk, which is to the right of the wider East Drive.

3. After the zoo, go left onto Wallach Walk.

4. Past the Willowdell Arch, make a left on East Drive.

5. Take the path on the right for access to The Mall.

6. Go to your right around The Lake.

7. Walk north on East Drive.

8. Go left and cross the Great Lawn.

9. Turn left (south) on West Drive.

10. Follow the path to and from Strawberry Fields.

11. Follow one of the footpaths off West Drive to Columbus Circle (Central Park West and West 59th Street).

CONNECTING THE WALKS

Walks 19 and 21 (Upper West Side and Central Park West) begin where this one ends.

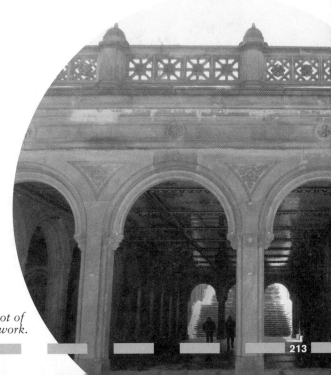

The Lower Passage to Bethesda Terrace is a riot of arches and gorgeous tilework.

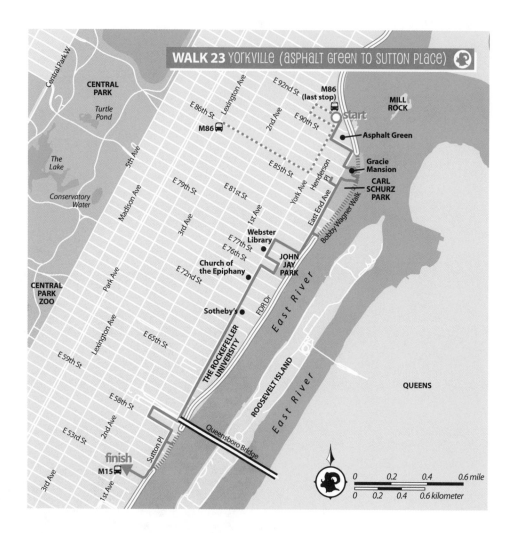

WALK 23 Yorkville (Asphalt Green to Sutton Place)

CENTRAL PARK

Turtle Pond

The Lake

Conservatory Water

CENTRAL PARK ZOO

Central Park W

Central Park W

5th Ave

Madison Ave

Park Ave

Lexington Ave

3rd Ave

2nd Ave

E 92nd St

E 90th St

E 86th St

E 85th St

E 81st St

E 79th St

E 77th St

E 76th St

E 72nd St

E 65th St

E 59th St

E 58th St

E 53rd St

Lexington Ave

2nd Ave

1st Ave

York Ave

Henderson Pl

East End Ave

Bobby Wagner Walk

M86 (last stop)

M86

start

Asphalt Green

Gracie Mansion

CARL SCHURZ PARK

MILL ROCK

Webster Library

Church of the Epiphany

JOHN JAY PARK

Sotheby's

FDR Dr.

THE ROCKEFELLER UNIVERSITY

East River

East River

ROOSEVELT ISLAND

QUEENS

Queensboro Bridge

finish

M15

Sutton Pl

1st Ave

2nd Ave

3rd Ave

0   0.2   0.4   0.6 mile

0   0.2   0.4   0.6 kilometer

23 YORKVILLE (ASPHALT GREEN TO SUTTON PLACE): A TREK INTO THE FAR EAST SIDE

BOUNDARIES: **E. 90th St., 1st Ave., E. 53rd St., East End Ave.**
DISTANCE: **3.3 miles**
SUBWAY: **4, 5, 6 to 86th St., then M86 bus to York Ave.**

Tourists, not to mention many New Yorkers, don't usually trek beyond First Avenue on the Upper East Side, especially because subway service is already three avenues away and most of the city's major attractions are elsewhere. But Yorkville is where you find Gracie Mansion, home to many New York City mayors, as well as the quiet and expansive Carl Schurz Park. John Jay Park, a bit farther south, has a wonderful swimming pool and is bordered by the magnificent apartments of Cherokee Place, a street many New Yorkers have never heard of. (They may even think you made this up!) This area also encompasses the moneyed residences of Sutton Place, as well as the think tank known as The Rockefeller University. And walking this far east affords you some prime views of the East River. Especially if the weather is pleasant, this can be a very enjoyable jaunt. Try to do the walk on a Wednesday, when you can take an inside tour of Gracie Mansion.

● On East 86th Street, take the eastbound M86 bus to East 91st Street and York Avenue. Walk back to York and make a right, then a left on East 90th Street. Past the sports field is an arched building. This used to be the municipal plant that made asphalt for city roads. In 1968 it ceased operations; other parts of the complex were torn down, but this peculiarly shaped container site was renovated into a city-run recreation center, Asphalt Green, which opened in 1984. Notice the street signs along York between East 90th and East 91st Streets, for George & Annette Murphy Square. (Dr. George Murphy, a professor at Cornell Medical College, led the group responsible for creating Asphalt Green.)

● At the end of East 90th Street, cross onto the sidewalk that skirts the FDR Drive; here, 90th Street bends right to become East End Avenue. Soon you will come upon Carl Schurz Park, named for the first German-born American elected to the US Senate. (This area was once Manhattan's neighborhood of choice for German immigrants.) Look out to the highway to see an overpass engraved with EAST RIVER DRIVE, the alternate name for the FDR Drive. At East 89th Street, take the stairs up into the park, then follow the paved path over the highway to the promenade along the East River, Bobby Wagner Walk. It offers a wonderful view: You can look across to Queens and north to the Robert F. Kennedy Bridge (originally the Triborough Bridge, which is what most people still call it). Randalls and Wards Islands are beneath the bridge; the channel between them was landfilled in the early 1960s, so they're really one island now. The arched bridge you see is the Hell Gate Bridge; from certain angles, you can see part of the South Bronx, too. To your left in Manhattan is the 90th Street Ferry Terminal.

- Take the footpath back across the highway and proceed to the large, fenced butter-yellow house with white-and-green trim. This is Gracie Mansion, the official residence of New York mayors since 1942 (although Michael Bloomberg lived in his own Upper East Side home during his term). Dating to the 1790s, the mansion is on the former site of a military fort. It's open occasionally for tours (see website for details) and for invitation-only events hosted by the mayor.

- Walk down to East End Avenue by following the footpath. Turn left and walk on East End to East 86th Street; to your right, notice the old redbrick town houses, some with oriels and mansard roofs; they're part of the Henderson Place Historic District (see below).

- Cross East End Avenue at East 86th and walk to the small street on your right, Henderson Place. Its 24 Queen Anne houses, built in 1883 "for persons of moderate means," make up a landmarked historic district. Terra-cotta trim, gables, and turrets give the homes a storybook feel. The sidewalk sports period-style street lamps.

- Go back to East End Avenue and turn right, passing Carl Schurz Park's playground across the street. Just before East 84th is The Chapin School, a private girls' school established in 1901. Stay on the right on East End in this somewhat sedate residential area. Pass East 82nd Street, here called Gracie Terrace.

- Make a left on East 81st Street and cross the pedestrian bridge over the FDR Drive, or, if you don't like heights, just look out from the end of East 81st. Here you have an excellent view of the western side of Roosevelt Island.

● Return to East End, turning left and following it to its end, at the pretty, pre-WWI apartment building at 542 E. 79th Street. To the left is an entrance to the FDR Drive. Head away from the river on East 79th, going slightly uphill. Notice buildings on the left side of the block in a similar style as #542.

● Turn left on York Avenue, which is a mix of commercial and residential structures. East 78th Street is the educational hub of this area, with PS 158 to your left and the New York Public Library's Webster branch on the right. The library, an Andrew Carnegie–funded facility that opened in 1906, is one of the oldest public libraries in the city and was built in the Renaissance Revival style. The school (1898) has neoclassical details; the arched triple-door entrance is quite stylish, as is a decorated round window near the roof.

● Turn left at East 77th Street. On the right is a white-brick building, such as was popular in the 1950s and 1960s, with a spartan modernist look. Farther down on the left is a stately old apartment complex with balconied windows—the Cherokee, built in 1912 as the East River Homes. Its four interconnected buildings were developed as "model tenements" for working-class families with at least one member suffering from tuberculosis. They were renamed in the 1980s and are now lovely co-op homes. Cherokee Place extends one block in each direction from East 77th (only the block to the left takes car traffic). The vast public space in front of it is John Jay Park, named for the revered New York statesman and first Supreme Court chief justice. This park started out as a public bathhouse in the early 1900s; the spacious playground, sports courts, and pools (two!) were built in the early 1940s. Even though it has a relaxed, neighborly vibe, you can hear highway traffic from the FDR Drive, just below.

Carl Schurz Park offers prime city views.

- Turn right and walk along Cherokee Place's pedestrian plaza, which features welded steel sculptures by Douglas Abdell. Cherokee Place ends at East 76th Street. Just to the left is the private, coed Town School, more than 100 years old. Turn right on East 76th.

- Turn left on York Avenue and walk to East 74th, where Church of the Epiphany is located on the right. The Norman Gothic–style building was completed in 1939, but the congregation has been around since the 1830s. Note the spiky weathervane atop the tower. Continue along York, and past East 72nd Street on your left is the head-quarters of Sotheby's, one of the world's largest auction houses, in a modern glass-and-steel structure. You can stop inside the gallery to peruse the pricey offerings.

- Proceed to East 70th to see NewYork-Presbyterian Weill Cornell Medical Center—a mostly gray, institutional collection of buildings, although the Harkness Building has a grouping of Gothic-inspired arches with a set-back entrance. New York Hospital was founded in 1771, making it the second-oldest hospital in the US.

- Continue along to East 68th Street, a true brain trust of science and medicine: On the right is Memorial Sloan-Kettering Cancer Center, and on the left is The Rockefeller University. Sloan-Kettering, as it's usually abbreviated, began in 1884 as the New York Cancer Hospital (see Walk 21 for the original building). Rockefeller is a graduate and postgraduate center for biomedical research, and its list of Nobel Prize winners, both teachers and alumni, is impressive. Founder's Hall is at the center of the cam-pus, but the buildings are set back, with extensive gardens in front. The newer build-ings are at the southern end of the campus, near East 64th Street. (When I was in high school, I went with a few classmates to a chemistry lecture at Rockefeller, and we were so baffled by the level of discourse that we left after a while, embarrassed.)

- Farther down York Avenue, at East 61st Street, is Twenty-Four Sycamores Park, a cheery playground in the shadow of the Queensboro Bridge. York Avenue gets steeper here. Cross East 59th Street carefully—it often seems to bottleneck here.

- Turn right at East 59th for a minor detour. From the right side of the street, you see the gradual ascent of the bridge. The Manhattan approach to the bridge, in fact, is supported on a series of Guastavino-tile vaults, which form the cathedral-like ceiling of the supermarket and event space located there.

- Turn left on First Avenue, then left again at East 58th Street. This block is a mix of big apartment buildings and walk-ups. York Avenue is known as Sutton Place here, and East 58th morphs into Sutton Square when you cross it. The namesake is Effingham B. Sutton, a real estate developer. Turn right on Sutton Place to head south. The buildings here, which shelter socialites and other notables, radiate money and privilege.

- Turn left at East 57th Street. This tiny spur has comfortable seating that affords views of the East River.

- Walk back to Sutton Place and continue left. At East 54th Street, Sutton Place narrows, and you come to a pretty sliver of a park. Here the street is more properly called Sutton Place South, and it dead-ends at East 53rd Street.

- Go right on East 53rd to First Avenue for an uptown bus, Second Avenue for a downtown bus, or Lexington Avenue for the E, M, or 6 train.

POINTS OF INTEREST

Asphalt Green asphaltgreen.org, 555 E. 90th St., 212-369-8890

Carl Schurz Park carlschurzparknyc.org, East End Avenue between East 90th and East 84th Streets, 212-459-4455

Gracie Mansion tinyurl.com/graciemansion, East End Avenue and East 88th Street, 212-570-4751

Webster Library nypl.org/locations/webster, 1465 York Ave., 212-288-5049

The Cherokee cherokee-nyc.com, East 77th to East 78th Street east of York Avenue

John Jay Park nycgovparks.org/parks/john-jay-park-and-pool, East 76th Street near FDR Drive, 212-794-6566

Church of the Epiphany epiphanynyc.org, 1393 York Ave., 212-737-2720

Sotheby's sothebys.com, 1334 York Ave., 212-606-7000

NewYork-Presbyterian Weill Cornell Medical Center nyp.org/facilities/weillcornell.html, York Avenue between East 70th and East 68th Streets, 212-746-5454

The Rockefeller University rockefeller.edu, 1230 York Ave., 212-327-8000

route summary

1. At the end of East 90th Street, take the FDR Drive sidewalk south (East 90th becomes East End Avenue).

2. Go into Carl Schurz Park at East 89th Street.

3. Cross over the FDR Drive to Bobby Wagner Walk, then return to the park.

4. Turn left on East End Avenue.

5. Cross on East 86th Street to Henderson Place, on your right.

6. Double back to East End Avenue.

7. If you wish, go across the East 81st Street pedestrian bridge and back on your way to the south end of East End Avenue.

8. Turn right on East 79th Street.

9. Turn left on York Avenue.

10. Turn left on East 77th Street.

11. Go right onto the pedestrian side of Cherokee Place.

12. Turn right on East 76th Street.

13. Turn left on York Avenue.

14. Turn right on East 59th Street.

15. Turn left on First Avenue.

16. Turn left on East 58th Street.

17. Turn right on Sutton Place, dipping in and out of East 57th Street on the left.

18. Turn right on East 53rd Street for public transit.

CONNECTING THE WALKS

Walk north six blocks to East 59th Street, then six avenues west to Fifth Avenue for Walk 22 (Central Park) or Walk 20 (Fifth Avenue).

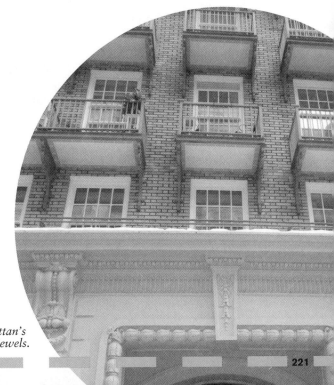

The Cherokee is one of Manhattan's unheralded residential jewels.

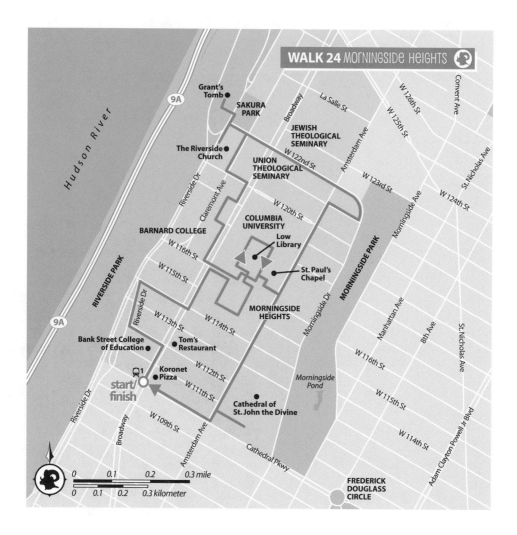

WALK 24 Morningside Heights

Hudson River

Grant's Tomb

SAKURA PARK

9A

Broadway

La Salle St

W 126th St

Convent Ave

JEWISH THEOLOGICAL SEMINARY

W 125th St

The Riverside Church

W 122nd St

Amsterdam Ave

W 123rd St

St. Nicholas Ave

UNION THEOLOGICAL SEMINARY

Riverside Dr

Claremont Ave

W 120th St

W 124th St

COLUMBIA UNIVERSITY

BARNARD COLLEGE

Low Library

MORNINGSIDE PARK

Morningside Ave

W 116th St

W 115th St

St. Paul's Chapel

RIVERSIDE PARK

MORNINGSIDE HEIGHTS

Morningside Dr

Manhattan Ave

8th Ave

St. Nicholas Ave

Riverside Dr

W 113th St

W 114th St

9A

W 116th St

Bank Street College of Education

Tom's Restaurant

W 112th St

Morningside Pond

W 115th St

Adam Clayton Powell Jr Blvd

1

Koronet Pizza

start/ finish

W 111th St

Cathedral of St. John the Divine

W 114th St

Riverside Dr

Broadway

W 109th St

Amsterdam Ave

Cathedral Pkwy

0   0.1   0.2   0.3 mile

0   0.1   0.2   0.3 kilometer

FREDERICK DOUGLASS CIRCLE

BOUNDARIES: **W. 110th St., Riverside Dr., W. 122nd St., Morningside Dr.**
DISTANCE: **2.8 miles**
SUBWAY: **1 to Cathedral Pkwy./110th St.**

Manhattan is full of glamorous and wonderful sights, but few neighborhoods can boast as many beautiful buildings mixed with historical and natural treasures as does Morningside Heights. It's home to the extraordinarily handsome campus of Columbia University, part of the venerated Ivy League and founded in 1754 as King's College. Barnard College— Columbia's undergraduate women's division, and my alma mater—is part of the Seven Sisters association of highly competitive all-female colleges.

Morningside Heights is also home to two of Manhattan's most significant churches: Riverside Church and the Cathedral of St. John the Divine. There are also a number of smaller gems not to be overlooked here, as well as the lovely Riverside Park. This area saw action during the American Revolution and over the years has continued to play host to intellectual and spiritual events of many types.

● **Exit from the 1 train at Cathedral Parkway and walk north on Broadway. College students enjoy filling up at Koronet Pizza, known for its gigantic slices ("slabs," some dub them). Look across Broadway and scrutinize a large faded ad on the redbrick building on West 111th Street; it appears to be for First National City Bank. Walk to the northeast corner of West 112th and possibly stop in for a meal or snack at Tom's Restaurant. Yes, it's the Tom's that was featured on** *Seinfeld* **and celebrated in Suzanne Vega's song "Tom's Diner." As an undergrad at Barnard College, I sometimes ordered omelets or grilled-cheese sandwiches here; many laud the French fries. See another very faded ad on the off-white brick building midblock on the other side of Broadway—that one's a mystery.**

● **Turn left and head west on West 112th. Within the Bank Street College of Education on your left are a highly thought-of graduate school, a progressive-minded primary school for kids in nursery school through eighth grade, a research division, and a publishing unit. As an undergraduate, I worked part-time in Bank Street's**

Back Story: Movie Madness

One day early in my sophomore year at Barnard College, a friend burst into my dorm suite and announced that a movie was being filmed "across the street," on the Columbia campus. She said she'd seen Dan Aykroyd and others shooting a scene. I dropped whatever it was I was doing, grabbed my camera, and ran over.
I watched along with an eager crowd as the actors went through their paces at a school building close to Broadway. Even with my decent SLR camera, my shots weren't the best, but in a few I could make out the actors' faces. The main thing was that it was an exciting interlude in a mundane day, witnessing A-listers making a film—*Ghostbusters*—at our home.

Columbia, and to a lesser extent Barnard and the surrounding schools, can be seen in several movies and TV shows, plus a few music videos. The 2013 indie flick *Kill Your Darlings* recounted Allen Ginsberg's days at Columbia in the 1940s; *The Nanny Diaries* also filmed scenes here.

Why Columbia? Sometimes the story is rooted in the school, but it's also the picturesque, classic look of the place that draws filmmakers. No other Manhattan college campus is as visually arresting.

after-school program and found the environment very welcoming. If you go inside this pleasant-looking, fairly modern building, you'll find an unusual sight on the first floor: A tree from the lower floor spreads its branches above and through a circular bench and fence. Once outside again, look at the plaque beside the main entrance, dedicated to Margaret Wise Brown, who wrote classic children's books such, as *Goodnight Moon* and *The Runaway Bunny.* She also worked at the Bank Street School when she began writing her renowned books. It should be noted that this school derives its name from its original location, on Bank Street in Greenwich Village. (My mother took classes at that site.)

● Continue west and skirt the edge of lengthy Riverside Park. The statue of Samuel J. Tilden at Riverside Drive, sculpted by William Ordway Partridge, is a solemn depiction of the former New York governor and presidential hopeful.

- Turn right on Riverside. At West 113th Street is a dramatic statue commemorating Hungarian president Louis Kossuth. It consists of three male figures and a flag.

- Riverside Drive is known for its sumptuous apartment buildings, and a particularly impressive specimen is #410. Pass through the arches and walk to the entrance; take a photo of the elaborate ironwork and stained glass.

- Make a right at West 114th and approach St. Hilda's & St. Hugh's, an Episcopal school for students through grade eight. The school's colorful crest is worth a glance, and the foundation stone of the building contains a relic from St. Hilda's Abbey in Yorkshire, England. This street is a bit steep, so pause and gaze at the apartment buildings on your right. The pretty fire escapes are set back and framed by arches; also admire the stone friezes about the windows. Revere Hall, at #622, has lovely terra-cotta detail; it was once home to movie mogul Cecil B. DeMille, as well as Barack Obama when he was a Columbia undergrad. Close to Broadway, a building entrance displays wistful, childlike faces.

- Turn left on Broadway, with Broadway Presbyterian Church at the corner. This Gothic church has sweeping windows above the entrance, as well as charming lamps and other decoration. The whole block on the other side is occupied by Alfred Lerner Hall, one of the newer buildings at Columbia University. It opened in 1999 as a replacement for Ferris Booth Hall, the quirky old student center that was considerably smaller; it has a sophisticated, if a bit foreboding, look. Lerner is home to the campus bookstore, the Roone Arledge Auditorium and Cinema, and the university's radio station, WKCR-FM, well known for its jazz programming (Phil Schaap's weekday *Bird Flight* showcases the music of Charlie Parker) as well as classical music of many eras, Indian ragas, bluegrass . . . and, on Saturdays, broadcasts of Columbia football games.

- Continue north on Broadway and turn right at West 116th for the legendary College Walk of Columbia University. Admire the neoclassical statues that flank the gates. College Walk, Columbia's older buildings, and the lawns were designed in the 1890s by noted architects McKim, Mead & White in the Beaux Arts style, adding up to a gracious, manicured layout. The eastward view is neatly balanced. The journalism school is based in the first building on your right, with a statue of a pensive Thomas Jefferson. Go right on the path next to it and pass Furnald Hall—a dormitory (my senior-year home) with a dark but comfy central hall that is the site of various student events such as dances and a cappella concerts—and then the main entrance of Lerner Hall. This side of Lerner is much more inviting: A glass wall reveals walkways and banners of student organizations. Coupled with the reflections from Furnald and the journalism buildings, this is a colorful, energetic scene.

- Turn left and gaze upon Butler Library. Named for a past university president, Nicholas Murray Butler, this is a hive of activity, study, and at times unfortunate napping. "The Stacks" are voluminous. The night before the organic-chemistry final, the marching band roams the campus, playing loud and obnoxious tunes and tromping through Butler. Find the plaque dedicated to the US Naval Reserve Midshipmen's School, from the 1940s. The lawn just in front of the library used to play host to a large Henry Moore sculpture (students would attempt to throw balls and Frisbees through a space in it), but that, alas, is gone. When he was a student here, future Yankee legend Lou Gehrig would play baseball on the lawns.

- Turn left, back toward College Walk, and you will see the Sundial, a pretty piece that is sometimes overlooked because students and neighborhood tykes sprawl all over it. (Note the bronze details of cherubs and such.) On the other side of the walk, ascend "The Steps," a prime meeting spot for the whole neighborhood. The plaza area is dotted with impressive fountains, lampposts, and decorative urns. Class photos, dance performances, fairs, filming—you name it, it takes place here. Halfway up the steps to Low Memorial Library, one of the main symbols of Columbia, is the beloved statue *Alma Mater,* designed by Daniel Chester French. People love to pose with her, and her scepter has been pilfered a few times.

- To the left of Low when facing it, you encounter Dodge Hall/Miller Theatre (closest to College Walk), Lewisohn Hall, and graceful Earl Hall (1900–02), one of the oldest campus buildings. A variety of activities take place here, including religious services, club meetings, and volunteer opportunities. Walk north, past Earl, and you'll see the Mathematics Building and fierce lion statues (Columbia's sports teams are the Lions); now make a right and stroll past Havemeyer, Uris, and Schermerhorn Halls. Make another right in this quadrant to see Avery Hall. Flanking Low Library on this side is St. Paul's Chapel—inside and out, one of the campus's masterpieces. It was built in 1904 to designs by I. N. Phelps Stokes, and it features vivid stained-glass windows designed by John La Farge. If you have time and the chapel is open, roam respectfully and be bowled over by the details. The basement has the Postcrypt, which has held acoustic music and spoken-word performances over the years (as an undergrad and even afterward, I frequented it and liked its cozy feel). Outside, don't miss the copy of Rodin's *The Thinker,* surrounded by trees.

● An overpass crosses above Amsterdam Avenue—walk it (it has a modest incline), and on the other side you will see some graduate-school buildings, such as International Affairs and the Law School (both modern buildings quite different from most on campus), the Italian Academy, and some statues, including *Three Way Piece: Points,* a Henry Moore creation we all called "The Tooth." (Well, it *does* resemble a molar.) These are part of Revson Plaza, a green oasis mounted above the roadway.

● Walk back to St. Paul's and down the steps to College Walk. Walk west across Broadway (College Walk becomes West 116th Street). Make a right and walk about a block to the main entrance of Barnard College, and turn left into the campus. My alma mater has a beautiful iron gate, and Barnard Hall has the same scholarly air as the main school buildings throughout the Columbia campus. But the feel of this all-women's campus is somewhat different, though it has changed in the last 20 years or so with the addition of another dormitory and a larger student center, among other things. (While Barnard students take classes at Columbia and vice versa, the two schools are independent institutions, with separate admissions, faculties, and endowments. Barnard women receive degrees signed by the presidents of both schools.)

● Walk to your right and follow the path north. You will see a bench with sayings by artist Jenny Holzer, along with the Barnard Greek Games statue. On your left is boxy Lehman Hall, with its library, and on the right is the orange-red Diana Center, finished in 2010. Much more compact than Columbia, the Barnard campus is an amusing mix of architectural styles. When you reach Milbank Hall, a neoclassical building, you'll most likely need to walk back to the school's main entrance to exit the campus. The exit will leave you on the west side of Broadway—turn left and walk to West 120th Street to cross Broadway. Across the street on your left will be Columbia's Teachers College, and Horace Mann Hall is that pretty redbrick building at the corner.

● Turn left on West 120th Street and marvel at Union Theological Seminary. Founded in 1836, this Gothic-style complex is stirring and full of detail. Look heavenward.

Then, at Claremont Avenue, make a right and see the spectacular Riverside Church. Don't be embarrassed to say "Wow!" as you study it up close and all around. It is marvelous.

- Slowly walk to your right on Claremont and absorb the glory of this interdenominational church. The windows are amazing. Depending on the time of year, the garden is very colorful. The *Madonna and Child* statue by Sir Jacob Epstein is touching.

- Make a left on West 122nd and look up (if you haven't been craning your neck too much already) to glimpse one of my favorite parts of The Riverside Church: the statue of the bugle-blowing angel that crowns the dome.

- Turn left onto Riverside Drive to see more of the church's statues, carvings, and decorative touches. The entrance is based on Chartres Cathedral in France. Take the time to go inside and marvel at all the stained-glass windows, the precision stonework, various pieces of art, and more. The Riverside Church is the tallest church in the United States and was designed by Allen, Pelton and Collens. The primary benefactor of this treasure was John D. Rockefeller Jr.

- When you finally pull yourself away from The Riverside Church, visit tranquil Sakura Park, across West 122nd Street. See the statue of Civil War general Daniel Butterfield, the pretty pavilion, and the Japanese stone lantern (*tori*), and look over the stone fence for a good view of upper Manhattan. Stately International House and a stone eagle above the entrance are at the northern part of the park.

- Out of the park, you can't help but see Grant's Tomb across Riverside Drive. Stroll around and take in the full measure of this national memorial. The eagle, columns, archway, and especially the dome are a secular, Classical complement to The Riverside Church. Note the two female figures that flank the sign reading LET US HAVE PEACE. You will notice on the paths and near benches a series of quirky and colorful tiled mosaics and figures. They don't quite mesh with the pomp of the tomb, but they have their own charm. If the tomb is open, get a good look at the interior. People like to Rollerblade around the tomb, children whiz by on scooters, small film crews occasionally walk around with their cameras and cables, and tour buses park across the street and the passengers come to ooh and aah.

- Walk along the tomb plaza, and on the lawn just across from Riverside Church are three plaques that commemorate the Battle of Harlem Heights, fallen soldiers of the Korean War, and a World War II chaplain. There is also a rock that had a plaque removed—I wonder what it recorded.

- Head east on West 122nd Street, this section of which is rightly dubbed Seminary Row. To your left you will see the Manhattan School of Music, followed by the Jewish Theological Seminary (JTS). With its entrance on the corner of Broadway and its center section constructed like a tower, JTS is the educational home of Conservative Judaism in the United States, granting undergraduate and graduate degrees and ordaining rabbis and cantors. The interior court is spacious and airy.

- Across the street on West 122nd are some handsome apartment buildings, such as Castle Court, which has artistic lampposts, and the Sarasota farther down the block. At #500 is Reldnas Hall (I suspect its namesake was actually Sandler). Cross Amsterdam Avenue and you will see one of the more unusually constructed public schools in New York: PS 36, which seems to rise from a rock formation.

- Continue to the end of West 122nd and onto Morningside Drive to see an atypical apartment building that curves with the road at #114. The Circle is considered a sought-after address (at least according to real estate websites).

- Peer down into Morningside Park on your left. It has peaceful sitting areas and steep staircases. Years ago, this was a dangerous park, and in the 1960s Columbia wanted to take it over and build a gym on the site. The community fought back, and

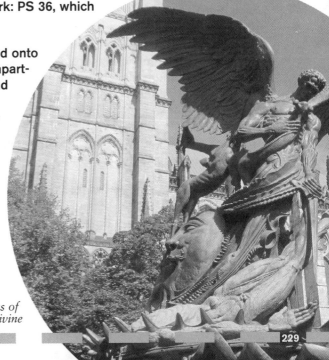

The Peace Fountain, centerpiece of the gardens of the Cathedral of St. John the Divine

since then it's been cleaned up and renovated, its statues delighting people and its playgrounds heavily used.

- Turn right on West 121st Street. Make a left on Amsterdam Avenue to get another view of Teachers College (to the right). As you stroll, you will also pass Plimpton Hall, a Barnard dorm; cheery restaurants; and, at West 118th, a stone house and a community garden. Continue walking south and pass the bland buildings comprising Mount Sinai St. Luke's Hospital.

- At the junction of Amsterdam Avenue and West 112th Street is another amazing religious site: the Cathedral of St. John the Divine. This still-unfinished house of worship may not bowl you over as much as the sky-high Riverside Church, but the front exterior is dizzying with detail. Windows, arches, statues (some of which are painted in pale colors), door panels, and more add to the overwhelming feeling of entering a living piece of art. Work on this Episcopal cathedral began in the 1890s, and something always seems to be getting added or renovated here. The interior seems endless, with paths, chapels, displays of artwork, relics, photos, and stained-glass windows. On a sunny day, light streams through the windows in celestial fashion. Among the many impressive items you'll find inside are a national AIDS memorial, the gorgeous baptismal font, a menorah, a replica of the Declaration of Independence wrought in metal, a 9/11 memorial statue, and a choirboys' memorial. You should also poke around in the gardens on the south side of the building. The Children's Sculpture Garden is fantastical, with bronze pieces designed by students as well as an allegorical sculpture in the center called the Peace Fountain, depicting the triumph of good over evil. And if you're lucky, you might see the famous peacocks that strut about the grounds. Be kind to them.

- When you exit the garden, walk across Amsterdam Avenue and contemplate ordering a treat at The Hungarian Pastry Shop. Even if you don't, admire the art on the outside walls. A couple of doors down, tempt yourself with the offerings at V&T Pizzeria. I recommend the vegetarian lasagna.

- Make a right at West 110th (here co-named Cathedral Parkway, as in St. John the Divine), catching a look at the red-gold oval sign on #501, which refers to George

Gershwin's days here. There are lovely apartment buildings all along this street, some with gargoyles. As you approach Broadway, see Congregation Ramath Orah, an Orthodox synagogue, on your left. Neo-Georgian in style, it was built as a church, so it's another example of the "flipped" religious properties that can be found throughout the city.

● The subway entrance is at Broadway.

POINTS OF INTEREST

Koronet Pizza koronetpizzany.com, 2828 Broadway, 212-222-1566

Tom's Restaurant tomsrestaurant.net, 2880 Broadway, 212-864-6137

Bank Street College of Education bankstreet.edu, 610 W. 112th St., 212-875-4400

Riverside Park riversideparknyc.org, Riverside Drive between West 72nd Street and St. Clair Place, 212-870-3070

Broadway Presbyterian Church bpcnyc.org, 601 W. 114th St., 212-864-6100

Columbia University columbia.edu, West 116th Street and Broadway, 212-854-1754

Barnard College barnard.edu, 3009 Broadway, 212-854-2033

Union Theological Seminary utsnyc.edu, 3041 Broadway, 212-662-7100

The Riverside Church theriversidechurchny.org, 490 Riverside Drive, 212-870-6700

Sakura Park nycgovparks.org/parks/sakura-park, Riverside Drive and West 122nd Street

Grant's Tomb nps.gov/gegr, West 122nd Street and Riverside Drive, 212-666-1640

Jewish Theological Seminary jtsa.edu, 3080 Broadway, 212-678-8000

Morningside Park nycgovparks.org/parks/morningside-park, Manhattan Avenue/ Morningside Avenue between West 110th and West 123rd Streets

Cathedral of St. John the Divine stjohndivine.org, 1047 Amsterdam Ave., 212-316-7540

The Hungarian Pastry Shop 1030 Amsterdam Ave., 212-866-4230

V&T Pizzeria vtpizzeriarestaurant.com, 1024 Amsterdam Ave., 212-666-8051

Congregation Ramath Orah ramathorah.org, 550 W. 110th St., 212-222-2470

route summary

1. From the Cathedral Parkway station, walk north on Broadway.
2. Turn left on West 112th Street.
3. Walk right on Riverside Dr.
4. Turn right on West 114th Street.
5. Turn left on Broadway.
6. Enter the Columbia University campus at West 116th Street, and make a circuit of the campus.
7. Exit back at Broadway, cross over, and tour the Barnard College campus.
8. Leave the campus at Broadway and go left.
9. Make a left on West 120th Street, then a right on Claremont Avenue.
10. Go around Riverside Church on West 122nd Street and Riverside Drive.
11. Go into Sakura Park across West 122nd Street.
12. Visit Grant's Tomb across Riverside Drive.
13. Walk east on West 122nd Street, which turns into Morningside Drive.
14. Make a right on West 121st Street.
15. Make a left at Amsterdam Avenue.
16. Make a right on West 110th Street and walk back to the starting point on Broadway.

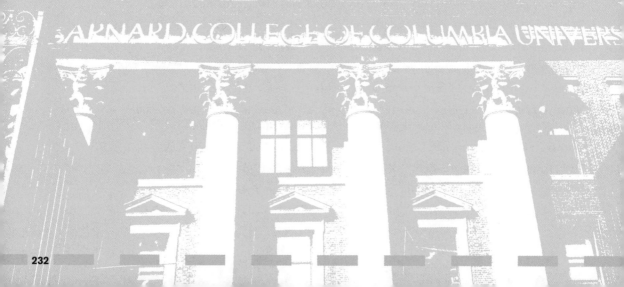

CONNECTING THE WALKS

Walk 10 blocks east to Lexington Avenue to start the next walk (Lower Harlem), or walk four blocks east to Frederick Douglass Boulevard and then six blocks north to West 116th Street for Walk 26 (Central Harlem).

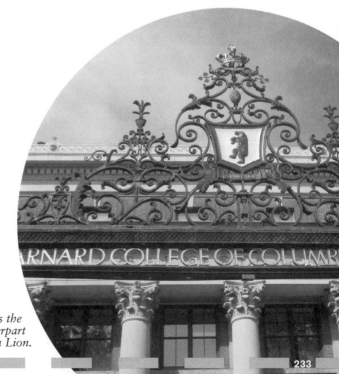

Barnard College's main entrance features the Barnard Bear, my alma mater's counterpart to the Columbia Lion.

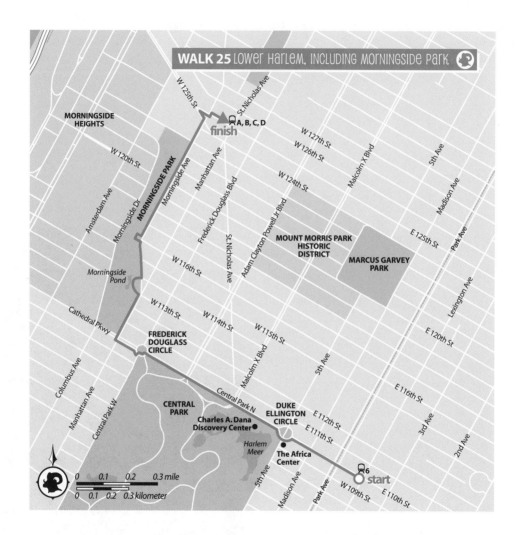

WALK 25 Lower Harlem, including Morningside Park

MORNINGSIDE HEIGHTS

W 125th St

St. Nicholas Ave

A, B, C, D
finish

W 127th St

W 126th St

W 124th St

Malcolm X Blvd

5th Ave

Madison Ave

W 120th St

Morningside Ave

Manhattan Ave

Frederick Douglass Blvd

St. Nicholas Ave

Adam Clayton Powell Jr. Blvd

MOUNT MORRIS PARK HISTORIC DISTRICT

MARCUS GARVEY PARK

E 125th St

Park Ave

Amsterdam Ave

Morningside Dr

MORNINGSIDE PARK

W 116th St

Morningside Pond

W 113th St

W 114th St

W 115th St

E 120th St

Lexington Ave

Cathedral Pkwy

FREDERICK DOUGLASS CIRCLE

Malcolm X Blvd

5th Ave

E 116th St

Columbus Ave

Manhattan Ave

Central Park W

Central Park N

CENTRAL PARK

Charles A. Dana Discovery Center

DUKE ELLINGTON CIRCLE

E 112th St

E 111th St

3rd Ave

2nd Ave

Harlem Meer

The Africa Center

5th Ave

Madison Ave

Park Ave

6
start

W 109th St

E 110th St

0   0.1   0.2   0.3 mile
0   0.1   0.2   0.3 kilometer

25 Lower Harlem, including Morningside Park

BOUNDARIES: **E. 110th St., Lexington Ave., W. 125th St., St. Nicholas Ave.**
DISTANCE: **1.5 miles**
SUBWAY: **6 train to 110th St.**

One of my favorite American poets, Langston Hughes, wrote, "I was in love with Harlem long before I got there, and I am still in love with it." Indeed, there is much to love—to see, to hear, to admire—in this epicenter of the African American experience.

Through the years, Harlem has been in the spotlight for many reasons—some positive (the Harlem Renaissance, ethnic arts and culture, beautiful architecture), others less so (poverty, crime, blight). Happily, the neighborhood has seen a huge resurgence over the past two decades.

The area most people consider Harlem (originally *Haarlem*, as rendered in Dutch) covers a large swath of northern Manhattan. This tour combines the 110th Street corridor and Morningside Park, a narrow strip of land that is one of the best-improved public parks in Manhattan.

● **One Hundred Tenth Street spans the island, from the FDR Drive on the east to Riverside Park on the west and, unlike the 50 streets immediately south of it, is not cut into by Central Park. It's named Central Park North where it borders the park from Fifth to Eighth Avenue (which is known as Central Park West or Frederick Douglass Boulevard this far uptown) and has the secondary name Cathedral Parkway to the west of that. The 6 train takes you to the stretch of East 110th that is co-named Tito Puente Way, for the beloved salsa musician whose signature song was "Oye Como Va." The honor is a nod to the immediate neighborhood, East Harlem, which is often referred to as Spanish Harlem.**

● **Look down East 110th for the elevated train tracks one block away (above Park Avenue), and walk toward them. These are the tracks for Metro North, the commuter railroad to Westchester County and upstate; they run underground from Grand Central Terminal to the 97th Street portal, then aboveground through East Harlem and the Bronx. On the left, at 120 E. 110th St., is the Clinton Community Center, which resembles an elementary school. Cross Park Avenue, which has three arched passageways** underneath the railroad tracks, two pedestrian and one vehicular. In cold weather, these pathways often accumulate icicles that resemble stalactites.

- To your left on the other side are the Lehman Village Houses, public housing named for Herbert Lehman, who served New York as both a governor and senator. (Lehman College in the Bronx is also named for him.) On the right corner, at Madison Avenue, is a community garden run by the 110th Street Block Association. Lexington, Park, and Madison Avenues look quite different here than they do farther south—but everything is relative, and these blocks are considerably nicer and safer than they were in the 1970s and '80s.

- Approaching Fifth Avenue, you come to Duke Ellington Circle, which celebrates the renowned jazz bandleader and composer. ("Take the A Train," "Satin Doll," and "Mood Indigo" are his most famous songs; I adore them.) To your left is a beige stone building with irregular windows and grillwork: The Africa Center. This museum and cultural center, the newest addition to Museum Mile—the collection of museums along Fifth Avenue that includes the Metropolitan Museum of Art and the Guggenheim—is still a work in progress, though it officially opened in September 2014 (check the website for the latest information). Signs indicate that this is also Frawley Circle, the street's name before it was rechristened for Ellington. Cross the circle carefully and walk up the steps. Way up on pillars is a statue of "Sir Duke" and his piano, with narrative plaques.

- Cross Fifth Avenue, which bisects the circle; the steps on each half-circle resemble seating for an auditorium. On your left is the northeast corner of Central Park. The Harlem Meer is the bucolic body of water you see, bordered by pathways and greenery. Originally a swamp, it was designed to be an attractive lake (*meer* is Dutch for "lake") and is an extension of the original Central Park.

- One Hundred Tenth Street is now Central Park North; it's also now West 110th Street, since you crossed Fifth Avenue. Central Park South, Central Park West, and Fifth Avenue (Central Park East, as it were) have long been fashionable addresses, and more and more these days, Central Park North homes are becoming desirable as well. Two Latino churches sit just off Fifth on your right, and at #31–33 Central Park N. is the Lincoln Correctional Facility. Don't worry about its mission—security is supertight, so have a closer look. There is a crest in the pediment above the entrance; try to make out the faded Jewish star in the center. This building was originally the Young Men's–Young Women's Hebrew Association of Harlem, a Jewish community organization. It later became housing for returning WWII veterans, and then a private school. On the park side is an entry path to the Charles A. Dana Discovery Center, a whimsical cottage where cultural and educational activities take place throughout the year.

● Continue to Malcolm X Boulevard, a.k.a. Lenox Avenue (Sixth Avenue south of Central Park), a wide street with a concrete median. To the left you have another nice view of the Harlem Meer, beyond which are the Lasker Rink and Pool. On the right, a few buildings over, is Second Canaan Baptist Church. Pass the entrance to the 110th Street subway station, served by the 2 and 3 trains, followed by 111 Central Park North, a sleek modern building with a loopy metal sculpture out front. This block has some lovely town houses in a variety of styles on the right, with the serene park on the left. Farther along to the right, at #137, is The Semiramis, an elegant apartment building with a distinctive bowed stone-and-brick facade; in the crest over the entrance is "1901," the year it was completed.

● The next avenue, which is Seventh below Central Park, is Adam Clayton Powell Jr. Boulevard. Powell was a minister, a member of the House of Representatives for this Harlem district, and the father of Adam Clayton Powell IV, also a politician. Like Lenox, this avenue is bisected by a concrete divider with trees and grass. Pass additional attractive and well-maintained apartment buildings on your right.

● Central Park North then curves into a traffic circle named for Frederick Douglass (as is the boulevard extending north from it). It's a counterpart to Duke Ellington Circle back at

The steep, picturesque northern edge of Central Park

the northeast end of the park; both circles correspond to Columbus Circle and Grand Army Plaza at the southwest and southeast ends of the park.

- Walk into Frederick Douglass Circle. Foremost is the statue of the esteemed abolitionist and writer. There are marble benches shaped like jigsaw puzzle pieces, along with trees and a stone wall with an eye-catching design. The 110th Street subway station for the B and C trains is nearby. Towers on the Park is a modern, handsome high-rise apartment complex on the circle. Continue along a short block of West 110th Street to Manhattan Avenue and the southeastern corner of Morningside Park. This avenue runs from West 100th to West 124th Street.

- Morningside Park today is an understated gem among New York City's parks, but for many years it had a bad reputation. When I was a student at nearby Barnard College in the 1980s, we were warned not to wander inside, although our rugby team played there often. The times I ventured in, the only fear I had was of slipping on broken or icy steps (the western side is steep). Years later, I've walked in the park, eaten lunch while sitting on a bench, watched people play soccer, seen children dart about in the playground, admired birds at the waterfall and arboretum. Peer into the park from the top of the stairs at the corner of Manhattan Avenue and West 110th (signed Cathedral Parkway here). In warm weather, it's lush and green; if there's snow, it looks quite rustic. A colorful playground is to your left. Looking west, you can see the back of the Cathedral of St. John the Divine and, to the right of it, buildings of Columbia University.

- Walk on Manhattan Avenue alongside the park, noting the apartment buildings across on the right. At West 112th stands a redbrick Beaux Arts row house with white trim and pretty dormers, including one that resembles a keyhole. From the plaza outside the park, descend the stairs. The athletic fields are located here, in one of the flatter parts of the park. Look across to the rough-hewn stone wall; you can make out a window or two—it's a bit mysterious. Follow the path to the right along the fields, and soon you'll see the kidney-shaped section of Morningside Pond. There is another segment of the pond just past it, along with the waterfall. Birds like to linger at this wonderful feature of the park. A winsome statue of a big bear peering down on a faun stands at the Seligman Fountain.

● Use the nearest exit from the park and go right on Morningside Avenue. At the triangle called Lafayette Square, you see where Morningside begins, splitting off from Manhattan Avenue to the north and west. Here is a robust statue of the Marquis de Lafayette and George Washington, shaking hands and clasping flags. Just across West 114th from the statue is a lovely brownstone (actually orange-red stone) apartment building called the Monterey, at #351. It was built around 1890.

● Walk back into the park to admire the Dr. Thomas Kiel Arboretum, to your right, and the Carl Schurz monument, to the left. Return to the east side of the park and exit onto Morningside Avenue, which is wider here than farther south. Go left. West 116th St. is also wider than most of the streets in the area because it has crosstown (two-way) traffic. Continue on Morningside, which affords you a good view of both the park and more attractive apartment buildings across the street on the right.

● Just past West 119th Street on the right is PS/IS 180, Hugo Newman College Preparatory School. Named for a career teacher and administrator, the school has a brightly painted mural and is set back from the sidewalk, with a playground out front. Continue your stroll, past more stylish apartments on your right and the verdant expanse of the park on your left. At West 121st is the ultramodern Church of the Master, a Presbyterian house of worship with huge windows.

● To the left, down West 123rd (the northern border of Morningside Park), is Columbia Secondary School for Math, Science, & Engineering. On the next block of Morningside Avenue to the right is the simple redbrick St. Luke's Baptist Church. Past West 124th Street, where a diagonal road called Hancock Place cuts through, is a tiny park, Roosevelt Triangle, with a bronze abstract sculpture called *Harlem Hybrid.* On the left corner across West 125th Street, see the Church of St. Joseph of the Holy Family, the oldest existing church in Manhattan above 44th Street. This Romanesque Revival redbrick church has been altered and enlarged since it was built in 1860. Go inside to admire the interior details.

● After you've visited the church, cross Morningside Avenue and walk east on West 125th Street. Pass the Manhattanville post office on your left and La Gree Baptist Church, in a grand turn-of-the-century former theater, on your right. (In 1806, the village of Manhattanville was established on this part of the island; Manhattanville continues to be used to name this part of Harlem.)

- At St. Nicholas Avenue, you can pick up the A, B, C, or D train.

POINTS OF INTEREST

Duke Ellington Circle tinyurl.com/dukeellingtoncircle, East 110th Street and Fifth Avenue

The Africa Center theafricacenter.org, 1 Museum Mile (1280 Fifth Ave.); check website for latest information

Charles A. Dana Discovery Center tinyurl.com/danadiscoverycenter, Central Park North between Fifth and Lenox Avenues, 212-860-1370

Frederick Douglass Circle tinyurl.com/frederickdouglassmemorial, Central Park West and Central Park North

Morningside Park nycgovparks.org/parks/morningside-park, Manhattan Avenue/Morningside Avenue between West 110th and West 123rd Streets

Church of the Master pcusa.org/congregations/5643, 81 Morningside Ave., 212-666-8200

Church of St. Joseph of the Holy Family stjosephoftheholyfamily.org, 405 W. 125th St., 212-662-9125

ROUTE SUMMARY

1. Walk west on East 110th Street from Lexington Avenue.
2. Proceed across Duke Ellington Circle and Fifth Avenue onto West 110th Street.
3. Turn right on Manhattan Avenue.
4. Enter Morningside Park at West 112th Street.
5. Leave the park on Morningside Street and go to Lafayette Square between West 114th and West 113th Streets.
6. Go back into the park; exit near West 116th Street on Morningside Avenue.
7. Walk north on Morningside.
8. Go right on West 125th Street to St. Nicholas Avenue for the subway.

CONNECTING THE WALKS

Go one block east to Frederick Douglass Boulevard and then nine blocks south to West 116th Street to start the next walk (Central Harlem).

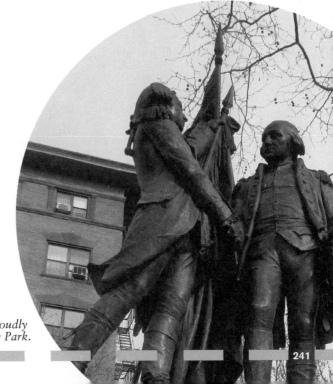

Washington and Lafayette stand proudly in the shadow of Morningside Park.

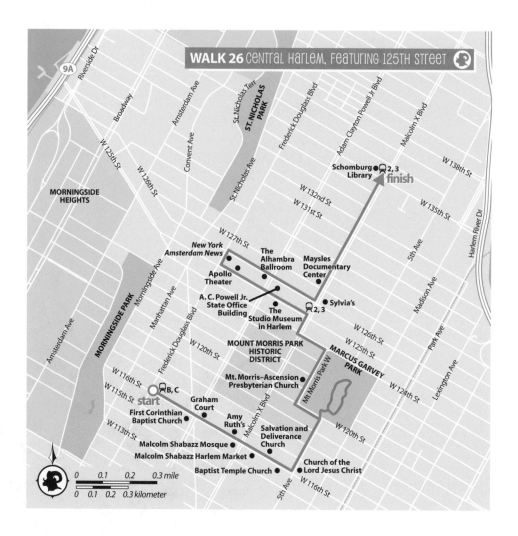

WALK 26 Central Harlem, featuring 125th Street

Riverside Dr
9A
Broadway
Amsterdam Ave
Convent Ave
St. Nicholas Terr
St. Nicholas Ave
Frederick Douglass Blvd
Adam Clayton Powell Jr Blvd
Malcolm X Blvd

W 138th St

ST. NICHOLAS PARK

W 125th St
W 126th St

MORNINGSIDE HEIGHTS

Schomburg Library ● 🚇 2, 3
finish

W 132nd St
W 131st St
W 135th St

Harlem River Dr

5th Ave
Madison Ave
Park Ave
Lexington Ave

W 127th St

New York Amsterdam News ●
The Alhambra Ballroom ●
Maysles Documentary Center ●

Apollo Theater ●

Morningside Ave
Manhattan Ave

A. C. Powell Jr. State Office Building ●
The Studio Museum in Harlem ●
🚇 2, 3 ● Sylvia's

MORNINGSIDE PARK

W 120th St

MOUNT MORRIS PARK HISTORIC DISTRICT

W 126th St
W 125th St

MARCUS GARVEY PARK

W 124th St

Amsterdam Ave

W 116th St
W 115th St start 🚇 B, C

Mt. Morris–Ascension Presbyterian Church ●

Mt Morris Park W

Graham Court ●

First Corinthian Baptist Church ●

W 113th St

Amy Ruth's ●

Malcolm X Blvd

Salvation and Deliverance Church ●

W 120th St

Malcolm Shabazz Mosque ●

Malcolm Shabazz Harlem Market ●

Baptist Temple Church ●

Church of the ● Lord Jesus Christ

5th Ave
W 116th St

0   0.1   0.2   0.3 mile
0   0.1   0.2   0.3 kilometer

26 Central Harlem, Featuring 125th Street: Harlem's Heart and Soul

BOUNDARIES: **W. 116th St., Frederick Douglass Blvd., W. 135th St., Lenox Ave.**
DISTANCE: **1.8 miles**
SUBWAY: **B or C to 116th St.**

Which institution truly defines the heart and soul of Harlem? The Studio Museum on 125th Street? The Apollo Theater, also on 125th Street? Or 125th Street itself?

Who embodies Harlem—the poets and artists of the Harlem Renaissance? The hip-hop musicians and rappers? Sylvia Woods, the restaurateur? Someone else?

Who's the quintessential Harlem resident: a colonial farmer, a newly wealthy assimilated Jew, an African American recently transplanted from the Deep South?

All of the above, my friends, all of the above. Harlem is stately older buildings, shiny new constructions, and dilapidated structures. Harlem is African American and Latino, with many whites and Asians as well, and in the past it had large Jewish and Italian communities. In the distant past, it was home to Native Americans and Dutch settlers. Harlem has a rich, varied history and a promising future. It had, and still has, various urban woes, but it also has many jewels and joys.

Harlem has ample subway service and several bus lines, as well as a station for the Metro North commuter railroad. It's bordered by Columbia University and City College, touched by Central Park, Morningside Park, and Thomas Jefferson Park, and blessed with Mount Morris/Marcus Garvey Park and smaller green spaces. It's home to many grand churches as well as small, modest ones.

Visit Harlem!

● **From the train station at Frederick Douglass Boulevard, walk east on West 116th Street. (Building numbers will be getting lower.) Toward the end of this block,**

Back Story: a singular showplace

Jazz chanteuse Ella Fitzgerald and heavy metal kings Metallica have something in common. Really, they do—they both graced the stage of Harlem's legendary Apollo Theater. The Apollo is best known for showcasing the music of African American performers, bringing audiences jazz, soul, funk, gospel, and hip-hop. But it has also reached further afield. Jimi Hendrix won an amateur contest here in 1964, and musicians have recorded live albums here—James Brown had a few.

But for all the acclaim it had from the 1930s through the 1960s, the Apollo began falling on bad times in the 1970s. It nearly closed a few times, but in 1983 it was rescued by the group Inner City Broadcasting and later by New York State. With its landmark status on the city and federal levels, the Apollo seems destined for many more years of entertaining people with music, dance, comedy, and occasional lectures.

a mix of residential and commercial sites, one interesting apartment house is #213, The Jerome. The building (from 1910) has a brick-and-quoin Beaux Arts design and ornate stonework over the windows; the name is inscribed elegantly over the entrance, which is flanked by twin Corinthian columns on each side.

● Continue to the corner. Two major roads cross here: The one going at a diagonal is St. Nicholas Avenue; the other is Adam Clayton Powell Jr. Boulevard. Before you cross Powell, take a look on the right at the First Corinthian Baptist Church, housed in a landmarked building from 1913 that was originally the Regent Theater. It's a neo-Venetian confection, rich in detail. Across Powell on the corner is the very stately Graham Court, once (and perhaps still) one of the premier apartment dwellings of central Harlem. Built 1899–1901, commissioned by an Astor, and designed by the same architects responsible for The Apthorp on the Upper West Side (see Walk 19), this is a beautiful building in the Italian Renaissance style; like The Apthorp, it has an atmospheric inner courtyard. The street corner is co-named for The Rev. Wyatt Tee Walker, a famous African American pastor and civil rights leader.

- Down the block on the left is Amy Ruth's, serving "home-style Southern cuisine." At the right corner of Malcolm X Boulevard (Lenox Avenue) is a somewhat modern building with a huge, deep-green dome. This is Malcolm Shabazz Mosque, named for the charismatic and controversial Malcolm X (he took on more than one religious name but was born Malcolm Little). The street level is made up of stores and businesses.

- As you cross the boulevard, notice that each corner has an entrance to the 116th Street station for the 2 and 3 subways. On the right side of the street, soon you will see the Malcolm Shabazz Harlem Market, a semienclosed set of stalls selling African foods, clothing, and crafts and offering services (hair braiding, for example). The entrance is flanked by two bright-green, -red, and -yellow towers.

  Many of the buildings on this block were built in the 1990s and after, but there are a few older buildings toward Fifth Avenue. A large white church with red accents, Salvation and Deliverance Church, was built in 1903 as Columbia Typewriter Company. It was then used as Cooper Junior High School, then the Institutional Synagogue (which moved to the Upper West Side), then Walker Memorial Baptist Church (which moved to the Bronx), and finally Salvation. *Whew.* Across the street is an old-new construction for the Baptist Temple Church. Originally built as Ohab Zedek synagogue (which started on the Lower East Side and later also moved to the Upper West Side), it's a hybrid building—the midsection collapsed in the early 2000s; the church rebuilt that part but kept the outer parts (where there are still two Jewish stars up top).

- Turn left on Fifth Avenue. The former Mount Morris Theatre, to your right, was turned into the Church of the Lord Jesus Christ of the Apostolic Faith. (As you can see, many Harlem churches are housed in former synagogues, theaters, banks . . .) Note the well-preserved lions' heads above the doors. Continue walking, and between East 119th and East 120th is 1481 Fifth Ave., a dramatic-looking 2000s building touted as boutique housing. The lower section is brown and cream brick; a statue of seated women is in front of the main entrance. The building looks right out onto Marcus Garvey Park, also known as Mount Morris Park. Fifth Avenue ends here but resumes four blocks north.

- Cross over to the park. It's very hilly in parts because of schist outcroppings. The colonial Dutch referred to this as Snake Hill; the British used the site as a fortification during the Revolutionary War; it opened as Mount Morris Park in 1840, and in 1973 it was renamed for Marcus Garvey, a black nationalist who was active in the 1920s and '30s. The Morris family has a long pedigree in New York State, and the Bronx has many places named for them (Morris Heights, Morris Park, Morris High School, Morrisania, among them). One of the most interesting things in the park is the cast-iron fire tower, which is no longer in use for summoning firefighters but is the last one of its kind standing in the United States. In addition, the park has sports fields, playgrounds, a swimming pool, and a recreation center. It also has a band shell where the annual Charlie Parker Jazz Festival takes place.

● After you've taken in the park, walk along West 120th Street with the park to your right, and notice the imposing brownstones lining the left side of the street.

● Make a right on Mount Morris Park West, within the Mount Morris Park Historic District, landmarked for its concentration of lovely brownstones, many of them renovated in the early 2000s. At West 122nd is Mount Morris–Ascension Presbyterian Church. This remarkable 1906 building has touches of Romanesque and Byzantine styles, a dome that draws the eye (you get a good view from across the street), and smaller details such as a medallion with Noah's Ark. At West 123rd there is an attractive corner town house with a lovely canopy arch over the entrance. This building has an unusual history: Dating to the late 1800s, it was the mansion of John Dwight, a founder of the company that created Arm & Hammer baking soda. In the early 1960s, the building was bought for use by the Commandment Keepers, an African American Jewish congregation. But they had internal squabbles about succession and fought over selling the building. If you look carefully, you will see some faded remainders of its Jewish past.

● At the end of Mount Morris Park West, turn left on West 124th Street. This block is a mix of old town houses and newer construction. Midblock on the right is a small community garden.

● At Lenox Avenue/Malcolm X Boulevard, make a right and walk to West 125th, the main street of Harlem, often referred to as "One Two Five." In the 1970s and '80s, there was considerable desolation here, coexisting with landmarks. But since the 1990s, this street (also named Dr. Martin Luther King Jr. Blvd.) has become a much more desirable destination; several major chain stores have moved in, banks and restaurants as well. On its eastern end, 125th Street feeds into the Robert F. Kennedy (Triborough) Bridge, which you can see if you look to your right.

● Make a left on West 125th. Near the end of the block are two prominent sites: On the left is The Studio Museum in Harlem, and on the right is the Adam Clayton Powell Jr. State Office Building. The museum, established in 1968, has an impressive collection of art and an artists-in-residence program. At 19 stories, the State Office Building (from the 1970s) is the tallest in Harlem. Its design and height have been both panned and praised. The spacious plaza surrounding it features an in-action statue of Powell himself. (In 2009, a large memorial was held in the plaza to honor the just-deceased Michael Jackson; I attended, and it was packed with people of all ages.)

● Across Adam Clayton Powell Jr. Boulevard on the left is a large white building, one of the tallest in Harlem. Originally Hotel Theresa and built in 1912–13, it is now an office building called Theresa Towers. The boulevard side has abundant terra-cotta ornamentation, as do the top floor and roof. In 1960, Fidel Castro stayed here while he was in town to speak to the UN General Assembly.

● Walk along the next block of West 125th Street for two historical theaters on your right. The first you will see is the Victoria from 1917, designed by Thomas Lamb, who built a number of famous cinemas around the country (including Broadway's Rivoli and Ziegfeld, both sadly demolished). It's currently vacant, but several plans for its redevelopment have been proposed. A bit farther up is the world-famous Apollo Theater, with its iconic vertical sign and marquee. Originally a burlesque house, it

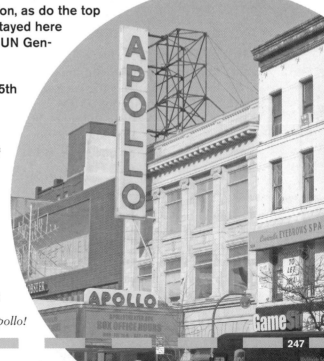

There's no time like showtime at the Apollo!

was renamed the Apollo in 1934, when it also opened its doors to black audiences and performers. Many, many jazz, gospel, R&B, pop, and rock acts have graced the stage, but one of its most famous (and scathing) features is the weekly Amateur Night, "where stars are born and legends are made." A performer can survive it and hit it big, or get booed badly!

● Walk forward to Frederick Douglass Boulevard and look across the street at the stores on the ground floor of the United House of Prayer for All People. One of them used to be a clothing store called Freddy's, which had been the focus of racial tension. In December 1995, a man went in and shot several people dead before setting the store on fire. This incident sparked a reevaluation of race relations in the neighborhood. Look down the boulevard to see the House of Prayer itself, which has two angel statues attached to it.

● Make a right at Frederick Douglass. Midblock is the home of the *New York Amsterdam News,* one of the oldest African American newspapers in the US. It was founded in 1909 and in the early 1940s moved to this building, which predates the paper's tenancy.

● Turn right at West 126th Street. Pass the modest Thomas Memorial Wesleyan Methodist Church on the right, and the much larger Trinity AME Church a bit farther down on the left. You also pass the back of the Apollo Theater, and on the left is PS 154M, the Harriet Tubman School. At the corner of Adam Clayton Powell Jr. Boulevard, look to the right. The Alhambra Ballroom, built in 1905, has previously been a theater, among other things. After some disheveled years, it was fixed up and is now a private event space. Across the boulevard is the side of the State Office Building. Walk the next block of West 126th, a long row of similar brownstones.

● Turn left on Lenox/Malcolm X. On the right, find Sylvia's, the city's most famous soulfood restaurant. The late Sylvia Woods opened it in 1962, and it's renowned for its Sunday gospel brunch. On the next block, across the avenue, is the Maysles Documentary Center and Cinema, established by Albert and David Maysles, the brothers who made the documentaries *Gimme Shelter* and *Grey Gardens,* among others. In this space, indie films are shown and courses in documentary filmmaking are held for children and adults.

● You can turn around and go to West 125th Street to catch the 2 or 3 train—or, if you're up for it, continue along to West 135th Street for the Schomburg Center for Research in Black Culture. Created in 1905 as a local library branch, the Schomburg Center has grown into a major research center that also holds exhibitions and performances, shows films, and runs many other cultural and educational activities. Harlem Hospital is across from the Schomburg Center, and the Harlem YMCA is around the corner on West 135th. There's also a 135th Street station for the 2 and 3.

POINTS OF INterest

First Corinthian Baptist Church fcbnyc.org, 1912 Adam Clayton Powell Jr. Blvd., 212-864-5976

Amy Ruth's amyruths.com, 113 W. 116th St., 212-280-8779

Malcolm Shabazz Mosque masjidmalcolmshabazz.com, 102 W. 116th St., 212-662-2200

Malcolm Shabazz Harlem Market 52 W. 116th St., 212-987-8131

Salvation and Deliverance Church salvationdeliverancehq.org, 37 W. 116th St., 212-722-5488

Baptist Temple Church 20 W. 116th St., 212-996-0334

Church of the Lord Jesus Christ of the Apostolic Faith tcljc.com, 1421 Fifth Ave., 212-369-3037

Marcus Garvey Park nycgovparks.org/parks/marcus-garvey-park, Mount Morris Park West between West 120th and West 124th Streets

Mount Morris–Ascension Presbyterian Church pcusa.org/congregations/10770, 16–20 Mt. Morris Park W., 212-831-6800

Adam Clayton Powell Jr. State Office Building ogs.ny.gov/bu/ba/acp.asp, 163 W. 125th St.

The Studio Museum in Harlem studiomuseum.org, 144 W. 125th St., 212-864-4500

Apollo Theater apollotheater.org, 253 W. 125th St., 212-531-5300

New York Amsterdam News amsterdamnews.com, 2340 Frederick Douglass Blvd., 212-932-7400

The Alhambra Ballroom alhambraballroom.net, 2116 Adam Clayton Powell Jr. Blvd., 212-222-6940

Sylvia's Restaurant sylviasrestaurant.com, 328 Malcolm X Blvd., 212-996-0660

Maysles Documentary Center and Cinema maysles.org/mdc, 343 Malcolm X Blvd., 212-537-6843

Schomburg Center for Research in Black Culture nypl.org/location/schomburg, 515 Malcolm X Blvd., 212-491-2200

route summary

1. Walk east on West 116th Street from Frederick Douglass Boulevard.
2. Turn left at Fifth Avenue.
3. Go into Mount Morris/Marcus Garvey Park, then return to Fifth Avenue.
4. Walk west on West 120th Street.
5. Turn right on Mount Morris Park West.
6. Turn left on West 124th Street.
7. Turn right on Lenox Avenue/Malcolm X Boulevard.
8. Turn left on West 125th Street.
9. Turn right on Frederick Douglass Boulevard.
10. Turn right on West 126th Street.
11. Turn left on Lenox Avenue.
12. Either walk south to West 125th Street or continue on to West 135th.

CONNECTING THE WALKS

No other walks are close by or easily arrived at.

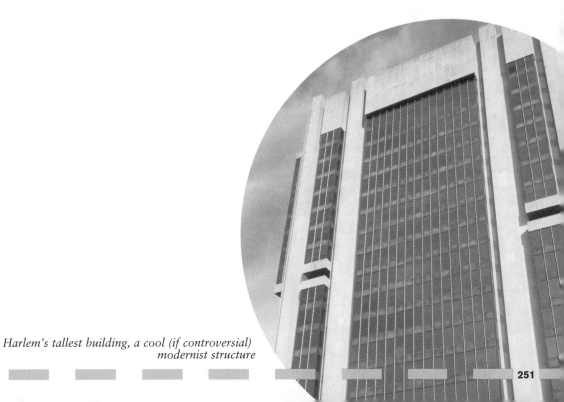

*Harlem's tallest building, a cool (if controversial)
modernist structure*

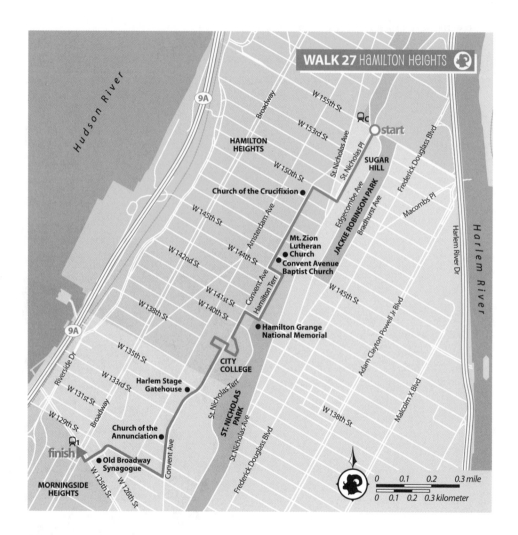

WALK 27 HAMILTON HEIGHTS

start

HAMILTON HEIGHTS

SUGAR HILL

Hudson River

9A

Broadway

W 155th St
W 153rd St
W 150th St

St. Nicholas Ave
St. Nicholas Pl

Frederick Douglass Blvd

Edgecombe Ave
Bradhurst Ave

Macombs Pl

Harlem River Dr

Harlem River

Church of the Crucifixion •

JACKIE ROBINSON PARK

W 145th St

Amsterdam Ave

W 144th St

Mt. Zion
Lutheran
• Church
Convent Avenue
Baptist Church

W 145th St

Convent Ave
Hamilton Terr

W 142nd St

W 141st St
W 140th St

W 138th St

Adam Clayton Powell Jr Blvd

Malcolm X Blvd

• Hamilton Grange
National Memorial

9A

W 135th St

CITY
COLLEGE

W 138th St

Riverside Dr

W 133rd St

Harlem Stage
Gatehouse •

St. Nicholas Terr

ST. NICHOLAS
PARK

Frederick Douglass Blvd

W 131st St

Broadway

W 129th St

Church of the
Annunciation •

Convent Ave

St. Nicholas Ave

finish

• Old Broadway
Synagogue

W 125th St
W 126th St

MORNINGSIDE
HEIGHTS

0   0.1   0.2   0.3 mile

0   0.1   0.2   0.3 kilometer

27 Hamilton Heights: Historic, Handsome, Hilly

BOUNDARIES: **W. 155th St., St. Nicholas Ave., W. 125th St., Broadway**
DISTANCE: **2 miles**
SUBWAY: **C to 155th St.**

Certain parts of Manhattan are always in the news, constantly being promoted. Other parts deserve the spotlight more often, and I'm happy to help them out. The neighborhood north of Harlem, Hamilton Heights, is home to a few treasures that have city, state, and national significance. Here you find Hamilton Grange, a home of early American statesman Alexander Hamilton. Also here is CCNY, City College of New York, a longtime intellectual powerhouse whose main campus is a stunning collection of buildings. The southern section of legendary Sugar Hill, with its magnificent houses, is the northern parcel of Hamilton Heights. In addition, you'll find notable and intriguing houses of worship, school buildings, and more.

- West 155th Street, the northern end of Hamilton Heights, is the southern boundary of Washington Heights (see the next walk). From the subway exit at West 155th and St. Nicholas Avenue, walk a block east on 155th to St. Nicholas Place; the street becomes elevated just past here and farther east feeds into the Macombs Dam Bridge to the Bronx. To the left is the road that merges about eight blocks away into Harlem River Drive (the northern extension of the FDR Drive). Also to the left is the edge of Highbridge Park.

- Baseball fans will like to know that they are just a few blocks south of Coogan's Bluff, just above West 158th, and the almost mystical John T. Brush Stairway, just south of West 157th, one of the few intact (albeit obscure) remnants of the Polo Grounds—the home field of Major League Baseball's New York Giants until they moved to San Francisco in 1958. The horseshoe-shaped stadium was also used by the Giants football team, and the New York Mets played there before Shea Stadium was built (the New York Jets did, too). The Polo Grounds stadium is gone, making the stairway kind of hard to find.

- Turn right (south) on St. Nicholas Place. This is part of Sugar Hill, an enclave favored by wealthy African Americans during the Harlem Renaissance of the 1920s. Its row houses and occasional freestanding houses were expansive and expensive, and some prime examples come into view when you reach West 153rd Street. On your right between West 153rd and West 152nd are some gems, especially the redbrick houses with decorative panels over the front doors. The next block isn't as fancy, but from West 151st to where St. Nicholas Place merges with St. Nicholas Avenue around West 149th, you'll find some very fine specimens. The houses at #16 and #14 have beautiful roofs and stonework; #10, a limestone palace built for circus magnate James Bailey, has a gorgeous extended staircase and turret. Just past West 150th are Fink House (8 St. Nicholas Place), a natty example of the Queen Anne style, and, next door, Baiter House (6 St. Nicholas Place), a French Renaissance beauty, narrower but still full of style and charm.

- Turn right on West 150th, then make a left on Convent Avenue (which derives its name from the nearby Convent of the Sacred Heart property). On the right at West 149th is the Episcopal Church of the Crucifixion, with massive columns and a spaceship-like roof. It was built in the late 1960s.

- Continue along Convent and admire the well-designed and -preserved town houses. At West 146th stands one of those sturdy brick New York Telephone Co. buildings. At West 145th there are a few significant houses of worship. Just to the left are Mount Zion Evangelical Lutheran Church and the School on the Hill—a building with delightful windows, lancets inside lancets. The church is small and has a stepped roofline. Across the street is the Convent Avenue Baptist Church. This white-marble neo-Gothic edifice was originally the Washington Heights Baptist Church, finished in 1899. Martin Luther King Jr.'s last public appearance in New York City was at this church, nine days before his assassination.

- The homes on Convent Avenue overflow with niceties, but by and large they harmonize well without trying to outdo each other. Some are in better shape than others, but in recent decades a "house proud" attitude has taken root, so that more and more of these are looking good (real estate prices have risen as well). At West 144th, take note of the former Lutheran Hospital of Manhattan, on the near left corner. A cornerstone reads NORMAN H. HUNT, INC. ARCHITECTS—not as famous as McKim, Mead & White, but they did a fine job here. Across the street is Greater Tabernacle Baptist Church, with a bowed front section.

- Make a left on West 144th, which ends at a short street called Hamilton Terrace. The white apartment buildings here, as a set, have gorgeous balconies and Renaissance-inspired details at the roofline. A humorous, nostalgic, and surprising sight is found by peering through the gap between the last house on the left on West 144th and the next one on Hamilton Terrace. A faded 1970s ad for WABC MUSIC RADIO 77 ALL HITS—ALL THE TIME is on an apartment-building wall, peeling but still quite legible in yellow, red, black, and white. (WABC was a major Top 40 music station in the 1960s and '70s but has been all-talk since 1982.)

- Turn right on Hamilton Terrace, where the house at #62 has been turned into the Children's Art Carnival. The house at #51, red brick with a cornice, has a different look from the others and is eye-catching. The road drops a bit, so be aware.

- Hamilton Terrace ends at West 141st Street, and on the right is the castlelike, reddish-brown stone of St. Luke's Episcopal Church (its front entrance is on Convent Avenue). Across the street from it is the white-brick, charm-free engineering school of City College. But more important here is the old yellow house on the hill: the landmarked Hamilton Grange National Memorial. Alexander Hamilton—lawyer, statesman, first Secretary of the Treasury, founder of the Federalist Party, aide to George Washington, the face of the $10 bill, and founder of the *New York Post*— lived in this house for two years before he was killed in a duel with Vice President Aaron Burr in 1804. The house was moved here, not far from its original location. Before entering, turn around and look out at the handsome town houses that descend toward St. Nicholas Avenue, with St. James Presbyterian Church and its proud tower at the corner.

The imposing Gothic entrance to City College

- If you tour the house, you can see the parlor, dining room, Hamilton's study, and an informational exhibit. Hamilton was certainly an intriguing figure of the early American republic—pro-business and definitely an urban, and urbane, citizen. Yet he was also emotional and rash, as his demise shows (he's buried at Trinity Church downtown; see Walk 3). Even if you don't go inside the house, walk around and see the grounds. You get a good view downward in many directions because of the elevation here. Then take West 141st back to Convent Avenue.

- Make a left on Convent and walk into City College, through the northern gate of the north campus. Savor this gate, replete with details; look for the three-faced Janus, longtime symbol of the college. The campus is made up of more than a dozen buildings, and the original five are neo-Gothic treats dating to 1902–07 and clad in Manhattan schist (excavated with the creation of the Broadway subway line) and white glazed terra-cotta. These older buildings feature grotesques—whimsical gargoyle-type statues—many of them reading books.

  The most magnificent building here is Shepard Hall, a C-shaped structure with a fantastic entrance and many other marvelous details outside. Politely ask the security officer if you can enter, especially if a gallery exhibit is going on (just show some ID). Inside are murals, gorgeous doors and windows, historical plaques, and sculptures and statues (including George Washington and a bust of Abraham Lincoln). One conference room has stained-glass windows of Aristotle, Socrates, and Plato. The main hall is breathtaking in its artistry: arches and pillars, stained-glass windows of various colleges around the country, flags, a lovely mural at the back of the stage, well-crafted hanging lights, a graceful pipe organ, and so much more.

  Next is Wingate Hall, its entrance flanked by lions holding crests. To one side of Wingate is Townsend Harris Hall, to another the open space within the quad, a flagpole in its center. Compton-Goethals Hall has a towerlike chimney that once provided venting for the campus's power and heating systems. Then examine Baskerville Hall. Continue along to see the much more modern Academic Center, with its bands of windows, and the Marshak Science Building, modern and dour. Walk a little more, and at West 135th Street is A. Philip Randolph High School. Not as grand as the oldest CCNY buildings, its neo-Gothic architecture is stately nonetheless and makes it fit in nicely with them. It was first built as the Training School for Teachers, and then for almost 50 years it served as the High School of Music and Art (which merged in the mid-1980s with the High School of the Performing Arts to become LaGuardia High School; see Walk 19). Beyond the high school is St. Nicholas Park, and below West 135th is the south campus of CCNY. Some of these buildings were constructed for Manhattanville College of the Sacred Heart and taken over by CCNY when that school moved to Westchester County.

● Continue along Convent Avenue as it curves. On your right, just past where Convent intersects West 135th Street, is a quirky old building with several charming circular windows, the Harlem Stage Gatehouse. It was built in the late 1880s as part of the Croton Aqueduct, a city water-distribution system built in the early 1800s. Since 2006, it has served as a performing-arts venue. Outside it are round marble seats engraved with quotes from W. H. Auden, Zora Neale Hurston, Lao Tzu, and others. Farther down Convent on the left is the bland brown-brick Aaron Davis Hall, another performing-arts space. Across from it at West 133rd Street is PS 161. Past 133rd on the left is the New York Structural Biology Center—serious stuff. Opposite this science center is the Church of the Annunciation, dedicated in 1907; Gothic in style, it has expansive windows and a three-door entrance. Across the avenue is Mott Hall School, PS/IS 223, a science and technology–focused school with a nationally ranked chess team. And to your left at West 130th Street is PS 129, John H. Finley School, a post-WWII building decked out with children's murals.

● Turn right on West 130th. Across Amsterdam Avenue to your right is a Y-shaped housing complex bisected by colored panels.

● Turn left on Amsterdam. At West 129th Street, with the Amsterdam bus depot on your left, turn right, passing the fortresslike Manhattanville Junior High School. Across the street is the Sheltering Arms Recreation Center, a public facility with two swimming pools and a field house.

● Past the school, West 129th makes an L-shaped bend left and becomes Old Broadway, a remnant of the colonial-era road first known as the Bloomingdale Road. (This is actually the southern spur; the other remaining section of Old Broadway is a few blocks north between West 131st and 133rd Streets.) To your left, after Old Broadway crosses West 126th, see quaint Old Broadway Synagogue, built in 1923, which calls to mind the small tenement synagogues of the Lower East Side. This congregation almost closed, but the rabbi kept it going by appealing to college students and faculty in the area; thus, it hangs on.

● Where the street ends at West 125th Street, turn right. One of the more remarkable stations of the subway system is the 1 stop at Broadway. It's the only elevated station of the 1 line in Manhattan, and boy, is it high up, spanning the Manhattan Valley ravine. You can take the train here or take a bus east and connect to other subway lines at their 125th Street stations.

POINTS OF INTEREST

Episcopal Church of the Crucifixion churchofthecrucifixion.org, 459 W. 149th St., 212-281-0900

Mount Zion Evangelical Lutheran Church 421 W. 145th St., 212-862-8680

Convent Avenue Baptist Church conventchurch.org, 420 W. 145th St., 212-234-6767

Hamilton Grange National Memorial nps.gov/hagr, 414 W. 141st St., 646-548-2310

City College of New York ccny.cuny.edu, 160 Convent Ave., 212-650-7000

Harlem Stage Gatehouse harlemstage.org, 150 Convent Ave., 212-281-9240

Church of the Annunciation theannunciation.net, 88 Convent Ave., 212-234-1919

Old Broadway Synagogue oldbroadwaysynagogue.blogspot.com, 15 Old Broadway, 212-662-9767

125th Street 1 Subway Station West 125th Street at Broadway

ROUTE SUMMARY

1. Walk east on West 155th Street from St. Nicholas Avenue.
2. Walk south on St. Nicholas Place.
3. Turn right on West 150th Street.
4. Go left on Convent Avenue.
5. Turn left on West 144th Street.
6. Turn right on Hamilton Terrace.

7. From Hamilton Grange, walk west on West 141st Street.

8. Turn left on Convent Avenue.

9. Walk into and around the City College campus.

10. From Convent Avenue, turn right on West 130th Street.

11. Turn left on Amsterdam Avenue.

12. Turn right on West 129th Street, which turns into Old Broadway.

13. Turn right on West 125th Street for the 1 train at Broadway.

CONNECTING THE WALKS

Walk south on Broadway for 15 blocks to West 110th Street to start Walk 24, Morningside Heights.

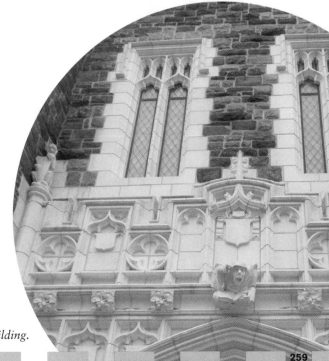

A scholarly gargoyle festoons a City College building.

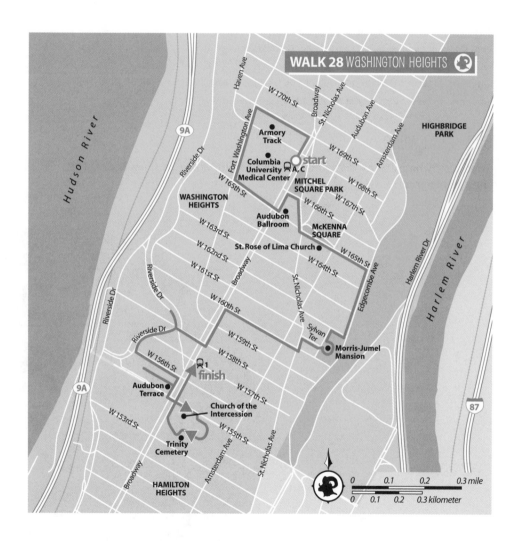

WALK 28 WASHINGTON HEIGHTS

Hudson River

Harlem River

HIGHBRIDGE PARK

9A

Haven Ave

W 170th St

Broadway

St. Nicholas Ave

Audubon Ave

Amsterdam Ave

Riverside Dr

Fort Washington Ave

Armory Track

W 169th St

start
A, C

W 168th St

Columbia University Medical Center

MITCHEL SQUARE PARK

W 167th St

W 165th St

WASHINGTON HEIGHTS

W 166th St

Audubon Ballroom

McKENNA SQUARE

W 163rd St

St. Rose of Lima Church

W 165th St

W 162nd St

W 164th St

Edgecombe Ave

Broadway

St. Nicholas Ave

Harlem River Dr

W 161st St

Riverside Dr

W 160th St

Riverside Dr

W 159th St

Sylvan Ter

Morris-Jumel Mansion

Riverside Dr

W 156th St

W 158th St

1
finish

W 157th St

87

9A

Audubon Terrace

Church of the Intercession

W 153rd St

W 155th St

Amsterdam Ave

St. Nicholas Ave

Trinity Cemetery

Broadway

HAMILTON HEIGHTS

0   0.1   0.2   0.3 mile
0   0.1   0.2   0.3 kilometer

28 WaSHINGTON HeiGHTS:
HeiGHTS OF HiSTOrY, MeDiCiNe, anD More

BOUNDARIES: **W. 169th St., Jumel Terrace, W. 155th St., Riverside Dr.**
DISTANCE: **2.2 miles**
SUBWAY: **A/C/1 to 168th St.**

There is a serious and even somber air to much of Washington Heights. Its western anchor is Columbia-Presbyterian's massive cluster of medical buildings. In the middle of the neighborhood is the Audubon Ballroom, the site of Malcolm X's assassination and now an educational center. The southern border is taken up by the Trinity Church cemeteries and the imposing Church of the Intercession. The eastern section is lighter-hearted, with the uniquely charming row houses of Sylvan Terrace and the aristocratic Morris-Jumel Mansion. Interspersed throughout "WaHi" are many prewar buildings, various schools and houses of worship, and small parks. It's also home to the Audubon Terrace museums and dramatic outdoor sculptures.

● From the subway stop on Broadway or St. Nicholas Avenue, walk north to West 169th Street and make a left. The large building on your left is the Armory Track facility. Built as the Fort Washington Armory in the early 1900s, it became a homeless shelter— the city's largest—in the 1980s, but it was renovated in the early 1990s and turned into a sports-and-recreation facility.

● Make a left on Fort Washington Avenue and take in the front of Armory Track, which has a Classical Revival design and well-kept brickwork. You can go inside to visit the National Track and Field Hall of Fame. Back out on the avenue, walk to your left, through the heart of the NewYork-Presbyterian/Columbia University Medical Center complex. It's an intimidating set of buildings that vary in style and were built at different times. Among the most interesting architecturally are the Milstein Hospital Building, built in the late 1980s, and the Harkness Pavilion, an Art Deco high-rise completed in 1928.

- At West 165th Street, look to your right to get a good view of Riverside Drive and even a bit of New Jersey across the river, but turn left. To your left at Broadway, the handsome, fortresslike tan building is Morgan Stanley Children's Hospital. Cross Broadway and you will see a building with extravagant ornamentation. This is the Audubon Ballroom, commissioned in 1912 by film producer William Fox (note the fox heads between the windows) and designed by architect Thomas Lamb. The nautical facade, the centerpiece of which is a terra-cotta Neptune in a ship over the entrance, is spectacular. On February 21, 1965, Malcolm X was shot to death here as he approached the podium to address the Organization of Afro-American Unity. The building, which later had to stave off demolition, now houses businesses and The Malcolm X and Dr. Betty Shabazz Memorial and Educational Center. Go inside to see the exhibits (including a life-size statue of Malcolm X).

- Once outside, turn right on Broadway and walk to the small, oddly shaped Mitchel Square Park. Its noteworthy elements include outcroppings of Manhattan schist and a World War I memorial sculpture by Gertrude Vanderbilt Whitney, showing a Marine tending to a wounded soldier as an Army private looks on. Originally called Audubon Park, it was renamed for John Purroy Mitchel, New York City's youngest mayor, who died in 1918 at age 39 while serving in World War I.

- Walk east along West 166th Street, away from the hospital; then turn right on angled St. Nicholas Avenue. You will come to McKenna Square, a dagger-shaped space with a set of decorative columns, cobblestone, and glass panels. It memorializes a local resident, William J. McKenna, who died of wounds suffered during World War I. Across the street is St. Rose of Lima, a Romanesque Revival Catholic church built in the first decades of the 1900s. The entrance is quite pretty; look carefully at the intricate brick design across the front. On the other side of the park are the local post office (with a pleasing brick design) and Gregorio Luperón High School, a cheery 2008 building that has a peculiar two-part shape. Luperón was a statesman in the Dominican Republic; this neighborhood has been home to many Dominican Americans over the past few decades.

- Walk one more block on West 165th to Edgecombe Avenue and Highbridge Park. This section has the Sunken Playground, a creatively designed spot. Across the street is MS 326, a handsome redbrick structure. Take a stroll through the play area or rest on a bench; then pick up Edgecombe Avenue and walk south, with the park to your left. Between West 164th and 163rd is a place to glance at but not join: the Edgecombe Correctional Facility. (It does have a vaguely pleasant entrance.) More inspiring are the rock outcroppings in the park; you also see these in Central Park and, farther uptown, Inwood Hill Park (see Walk 30).

- Make a right on West 162nd Street, and you'll start to see beautiful old row houses. Make a left at Jumel Terrace for a special treat. Look for the entrance to the Morris-Jumel Mansion set back in Roger Morris Park. General George Washington headquartered here for the battle of Hamilton Heights. The house, dating to 1765 but restored, is on a cliff, so take the stairs and investigate. The garden is sweet, with teardrop-shaped patches, and the house is lavishly decorated. Walk around even if you can't enter. Then walk on slender Sylvan Terrace, a pedestrian-only street off Jumel Terrace. This lot of 20 gorgeous wooden row houses, with their matching pediments, windows, and staircases, is a gem worthy of daydreams. The western end has a tiny Greenstreets patch. These houses were built in 1882–83 and rented out to laborers and working-class civil servants. They were carefully restored starting in 1979 and are some of the very few remaining wood-frame houses in Manhattan.

- Turn left on St. Nicholas Avenue, then right on West 160th. Cross Amsterdam Avenue, where the lively brick building on your left is the Duke Ellington School, PS 4. Its facade resembles a patchwork quilt of brick and window, and the small park across the street is watched over by a wall mural exhorting SAY NO TO DRUGS and other uplifting messages.

The wooden row houses of Sylvan Terrace are a Manhattan rarity.

- Continue walking along West 160th, admiring the old housing stock, the street murals, etc., and at Broadway make a left.

- Make a right on West 158th Street. When you reach Riverside Drive, cross and bear right to see 815 Riverside, with its pretty layered brickwork. Turn around, head back across West 158th, and bear left on "RSD" to see more of its gorgeous, lesser-known apartment buildings. Their decoration and style differ, and architecture buffs will especially enjoy traipsing around here. Among the nicest buildings are #809 (with its green-tile roof and courtly doorways); #800, The Grinnell (large and elegant); and especially #790, The Riviera, which has a recessed entrance and an ornamental fountain with a carved lion's head. Stay to your left on Riverside and make a left on West 156th Street.

- A GOOD BOOK IS THE PRECIOUS LIFE BLOOD OF A MASTER SPIRIT—that's the first inscription you encounter on a series of regal buildings along West 156th. This is just part of the magnificent, inspirational, yet often-overlooked Audubon Terrace Historic District . . . magnificent because of its lavishly built Beaux Arts and American Renaissance structures, inspirational because of the arts and other cultural resources found here, and overlooked because these sites don't have the tourist cachet of many others in Manhattan. Avail yourself of them and you will be rewarded. First you see the back of the American Academy of Arts and Letters (where you find the above quote), then the Church of Our Lady of Esperanza, seemingly an import from Europe; closer to Broadway, you come to the former American Geographic Society, now used by Boricua College.

- Turn right on Broadway and walk to the elaborately gated entrance partway down the block. Picture-perfect. You hardly believe you're still in the New World as you ascend the steps. Up and to your right, in the plaza, are heroic statues. On the buildings all around are names of esteemed artists, writers, and thinkers of the classic canon. The most accessible building here, on the left, is the Hispanic Society of America, a moderately sized museum with treasures of Spanish art and craft. Quiet, a bit dark, and rarely crowded, it houses paintings by Goya, El Greco, Velázquez, and others.

- From the outside you can admire the former home of the American Numismatic Society and the buildings of the American Academy of Arts and Letters (public hours are very restricted). Study their details, especially the doors, chock-full of symbols and references to history and art. These buildings were designed by esteemed architects.

● When you've had your fill of Audubon Terrace and its riches, proceed down Broadway. Past West 155th Street, a large cemetery is on your right as well as on your left, past the church. This is the Church of the Intercession, opened in 1915 and designed in the Gothic Revival style by Bertram Goodhue. The church is linked to historic Trinity Church downtown, which is why this is Trinity Cemetery. (Originally independent, Intercession became a Trinity chapel for financial reasons but later became its own church again.) Walk to your left along West 155th and find an entrance; go inside and absorb the beautiful stained-glass windows, the arches, even the artwork on floor stones. There's a nice little garden to check out, too. Look across to the north side of West 155th to see North Presbyterian Church, which seems to match Intercession stylistically.

Enter the graveyard and explore respectfully. Look for John James Audubon's prominent stone, a large cross with his likeness in a raised engraving. So much of this area pays tribute to the famed naturalist because his estate was located in the area. Many notable New Yorkers are buried in both these cemeteries, including politicians (among them Ed Koch), writer Clement Clarke Moore, and actor Jerry Orbach. The section beside the church is easier to navigate than the cemetery across Broadway, but if you have time you can explore both sides.

● Although it's a bit of a hike from here, I will mention that the Polo Grounds ballpark was located three lengthy blocks to the east along West 155th Street, which was its southern border. Public housing named for the Polo Grounds replaced the stadium, which was torn down in the 1960s and was once home to the Giants baseball team. The football Giants, as well as the Yankees, Mets, and Jets, also played there at one time or another. A tiny remnant is the John T. Brush Stairway, near West 158th Street (it's difficult to find).

● From Trinity Cemetery, walk back up Broadway to West 157th Street for the 1 train or east on West 155th to St. Nicholas Avenue for the C.

POINTS OF INTEREST

Armory Track/National Track and Field Hall of Fame armorytrack.com, 216 Fort Washington Ave., 212-923-1803

The Shabazz Center (Audubon Ballroom) theshabazzcenter.net, 3940 Broadway, 212-568-1341

Mitchel Square Park nycgovparks.org/parks/mitchel-square, bounded by Broadway, St. Nicholas Avenue, West 166th Street, and West 167th Street

McKenna Square nycgovparks.org/parks/mckenna-square, West 165th Street between Audubon and Amsterdam Avenues

Highbridge Park nycgovparks.org/parks/highbridge-park, Edgecombe Avenue between West 155th and Dyckman Streets

St. Rose of Lima Church stroseoflimachurchnyc.org, 510 W. 165th St., 212-568-0091

Morris-Jumel Mansion morrisjumel.org, 65 Jumel Terrace, 212-923-8008

Sylvan Terrace Off Jumel Terrace between West 160th and West 162nd Streets

Audubon Terrace audubonparkny.com, Broadway at West 155th and 156th Streets

Hispanic Society of America hispanicsociety.org, 613 W. 155th St., 212-926-2234

Church of the Intercession intercessionnyc.org, 550 W. 155th St., 212-283-6200

Trinity Cemetery trinitywallstreet.org/content/cemetery, 770 Riverside Drive, 212-368-1600

route summary

1. Walk north on Broadway from West 168th Street.
2. Stroll left on West 169th Street.
3. Turn left on Fort Washington Ave.
4. Turn left on West 165th Street.
5. Go left on Broadway.
6. Turn right on West 166th Street.
7. Go right on St. Nicholas Avenue to McKenna Square.
8. Turn east on West 165th Street to Highbridge Park.
9. Go south on Edgecombe Avenue.
10. Turn right on West 162nd Street.
11. Turn left on Jumel Terrace.
12. Go onto the grounds of the Morris-Jumel Mansion.
13. Walk on Sylvan Terrace.
14. Turn left on St. Nicholas Avenue.
15. Turn right on West 160th Street.

16. Stroll left on Broadway.

17. Turn right on West 158th Street.

18. Make a quick jog right on Riverside Drive, then reverse direction, keeping left on Riverside.

19. Turn left on West 156th Street.

20. Turn right on Broadway.

21. Go into the Audubon Terrace complex.

22. Continue south on Broadway.

23. Turn left on West 155th Street for the church and cemetery.

24. Go north on Broadway or east on West 155th Street for the train.

CONNECTING THE WALKS

To start the previous walk (Hamilton Heights), go two blocks east on West 155th Street to St. Nicholas Avenue.

A quote from Emerson lends a scholarly air to a doorway at the American Academy of Arts and Letters, part of the Audubon Terrace complex of museums and learned societies.

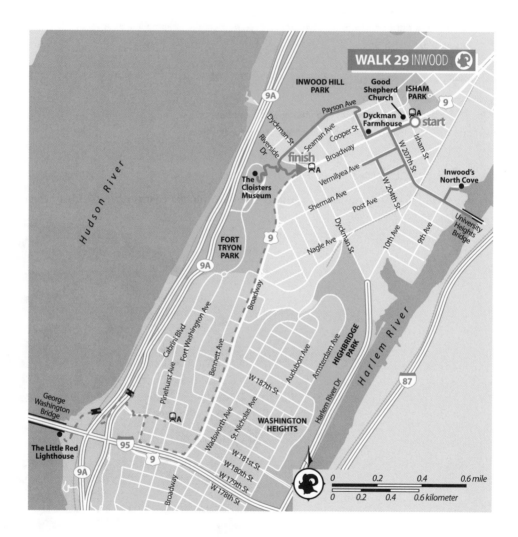

WALK 29 INWOOD

INWOOD HILL PARK

Good Shepherd Church

ISHAM PARK

Payson Ave

Dyckman St

Riverside Dr

9A

Seaman Ave

Cooper St

Dyckman Farmhouse

start

9

Isham St

W 207th St

finish

Broadway

A

The Cloisters Museum

Vermilyea Ave

W 204th St

Inwood's North Cove

Sherman Ave

Post Ave

University Heights Bridge

FORT TRYON PARK

9

Nagle Ave

Dyckman St

10th Ave

9th Ave

Hudson River

Broadway

Harlem River

Cabrini Blvd

Fort Washington Ave

HIGHBRIDGE PARK

9A

Pinehurst Ave

Bennett Ave

Audubon Ave

Amsterdam Ave

Harlem River Dr

87

George Washington Bridge

W 187th St

Wadsworth Ave

St. Nicholas Ave

WASHINGTON HEIGHTS

A

95

9

The Little Red Lighthouse

W 181st St

W 180th St

W 179th St

W 178th St

Broadway

9A

0   0.2   0.4   0.6 mile

0   0.2   0.4   0.6 kilometer

29 INWOOD: DIFFErENT DrUMMer

BOUNDARIES: **Payson Ave., W. 207th St., 9th Ave., The Cloisters (extension goes south to W. 179th St. and west to Hudson River)**
DISTANCE: **2.2 miles, or 5.7 miles with Little Red Lighthouse extension**
SUBWAY: **A to 207th St.**

Much of Manhattan is set on a grid of right-angled intersections, with major thoroughfares following different paths (Broadway and St. Nicholas Avenue are the two longest exceptions, the Bowery a shorter one). But there are neighborhoods that vary greatly from this carefully planned design—those at Manhattan's southernmost and northernmost tips, and, to a lesser extent, the West Village. Inwood is somewhat between extremes: It's set on a grid, but one that's at odds with the areas south of it. And besides that, it's very near some of the hilliest parts of Manhattan.

There is a certain defiant, individualistic streak to be found in Inwood. Its personality is a mix of the rugged and refined, the artistic and the unpolished. It has an undeniable Latino flavor, a growing artsy-craftsy contingent, and a mix of other ethnicities. Native Americans played a significant role here, which is still present, if more subtle. Inwood has Fort Tryon Park and the over-the-top romanticism of The Cloisters, a re-created French castle filled with art and decorative pieces. Nature, commerce, art, religion, and much more mingle here in delightful fashion.

This walk includes a special add-on: a visit to the Little Red Lighthouse, the star of a classic children's book. You can walk there from the end of this tour, or take the subway or bus. It's not the only lighthouse in New York City, but it is unique to Manhattan.

● **Exit the last stop on the A line onto Broadway. A street sign commemorates it as INWOOD'S HEROES OF 9/11 WAY. At 4967 Broadway, behold the Romanesque Revival Church of the Good Shepherd. It was built on land purchased from the Isham family (as in Isham Street, bordering it). The second church built for this Catholic parish, this one dates to the 1930s. A cross made of steel retrieved from the World Trade Center site stands in the churchyard; memorial stones on the ground bear the names of locals who died during 9/11. Go inside and take in the lovely stained-glass windows, light fixtures, and tiled mosaics.**

- Leaving the church, turn right and walk west on Broadway to West 207th Street, then head left. This is a bustling commercial strip, full of local businesses as well as some chain outposts.

- Make a right on Vermilyea Avenue and stroll one of the nicer residential blocks of the area. At #120 is a handsome redbrick apartment building. Across the street, at #111, is a Latino Seventh-day Adventist church that was built as the Inwood Hebrew Congregation. The church has retained much from the synagogue days, inside and out.

- Cross West 204th Street. On this block is the local post office building, simple but stately. Next door is the rustic Mount Washington Presbyterian Church. Note the handsome doors and the church name spelled out in Old English script. Look up to see the bell tower.

- Return to West 204th and head right. At the corner of Sherman Avenue is an elementary school, Washington Heights Academy. This modern building features a stirring wall design of tree shadows called *Trace,* by artist Wennie Huang.

- Turn left on Sherman Avenue, a shopping magnet for the neighborhood, with storefronts and street vendors alike.

- Turn right on West 207th Street. At Post Avenue you will see an attractive redbrick building repurposed as the Audubon Partnership for Economic Development; check out the pedimented entrance and Palladian windows. Then approach the elevated-train station at 10th Avenue, built in 1906; notice the sunburst motif surrounded by small urns.

- Continue on West 207th, and after almost two blocks you'll be on the University Heights Bridge. In a city with huge, stellar bridges, the University Heights Bridge is a modest affair, but it has its charms. Walk under the canopies. Check out the metalwork, including floral and star medallions. The bridge spans the Harlem River, specifically the part known as Sherman Creek. You can look over at (and walk into) the Bronx. On the Manhattan side and to the left, train buffs will enjoy the view of the large train MTA train yard.

- Turn around and make a right on Ninth Avenue, which curves farther right. Walk into the parking lot to see Inwood's North Cove, a wetlands and bird sanctuary. On one visit, I saw dozens of geese padding around. Behind you is the Ninth Avenue Unit Shop. Peek inside to see what the transit workers do and the equipment they use.

- Walk back to West 207th and peruse the business district again (maybe buy a snack or drink).

- Make a left on Broadway. Between West 207th and 204th—yes, they're consecutive streets—is perhaps the most historically significant place in the neighborhood: the Dyck-man Farmhouse and garden. Sitting on a ledge, it's the oldest remaining farmhouse in Manhattan. The earliest parts were built around 1784, and the style is Dutch Colonial.

- Make a right and walk along West 204th. Here you'll find Art Deco apartment buildings, well kept and brimming with elegant details. The one at #687 is particularly stylish; check out the two-tone brickwork and the geometric entrance design.

- Make a right on Seaman Avenue and admire #116 with its layered brickwork. Make a left on Payson Avenue, which curves and skirts Inwood Hill Park. Admire the apartment buildings and houses on your left, plus the park on your right. The building at #119 has a pretty frieze of a flowerpot over its entrance; #109 has a smudged-over sign about the door, indicating that it once housed a convent. Payson ends at Riverside Drive and Fort Tryon Park. There's a pretty Mormon church here, too, built in 2000 in a retro-Colonial style.

- Turn left on Riverside and walk until it merges with Broadway, passing the

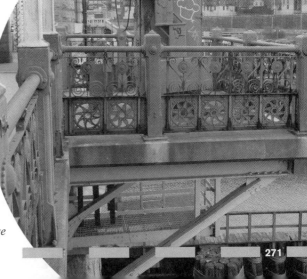

The University Heights Bridge

Riverside-Inwood Neighborhood Garden (RING)/Lt. William Tighe Triangle. Then turn right on Broadway and enter impressive Fort Tryon Park, with the Anne Loftus Playground at the entrance. As of this writing, the play area has one of the older climbing structures in town, the throwback metal-rod "monkey bars," which have largely been replaced throughout the city. (More-recent play equipment is also present.)

● Look for signs that direct you to The Cloisters, which is devoted to the art and architecture of medieval Europe. It's a bit of a hike (if you want, you can pick up the MTA M4 bus that goes up to the parking lot), but if you hoof it, you can admire the rocks and nature along the path. Go high up enough that you can gaze down at the Hudson River and Henry Hudson Parkway. The stone castle of The Cloisters is truly a wondrous sight in Manhattan. Its museum is replete with religious art, tapestries, elaborate furniture, and ritual items, and the buildings have courtyards. If you merely desire to take a peek, do so and then roam outside. In warm weather, the grounds outside The Cloisters are prime picnic pickings. There's a lovely garden and playground, too. The nearest subway is the A, at Dyckman Street and Broadway.

EXTENSION TO THE LITTLE RED LIGHTHOUSE:

If you have more energy and the weather is nice, this is a fun journey. The lighthouse is a gem that most people wouldn't believe is in Manhattan.

● Take Broadway south to West 179th Street and make a right. Stay on the north side of the street, across from the George Washington Bridge Bus Station. On your right, you pass Congregation Shaare Hatikvah, a postwar synagogue of tan brick, and the heavy stone building of Holyrood Episcopal Church (the entrance is grand). At Pinehurst Avenue, you'll see the Washington Heights Congregation, a synagogue with charming turretlike features.

● Turn right at Cabrini Boulevard, where you'll see George Washington Bridge Park. Here you skirt the approaches to the bridge, so be mindful.

● Turn left on West 181st Street. At Haven Avenue, there is a sign for Plaza Lafayette, which harks back to an older street name. A small, pretty park bisects the street.

- Turn right on Riverside Drive, then make a left onto the pedestrian overpass above the Henry Hudson Parkway. It's an intriguing walk that affords you a great view of the highway, the river, and the bridge. Walk down onto the Hudson River Greenway path, which is frequented by bicyclists. You'll see an old, unused staircase that's built into the highway's stone retaining wall.

- Bear left, staying on the official path. It's circuitous and somewhat up-and-down. You'll walk under a small overpass; you'll also see freight-train tracks. Continue walking so that you're basically in the shadow of the George Washington Bridge. This is a magnificent sight; looking onto the bridge from the ground level is impressive. Walk until you see display signs for the lighthouse—which is easy to spot because it's bright red. Originally known as Jeffrey's Hook Lighthouse and built in 1880, this structure still stands because activists wanted it saved even with the construction of the big bridge. Originally it stood sentry in Sandy Hook, New Jersey, but in 1921 it was moved to Manhattan and reassembled by the Coast Guard. The lighthouse was also paid tribute in the 1942 children's book *The Little Red Lighthouse and the Great Gray Bridge,* by Hildegarde Swift.

  This park area is also known as Fort Washington Point. Walk all around the lighthouse, get close to the rocks by the river, see the bridge's shadow in the river. Take it all in! When you've had your fill, retrace your steps back to Riverside Drive. If you have energy to burn and want more adventure, you can walk on the pedestrian path of the George Washington Bridge. (Access is from Cabrini Boulevard and West 177th Street, but check panynj.gov if there's a rerouting due to construction.) Otherwise, walk back onto West 181st Street and make a left at Fort Washington Avenue to get the A train.

POINTS OF INTEREST

Church of the Good Shepherd goodshepherdnyc.org, 4967 Broadway, 212-567-1300

Mount Washington Presbyterian Church 84 Vermilyea Ave., 212-567-0442

University Heights Bridge nycroads.com/crossings/university-heights, West 207th Street and Ninth Avenue

Inwood's North Cove nycwetlands.org, Ninth Avenue at the Harlem River

Dyckman Farmhouse Museum dyckmanfarmhouse.org, 4881 Broadway, 212-304-9422

Fort Tryon Park forttryonparktrust.org, Broadway at Dyckman Street, 212-795-1388

The Cloisters metmuseum.org/visit/visit-the-cloisters, Fort Tryon Park, 212-923-3700

EXTENSION

Little Red Lighthouse tinyurl.com/littleredlighthousenyc, Fort Washington Park/Hudson River Greenway, 212-408-0100

route summary

1. Commence at Isham Street and Broadway.
2. Walk south on Broadway.
3. Turn left on West 207th Street.
4. Walk right on Vermilyea Avenue, past West 204th Street, then turn around.
5. Stroll south on West 204th Street.
6. Turn left on Sherman Avenue.
7. Turn right on West 207th Street and walk to the University Heights Bridge.
8. Walk north on Ninth Avenue to Inwood's North Cove.
9. Double back onto West 207th Street.
10. Make a left on Broadway.
11. Turn right on West 204th Street.
12. Go right on Seaman Avenue.
13. Turn left on Payson Avenue.
14. Turn left on Riverside Drive and follow it to Broadway.
15. Go into Fort Tryon Park, following the signs and path to The Cloisters.
16. Return to Broadway for the train at Dyckman Street.

EXTENSION

17. Go south on Broadway and, at West 179th Street, turn right.
18. Turn right on Cabrini Boulevard.
19. Turn left on West 181st Street.
20. Turn right on Riverside Drive.

21. Turn left onto the pedestrian overpass and follow it into the park, following the signs to the lighthouse.

22. Backtrack to West 181st Street and Fort Washington Avenue for the subway or to Cabrini Boulevard and West 177th for the bridge.

CONNECTING THE WALKS

From the lighthouse, walk on West 181st Street about 4 blocks east to Broadway, then walk 13 blocks south to West 168th Street to start Walk 28 (Washington Heights).

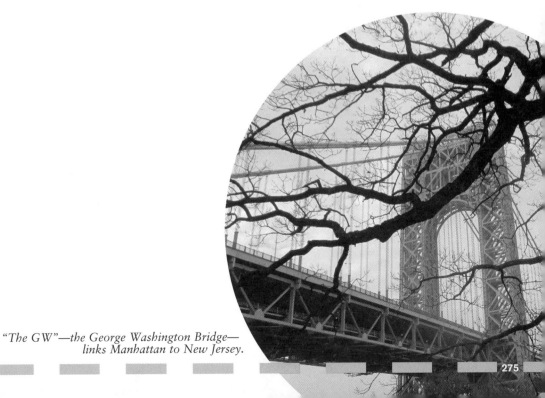

"The GW"—the George Washington Bridge—
links Manhattan to New Jersey.

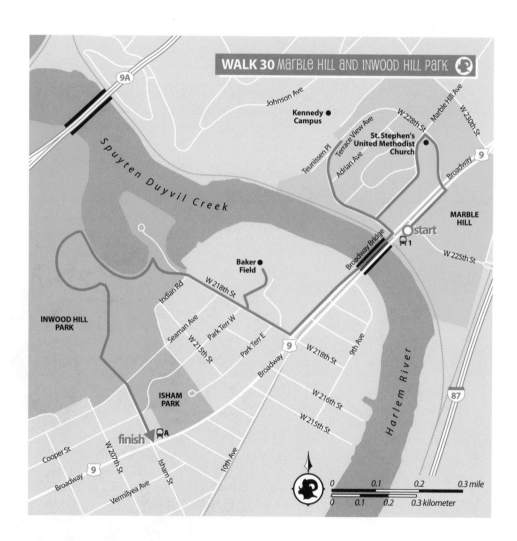

WALK 30 MARBLE HILL AND INWOOD HILL PARK

Johnson Ave

Kennedy Campus

Terrace View Ave

W 228th St

Marble Hill Ave

W 230th St

Teunissen Pl

St. Stephen's United Methodist Church

Adrian Ave

Broadway

9

Spuyten Duyvil Creek

MARBLE HILL

start

1

W 225th St

Broadway Bridge

Baker Field

W 218th St

Indian Rd

Seaman Ave

Park Terr W

Park Terr E

9

W 218th St

9th Ave

Harlem River

INWOOD HILL PARK

W 215th St

Broadway

W 216th St

87

ISHAM PARK

W 215th St

finish A

Cooper St

W 207th St

10th Ave

Broadway

9

Isham St

Vermilyea Ave

0   0.1   0.2   0.3 mile

0   0.1   0.2   0.3 kilometer

30 Marble Hill and Inwood Hill Park: The Tip-Top of Manhattan

BOUNDARIES: **W. 228th St., Broadway, W. 207th St., Inwood Hill Park**
DISTANCE: **1.5–2.5 miles, depending on your route in the park**
SUBWAY: **1 to 225th St.**

Is there a place in Manhattan that *isn't* in Manhattan? Does that question even make sense?

Yes and yes. The northernmost part of Manhattan, Marble Hill, is physically in the Bronx. Walking around here, you're not on the island of Manhattan, but you're still in the *borough* of Manhattan. Marble Hill was severed from the island and "sewed on" to the Bronx in 1895 as part of a public-works project related to water traffic. So while this area seems like it should be "South Riverdale" in the Bronx, it is indeed Manhattan.

After taking in the sights of Marble Hill, cross the Broadway Bridge and wander around Inwood, the section of Manhattan (island) that is farthest north. The highlight here is the astonishing natural beauty of large Inwood Hill Park. Don't think that if you've seen one big urban park, you've seen them all. Much of Inwood Hill is natural—unlike New York City's many planned and human-made parks—and thus more amazing. It can be a bit confusing, too, so depending on your sense of adventure, you may hike deep into the woods or just skirt the border. However you do it, a walk in this park is memorable.

● **Before you descend from the elevated 1 train, walk the length of the platform for some fine views. At the front (for northbound trains), you see well-tended apartment buildings and greenery. To the left (southbound), you see smaller homes and gardens. Walk toward the back of the uptown platform (or the front of the southbound platform, if on that side) and admire the industrial coolness of the Broadway Bridge. Look to your left to see the curve of the Harlem River. The Metro North railroad train tracks hug the shoreline. The view brings together the Bronx and Manhattan. Go downstairs and note the old-fashioned decorative touches to the banisters.**

- Walk north and east (away from the river) on Broadway, past the commercial strip, and make a left onto West 228th Street. Look to your left at the set of stairs between two apartment buildings. This is the narrow and steep Marble Hill Lane, just one indicator of the hilliness in the area; the streets can be twisty, too. On your right, at the corner of Marble Hill Avenue, look down at the field of Marble Hill Playground. Across the street is the cheerfully cottagelike St. Stephen's United Methodist Church, dedicated in 1897. It has precious woodwork, solid stonework, and fetching windows with intricate detailing. A large window on the avenue side even has a Jewish star in the middle, surrounded by crosses. Although the color is faded from some of the stained glass, these are stellar windows. A weathered plaque commemorates the Wading Place and the Kings Bridge (which lent its name to a neighborhood in the Bronx).

- With the church on your left, walk along Marble Hill Avenue and admire the private homes as well as the huge weeping willow tree. At #70 is a prewar apartment building with a recessed courtyard and terra-cotta flights of fancy over the entrance and at the roofline. At the corner of Marble Hill Avenue and Fort Charles Place is a white-and-brown house from 1894, with a half-timbered design and gingerbread woodwork over the porch—sort of a Swiss chalet in the city.

- Make a right on West 225th Street to see the Marble Hill station for the Metro North commuter railroad. A derailment here on December 1, 2013, left four people dead.

- Continue along and admire the unusual brown-brick apartment building at #129. With its corner casement windows, it has a staggered look to it, and an Art Deco sensibility.

- West 225th turns into Terrace View Avenue at Teunissen Place, and you'll see the Kennedy Campus, which houses eight different public schools (including two charter schools). Formerly John F. Kennedy High School, the campus comprises a boxy early-1970s building with large sports fields.

- Retrace your steps to West 225th and continue to Broadway; while doing so, look out at the river and appreciate it. You may also see and hear trains on their routes.

- At Broadway, make a right and walk onto the Broadway Bridge. I really enjoy strolling over this short span; hope you do, too. On the northern tip of Manhattan, pass a humdrum medical facility on your right and then the Columbia University sports complex, more commonly called Baker Field.

- Turn right on West 218th Street and walk beside the athletic center. If you have time, enter so you can explore the fields and facilities. You'll see the lion logo, for the team mascot. Admire the lion statue and its plaques honoring George F. Baker. From the football-stadium stands, you get a nice panorama of the Bronx and the Henry Hudson Bridge. Try to find the C of bushes behind the field.

- Make your way back to West 218th and hang a right. Note the elaborate metal gate with the bronze medallion; it depicts the *Alma Mater* statue found in the center of the Columbia campus. Also glimpse the flat statues in the gate, of a football player and a rower. Continue along to see the Boathouse Marsh. The school's rowing teams use the white house that's now surrounded by a small nature preserve. You can walk onto the deck, which has benches. Look at the rock wall across the Spuyten Duyvil Creek and notice a painted C: The so-called Big C Rock is regularly touched up by the crew teams. (Notice how the C reflects so well on the water.)

- Walk more on West 218th, passing Indian Road and the welcoming coffeehouse at the corner. Farther along, your path takes you into Inwood Hill Park on an outcropping of land that fronts Spuyten Duyvil Creek between the Hudson and Harlem Rivers (the creek separates Marble Hill from the rest of Manhattan). This Dutch name probably means "Spitting Devil" or "Spewing Devil," and this waterway has had a history of being rough, although it usually looks pretty gentle these days. Take in the rocks, trees, smalls animals lurking about, the flow of the water, a wide variety of forest plants, and lichens on logs. Depending on the time of year, the foliage is spectacular.

- Walk over to the Inwood Hill Boat Dock. In a smattering of spots along the path stand plastic-coated display boards with explanations of the nature and history here. If you stay fairly close to the water, you won't get confused, but if you do decide to troop farther into the woods, there are paths to follow. Kids like to hunt for Shorakkopoch Rock—marked with a plaque, it supposedly marks the spot where Peter Minuit bought Manhattan from the Lenape Indians. But in order to come upon it and the nearby Native American caves, you may need guidance from locals who are familiar with the spots. If you want to play it safe, walk the footpaths that surround the sports fields, then go back to the street on the south side of the park, Seaman Avenue.

● Turn onto Isham Street, which is east of (and parallel to) West 207th Street, and pass Isham Park. Smaller than Inwood Hill Park, this is a pleasant but more typical city park. After passing Good Shepherd School, you end up at Broadway in front of the Church of the Good Shepherd.

The 207th Street A train station is here, too—and it's worth more than a passing glance inside. AT THE START and AT LONG LAST are the glittering coming-and-going messages on the white-tiled walls, because this is the first—or last, depending on which way you're going—stop of the A line, which runs the length of Manhattan, then goes across Brooklyn and into Queens. Numerous tiles bear quotes about the neighborhood from various residents over the years. A kind of oral-history project, they're among the most unusual and thoughtful installations in any New York City subway station. From here, take the train south.

POINTS OF INTEREST

St. Stephen's United Methodist Church 146 W. 228th St., 718-562-8692

Broadway Bridge tinyurl.com/broadwaybridge, Broadway between West 220th and West 225th Streets

Baker Athletics Complex, Columbia University gocolumbialions.com, 533 W. 218th St., 889-546-6711

Inwood Hill Park nycgovparks.org/parks/inwood-hill-park, West 218th Street at Indian Road, 212-639-9675

Isham Park nycgovparks.org/parks/isham-park, bounded by Isham Street, Broadway, Seaman Avenue, and Indian Road

207th Street A Station tinyurl.com/207thstsubway, Broadway at Isham Street

ROUTE SUMMARY

1. From the 1 station at West 225th Street, walk north on Broadway.
2. Turn left on West 228th Street.

3. Turn left on Marble Hill Avenue.

4. Turn right on West 225th Street.

5. Turn right on Terrace View Avenue, then double back onto West 225th.

6. Turn right on Broadway and cross the bridge.

7. Turn right on West 218th Street, visiting the Columbia sports complex en route.

8. Go into Inwood Hill Park at Spuyten Duyvil Creek.

9. Exit the park onto Seaman Avenue.

10. Walk south on Isham Street.

11. Catch the train at the 207th Street station on Broadway.

CONNECTING THE WALKS

The previous walk (Inwood) starts where this one ends.

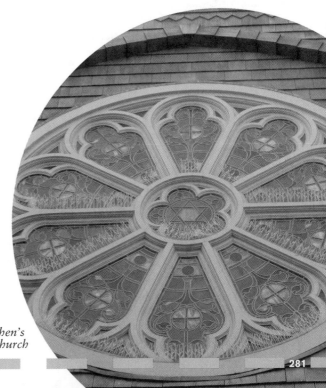

*The lovely rose window of St. Stephen's
United Methodist Church*

Appendix 1: Walks by Theme

Architectural Gems

The Bowery, Little Italy, and Soho (Walk 7)
Central Park West (Walk 21)
Chelsea and Madison Square Park (Walk 12)
Civic Center and Chinatown (Walk 5)
42nd Street (Walk 15)
Hamilton Heights (Walk 27)
Lower Midtown/Garment District (Walk 14)
Rockefeller Center (Walk 17)
Washington Heights (Walk 28)
Yorkville (Asphalt Green to Sutton Place) (Walk 23)

Around Campus

Battery Park City and Tribeca (Walk 2)
Central Greenwich Village (Walk 9)
East Village (Walk 8)
Hamilton Heights (Walk 27)
Lenox Hill (Walk 18)
Lower Midtown/Garment District (Walk 14)
Morningside Heights (Walk 24)
Upper West Side (Walk 19)

Arts and Culture

Bowling Green and the Battery (Walk 1)
Central Harlem (Walk 26)
Central Park West (Walk 21)
Fifth Avenue (Walk 20)
Inwood (Walk 29)
Rockefeller Center (Walk 17)
Upper West Side (Walk 19)
Wall Street/Financial District (Walk 3)
Washington Heights (Walk 28)

Entertainment Centers

Lower Midtown/Garment District (Walk 14)
Rockefeller Center (Walk 16)
Times Square/Theater District (Walk 16)

Ethnic Heritage

Central Harlem (Walk 26)
Civic Center and Chinatown (Walk 5)
Lower East Side (Walk 6)
Lower Harlem (Walk 25)
Washington Heights (Walk 28)

Historical Treasures

Bowling Green and the Battery (Walk 1)
Central Greenwich Village (Walk 9)
East Village (Walk 8)
42nd Street (Walk 15)
Hamilton Heights (Walk 27)
Inwood (Walk 29)

Lower East Side (Walk 6)
Morningside Heights (Walk 24)
Wall Street/Financial District (Walk 3)
Washington Heights (Walk 28)

Parks, Playgrounds, Nature

Battery Park City and Tribeca (Walk 2)
Bowling Green and the Battery (Walk 1)
Central Greenwich Village (Walk 9)
Central Harlem (Walk 26)
Central Park (Walk 22)
Chelsea and Madison Square Park
   (Walk 12)
City Hall and South Street Seaport
   (Walk 4)
Civic Center and Chinatown (Walk 5)
42nd Street (Walk 15)
High Line (Walk 13)
Lower East Side (Walk 6)
Lower Harlem (Walk 25)
Marble Hill and Inwood Hill Park
   (Walk 30)
Morningside Heights (Walk 24)
Union Square, Gramercy Park, and
   Stuyvesant Square (Walk 11)
West Village (Walk 10)
Yorkville (Asphalt Green to Sutton Place)
   (Walk 23)

Sacred Spaces

Central Harlem (Walk 26)
Central Park West (Walk 21)
City Hall and South Street Seaport (Walk 4)
Fifth Avenue (Walk 20)
Lower East Side (Walk 6)
Lower Midtown (Walk 14)
Morningside Heights (Walk 24)
Wall Street/Financial District (Walk 3)
West Village (Walk 10)

Shopping Central

Battery Park City and Tribeca (Walk 2)
42nd Street (Walk 15)
Lenox Hill (Walk 18)
Lower Midtown/Garment District (Walk 14)
Rockefeller Center (Walk 17)
Upper West Side (Walk 19)

Wining, Dining, and Noshing

The Bowery, Little Italy, and Soho (Walk 7)
Central Harlem (Walk 26)
Civic Center and Chinatown (Walk 5)
East Village (Walk 8)
Lenox Hill (Walk 18)
Lower East Side (Walk 6)
Times Square/Theater District (Walk 16)
West Village (Walk 10)

Appendix 2: POINTS OF INTEREST

cemeteries

Chatham Square Cemetery, Congregation Shearith Israel shearithisrael.org/content/chatham-square-cemetery, 55 St. James Place (Walk 5)

New York City Marble Cemetery nycmc.org, East Second Street between First and Second Avenues, 917-780-2893 (Walk 8)

New York City Vietnam Veterans Memorial Plaza vietnamveteransplaza.com, 55 Water St., 212-471-9496 (Walk 1)

New York Marble Cemetery marblecemetery.org, East Second Street between Second Avenue and the Bowery, 410-586-1321 (Walk 8)

Second Cemetery of Congregation Shearith Israel shearithisrael.org/content/eleventh-street-cemetery, 72 W. 11th St. (Walk 9)

Third Cemetery of Congregation Shearith Israel shearithisrael.org/content/twenty-first-street-cemetery, 110 W. 23rd St. (Walk 12)

Trinity Cemetery trinitywallstreet.org/content/cemetery, 770 Riverside Drive, 212-368-1600 (Walk 28)

educational and cultural centers

The Africa Center theafricacenter.org, 1 Museum Mile (1280 Fifth Ave.); check website for latest information (Walk 25)

American Irish Historical Society aihs.org, 991 Fifth Ave., 212-288-2263 (Walk 20)

Anthology Film Archives anthologyfilmarchives.org, 32 Second Ave., 212-505-5181 (Walk 8)

Asia Society asiasociety.org, 725 Park Ave., 212-288-6400 (Walk 18)

Bank Street College of Education bankstreet.edu, 610 W. 112th St., 212-875-4400 (Walk 24)

Barnard College barnard.edu, 3009 Broadway, 212-854-2033 (Walk 24)

Borough of Manhattan Community College bmcc.cuny.edu, 199 Chambers St., 212-220-8000 (Walk 2)

Carnegie Hall carnegiehall.org, 881 Seventh Ave., 212-247-7800 (Walk 16)

Center for Architecture cfa.aiany.org, 536 LaGuardia Place, 212-683-0023 (Walk 9)

Center for Jewish History cjh.org, 15 W. 16th St., 212-294-8301 (Walk 12)

Charles A. Dana Discovery Center tinyurl.com/danadiscoverycenter, Central Park North between Fifth and Lenox Avenues, 212-860-1370 (Walk 25)

City College of New York ccny.cuny.edu, 160 Convent Ave., 212-650-7000 (Walk 27)

Columbia University columbia.edu, West 116th Street and Broadway, 212-854-1754 (Walk 24)

Cooper Union cooper.edu, 30 Cooper Square, 212-353-4100 (Walk 8)

Fashion Institute of Technology fitnyc.edu, 227 W. 27th St., 212-217-7999 (Walk 14)

Fordham University–Lincoln Center Campus tinyurl.com/fordhamlincolncenter, West 60th to West 62nd Street between Columbus and Amsterdam Avenues, 212-636-6000 (Walk 19)

The General Theological Seminary gts.edu, 440 W. 21st St., 212-243-5150 (Walk 12)

Hispanic Society of America hispanicsociety.org, 613 W. 155th St., 212-926-2234 (Walk 28)

Hudson Park Library nypl.org/locations/hudson-park, 66 Leroy St., 212-243-6876 (Walk 10)

Hunter College hunter.cuny.edu, 695 Park Ave., 212-772-4000 (Walk 18)

Jefferson Market Library nypl.org/locations/jefferson-market, 425 Sixth Ave., 212-243-4334 (Walks 9 and 10)

Jewish Community Center Manhattan jccmanhattan.org, 334 Amsterdam Ave., 646-505-4444 (Walk 19)

Jewish Theological Seminary jtsa.edu, 3080 Broadway, 212-678-8000 (Walk 24)

John Jay College of Criminal Justice www.jjay.cuny.edu, 899 10th Ave., 212-663-7867 (Walk 19)

Kosciuszko Foundation thekf.org, 15 E. 65th St., 212-734-2130 (Walk 20)

LaGuardia High School laguardiahs.org, 100 Amsterdam Ave., 212-496-0700 (Walk 19)

Little Red School House & Elisabeth Irwin High School lrei.org, 272 Sixth Ave., 212-477-5316 (Walk 9)

Muhlenberg Library nypl.org/locations/muhlenberg, 209 W. 23rd St., 212-924-1585 (Walk 12)

Murry Bergtraum High School for Business Careers tinyurl.com/bergtraumhs, 411 Pearl St., 212-964-9610 (Walk 5)

The New School newschool.edu, 68 Fifth Ave., 212-229-5108 (Walk 9)

New York Public Library, Main Branch nypl.org/locations/schwarzman, Fifth Avenue and West 42nd Street, 917-275-6975 (Walk 15)

New York Studio School of Drawing, Painting & Sculpture nyss.org, 8–14 W. Eighth St., 212-673-6466 (Walk 9)

New York University nyu.edu, 70 Washington Square S., 212-998-1212 (Walk 9)

The Paley Center for Media paleycenter.org, 25 W. 52nd St., 212-621-6600 (Walk 17)

PS 001 Alfred E. Smith tinyurl.com/ps001alfredesmith, 8 Henry St., 212-267-4133 (Walk 5)

PS 234 ps234.org, 292 Greenwich St., 212-233-6034 (Walk 2)

The Rockefeller University rockefeller.edu, 1230 York Ave., 212-327-8000 (Walk 23)

Schomburg Center for Research in Black Culture nypl.org/location/schomburg, 515 Malcolm X Blvd., 212-491-2200 (Walk 26)

Science, Industry and Business Library nypl.org/locations/sibl, 188 Madison Ave., 917-275-6975 (Walk 14)

Seward Park Library nypl.org/locations/seward-park, 192 E. Broadway, 212-477-6770 (Walk 6)

Seward Park High School Campus sewardparkhs.com, 350 Grand St., 212-673-2650 (Walk 6)

The Shabazz Center (Audubon Ballroom) theshabazzcenter.net, 3940 Broadway, 212-568-1341 (Walk 28)

Sony Wonder Technology Lab sonywondertechlab.com, 550 Madison Ave., 212-833-8100 (Walk 17)

Stuyvesant High School stuy.edu, 345 Chambers St., 212-312-4800 (Walk 2)

Ukrainian Institute of America ukrainianinstitute.org, 2 E. 79th St., 212-288-8660 (Walk 20)

Union Theological Seminary utsnyc.edu, 3041 Broadway, 212-662-7100 (Walk 24)

University Settlement at the Houston Street Center hsc.universitysettlement.org/hsc, 273 Bowery, 212-475-5008 (Walk 7)

Webster Library nypl.org/locations/webster, 1465 York Ave., 212-288-5049 (Walk 23)

enTerTainmenT, nightlife, and performing arTs

Angelika Film Center angelikafilmcenter.com/nyc, 18 W. Houston St., 212-995-2570 (Walk 9)

Apollo Theater apollotheater.org, 253 W. 125th St., 212-531-5300 (Walk 26)

Beacon Theatre beacontheatre.com, 2124 Broadway, 212-465-6500 (Walk 19)

Blue Note bluenote.net, 131 W. Third St., 212-475-8592 (Walk 9)

The Bowery Ballroom boweryballroom.com, 6 Delancey St., 212-260-4700 (Walk 7)

The Bowery Electric theboweryelectric.com, 327 Bowery, 212-228-0228 (Walk 8)

Cafe Wha? cafewha.com, 115 MacDougal St., 212-254-3706 (Walk 9)

Cherry Lane Theatre cherrylanetheatre.org, 38 Commerce St., 212-989-2020 (Walk 10)

Comedy Cellar comedycellar.com, 117 MacDougal St., 212-254-3480 (Walk 9)

Copacabana copacabanany.com, 268 W. 47th St., 212-221-2672 (Walk 16)

Don't Tell Mama donttellmamanyc.com, 343 W. 46th St., 212-757-0788 (Walk 16)

Ed Sullivan Theater edsullivan.com/ed-sullivan-theater, 1697 Broadway, 212-975-4755 (Walk 16)

Electric Lady Studios electricladystudios.com, 52 W. Eighth St., 212-677-1366 (Walk 9)

Film Forum filmforum.org, 209 W. Houston St., 212-727-8110 (Walk 10)

Groove clubgroovenyc.com, 128 W. Third St., 212-254-9393 (Walk 9)

Harlem Stage Gatehouse harlemstage.org, 150 Convent Ave., 212-281-9240 (Walk 27)

IFC Center ifccenter.com, 323 Sixth Ave., 212-924-7771 (Walk 10)

Irving Plaza irvingplaza.com, 17 Irving Place, 212-777-6800 (Walk 11)

Kraine Theater horsetrade.info, 85 E. Fourth St., 212-777-6088 (Walk 8)

La MaMa Experimental Theatre Club lamama.org, 74A E. Fourth St., 646-430-5374 (Walk 8)

(Le) Poisson Rouge lepoissonrouge.com, 158 Bleecker St., 212-505-FISH (3474) (Walk 9)

Lincoln Center for the Performing Arts lincolncenter.org, Columbus Avenue between West 62nd and West 65th Streets, 212-875-5456 (Walk 19)

Lucille Lortel Theatre lortel.org/llt_theater, 121 Christopher St., 212-924-2817 (Walk 10)

Madison Square Garden thegarden.com, 4 Penn Plaza, 212-465-6741 (Walk 14)

Manhattan Center mcstudios.com, 311 W. 34th St., 212-564-1072 (Walk 13)

Maysles Documentary Center and Cinema maysles.org/mdc, 343 Malcolm X Blvd., 212-537-6843 (Walk 26)

Mercury Lounge mercuryloungenyc.com, 217 E. Houston St., 212-260-4700 (Walk 8)

New York Theatre Workshop nytw.org, 79 E. Fourth St., 212-780-9037 (Walk 8)

Players Theatre theplayerstheater.com, 115 MacDougal St., 212-475-1449 (Walk 9)

The Pyramid Club thepyramidclub.com, 101 Ave. A, 212-228-4888 (Walk 8)

Radio City Music Hall radiocity.com, 1260 Sixth Ave., 212-465-6741 (Walks 16 and 17)

Rod Rodgers Dance Company rodrodgersdance.org, 62 E. Fourth St., 212-674-9066 (Walk 8)

SOB's sobs.com, 204 Varick St., 212-243-4940 (Walk 10)

The Stonewall Inn thestonewallinnyc.com, 53 Christopher St., 212-488-2705 (Walk 10)

Sunshine Cinema tinyurl.com/sunshinecinema, 143 E. Houston St., 212-260-7289 (Walk 8)

Theater for the New City theaterforthenewcity.net, 155 First Ave., 212-254-1109 (Walk 8)

Theatre 80 St. Mark's theatre80.wordpress.com, 80 St. Mark's Place, 212-388-0388 (Walk 8)

Times Square timessquarenyc.org, bounded by West 42nd Street, Broadway, Seventh Avenue, and West 47th Street (Walks 15 and 16)

Village Vanguard villagevanguard.com, 178 Seventh Ave. S., 212-255-4037 (Walk 10)

Flora and Fauna

Bogardus Garden bogardusgarden.org, bounded by Hudson Street, West Broadway, and Reade Street (Walk 2)

Central Park Zoo centralparkzoo.com, West 64th Street and Fifth Avenue, 212-439-6500 (Walk 22)

Elizabeth Street Garden elizabethstreetgarden.org, bounded by Mott, Elizabeth, Prince, and Spring Streets (Walk 7)

Inwood's North Cove nycwetlands.org, Ninth Avenue at the Harlem River (Walk 29)

Liz Christy Community Garden lizchristygarden.us, Bowery and Houston Street (Walk 8)

FOOD and DrINK

Alleva allevadairy.com, 188 Grand St., 212-226-7990 (Walk 7)

Amy Ruth's amyruths.com, 113 W. 116th St., 212-280-8779 (Walk 26)

Arturo's 106 W. Houston St., 212-677-3820 (Walk 9)

Beauty Bar thebeautybar.con, 231 E. 14th St., 212-539-1389 (Walk 11)

Ben's Pizzeria 123 MacDougal St., 212-677-0976 (Walk 9)

Big Gay Ice Cream biggayicecream.com, 125 E. Seventh St., 212-533-9333 (Walk 8)

Blue Water Grill bluewatergrillnyc.com, 31 Union Square W., 212-675-9500 (Walk 11)

Burp Castle burpcastlenyc.wordpress.com, 41 E. Seventh St., 212-982-4576 (Walk 8)

Caffè Reggio caffereggio.com, 119 MacDougal St., 212-475-9557 (Walk 9)

Caliente Cab Co. calientecabco.com, 61 Seventh Ave. S., #1, 212-243-8517 (Walk 10)

Caravan of Dreams caravanofdreams.net, 405 E. Sixth St., 212-254-1613 (Walk 8)

Dublin House dublinhousenyc.com, 225 W. 79th St., 212-874-9528 (Walk 19)

Dylan's Candy Bar dylanscandybar.com, 1011 Third Ave., 646-735-0078 (Walk 18)

Eataly eataly.com, 200 Fifth Ave., 212-229-2560 (Walk 12)

Economy Candy economycandy.com, 108 Rivington St., 212-254-1531 (Walk 6)

Ferrara ferraranyc.com, 195 Grand St., 212-226-6150 (Walk 7)

Fine & Schapiro fineandschapiro.com, 138 W. 72nd St., 212-877-2721 (Walk 19)

House of Vegetarian 68 Mott St., 212-226-6572 (Walk 5)

Houston Hall houstonhallny.com, 222 W. Houston St., 212-675-9323 (Walk 10)

The Hungarian Pastry Shop 1030 Amsterdam Ave., 212-866-4230 (Walk 24)

International Culinary Center/L'Ecole Restaurant lecolenyc.com, 462 Broadway, 212-219-3300 (Walk 7)

John's of Bleecker Street johnsbrickovenpizza.com, 278 Bleecker St., 212-243-1680 (Walk 10)

Katz's Delicatessen katzsdelicatessen.com, 205 E. Houston St., 212-254-2246 (Walk 8)

Koronet Pizza koronetpizzany.com, 2828 Broadway, 212-222-1566 (Walk 24)

Lindy's 825 Seventh Ave., 212-767-8343 (Walk 16)

Lombardi's Pizza firstpizza.com, 32 Spring St., 212-941-7994 (Walk 7)

Mamoun's Falafel mamouns.com, 119 MacDougal St., 212-674-8685 (Walk 9)

McNulty's mcnultys.com, 109 Christopher St., 212-242-5351 (Walk 10)

McSorley's Old Ale House 15 E. Seventh St., 212-473-9148 (Walk 8)

Minetta Tavern minettatavernny.com, 113 MacDougal St., 212-475-3850 (Walk 9)

Moishe's Bake Shop moishesbakeshop.com, 115 Second Ave., 212-505-8555 (Walk 8)

Momofuku Ko momofuku.com/new-york/ko, 8 Extra Place, 212-203-8095 (Walk 8)

Murray's Cheese Shop murrayscheese.com, 254 Bleecker St., 212-243-3289 (Walk 10)

Nom Wah Tea Parlor nomwah.com, 13 Doyers St., 212-962-6047 (Walk 5)

Old Homestead Steakhouse theoldhomesteadsteakhouse.com, 56 Ninth Ave., 212-242-9040 (Walk 12)

The Original Chinatown Ice Cream Factory chinatownicecreamfactory.com, 65 Bayard St., 212-608-4170 (Walk 5)

The Original Vincent's tinyurl.com/originalvincents, 119 Mott St., 212-226-8133 (Walk 5)

Parisi Bakery parisibakery.com, 198 Mott St., 212-226-6378 (Walk 7)

Pete's Tavern petestavern.com, 129 E. 18th St., 212-473-7676 (Walk 11)

Porto Rico Importing Co. portorico.com, 201 Bleecker St., 212-453-5908 (Walk 9)

Restaurant Row restaurantrownyc.com, West 46th Street between Eighth and Ninth Avenues (Walk 16)

Russ & Daughters russanddaughters.com, 179 E. Houston St., 212-475-4880 (Walk 8)

Sardi's sardis.com, 234 W. 44th St., 212-302-0865 (Walk 16)

Serendipity 3 serendipity3.com, 225 E. 60th St., 212-838-3531 (Walk 18)

Sylvia's Restaurant sylviasrestaurant.com, 328 Malcolm X Blvd., 212-996-0660 (Walk 26)

Tavern on the Green tavernonthegreen.com, West 67th Street and Central Park West, 212-877-8684 (Walks 21 and 22)

Tom's Restaurant tomsrestaurant.net, 2880 Broadway, 212-864-6137 (Walk 24)

Union Square Cafe unionsquarecafe.com, 21 E. 16th St., 212-243-4020 (Walk 11)

V&T Pizzeria vtpizzeriarestaurant.com, 1024 Amsterdam Ave., 212-666-8051 (Walk 24)

Yonah Schimmel Knish Bakery knishery.com, 137 E. Houston St., 212-477-2858 (Walk 8)

GOVErNMeNT INSTITUTIONS

Adam Clayton Powell Jr. State Office Building ogs.ny.gov/bu/ba/acp.asp, 163 W. 125th St. (Walk 26)

City Hall nyc.gov, City Hall Park, 212-639-9675 (Walks 4 and 5)

Federal Reserve Bank of New York ny.frb.org, 33 Liberty St., 212-720-5000 (Walk 3)

James A. Farley Building, US Post Office usps.com, 421 Eighth Ave., 212-330-3296 (Walk 14)

Manhattan Municipal Building manhattanbp.nyc.gov, 1 Centre St., 212-669-8300 (Walk 5)

New York State Supreme Court nycourts.gov, 60 Centre St., 646-386-3600 (Walk 5)

Surrogate's Court Building nycourts.gov/courts/1jd/surrogates, 31 Chambers St., 646-386-5000 (Walk 5)

Thurgood Marshall US Courthouse ca2.uscourts.gov, 40 Foley Square, 212-857-8500 (Walk 5)

United Nations visit.un.org, 405 E. 42nd St., 212-963-4475 (Walk 15)

HISTOrICAL LANDMArKS

Audubon Terrace audubonparkny.com, Broadway at West 155th and 156th Streets (Walk 28)

Castle Clinton nps.gov/cacl, Battery Park (Walk 1)

Dyckman Farmhouse Museum dyckmanfarmhouse.org, 4881 Broadway, 212-304-9422 (Walk 29)

FDNY Engine 55 363 Broome St. (Walk 7)

Federal Hall nps.gov/feha, 26 Wall St., 212-825-6990 (Walk 3)

Gracie Mansion tinyurl.com/graciemansion, East End Avenue and East 88th Street, 212-570-4751 (Walk 23)

Hamilton Grange National Memorial nps.gov/hagr, 414 W. 141st St., 646-548-2310 (Walk 27)

Little Red Lighthouse tinyurl.com/littleredlighthousenyc, Fort Washington Park/Hudson River Greenway, 212-408-0100 (Walk 29)

Morris-Jumel Mansion morrisjumel.org, 65 Jumel Terrace, 212-923-8008 (Walk 28)

St. Paul's Chapel trinitywallstreet.org/content/st-pauls-chapel, 209 Broadway, 212-602-0800 (Walk 4)

Sylvan Terrace Off Jumel Terrace between West 160th and West 162nd Streets (Walk 28)

The Arsenal tinyurl.com/arsenalcentralpark, East 64th Street and Fifth Avenue, 212-408-0100 (Walk 20)

Trinity Church trinitywallstreet.org, 74 Trinity Pl., 212-602-0800 (Walk 3)

HOTELS

The Bowery Hotel theboweryhotel.com, 335 Bowery, 212-505-9100 (Walk 8)

Carlton Hotel carltonhotelny.com, 88 Madison Ave., 212-532-4100 (Walk 14)

The Carlyle rosewoodhotels.com/carlyle, 35 E. 76th St., 212-744-1600 (Walk 18)

Dream Downtown dreamhotels.com/downtown, 355 W. 16th St., 212-229-2559 (Walk 12)

Hotel Chelsea *(reopens 2016)* chelseahotels.com, 222 W. 23rd St. (Walk 12)

Hotel Edison & Edison Ballroom edisonhotelnyc.com, 228 W. 47th St., 212-840-5000 (Walk 16)

The Knickerbocker Hotel theknickerbocker.com, 6 Times Square, 212-204-4980 (Walk 15)

Leo House leohousenyc.com, 332 W. 23rd St., 212-366-0100 (Walk 12)

The Lucerne Hotel thelucernehotel.com, 201 W. 79th St., 212-875-1000 (Walk 19)

The Maritime Hotel themaritimehotel.com, 363 W. 16th St., 212-242-4300 (Walk 12)

The Marlton Hotel (Marlton House) marltonhotel.com, 5 W. Eighth St., 212-321-0100 (Walk 9)

Nolitan Hotel nolitanhotel.com, 30 Kenmare St., 212-925-2555 (Walk 7)

The Peninsula New York newyork.peninsula.com, 700 Fifth Ave., 212-956-2888 (Walk 17)

The Plaza Hotel theplazany.com, 768 Fifth Ave., 212-759-3000 (Walk 20)

The St. Regis New York stregisnewyork.com, 2 E. 55th St., 212-753-4500 (Walk 17)

The Standard High Line standardhotels.com/high-line, 848 Washington St., 212-645-4646 (Walk 13)

Wyndham New Yorker Hotel newyorkerhotel.com, 481 Eighth Ave., 212-971-0101 (Walk 13)

Medical Centers

Lenox Hill Hospital lenoxhillhospital.org, 100 E. 77th St., 212-434-2000 (Walk 18)

New York-Presbyterian Weill Cornell Medical Center nyp.org/facilities/weillcornell.html, York Avenue between East 70th and East 68th Streets, 212-746-5454 (Walk 23)

Memorials and Monuments

African Burial Ground National Monument nps.gov/afbg, 290 Broadway, 212-637-2019 (Walk 5)

Columbus Circle tinyurl.com/columbuscirclenyc, West 59th Street and Central Park West (Walk 21)

Duffy Square nycgovparks.org/parks/father-duffy-square/history, West 46th Street at Broadway (Walk 16)

Duke Ellington Circle tinyurl.com/dukeellingtoncircle, East 110th Street and Fifth Avenue (Walk 25)

FDNY Memorial Wall fdnytenhouse.com/fdnywall, 124 Liberty St. (Walk 3)

Frederick Douglass Circle tinyurl.com/frederickdouglassmemorial, Central Park West and Central Park North (Walks 21 and 25)

General Worth Square nycgovparks.org/parks/worth-square, Fifth Avenue at West 23rd Street (Walk 12)

Grant's Tomb nps.gov/gegr, West 122nd Street and Riverside Drive, 212-666-1640 (Walk 24)

Greeley Square nycgovparks.org/parks/greeley-square-park, bounded by Broadway, Sixth Avenue, and West 32nd Street (Walk 14)

Irish Hunger Memorial bpcparks.org/whats-here/parks/irish-hunger-memorial, Vesey Street and North End Avenue, 212-267-9700 (Walk 2)

Kimlau Square nycgovparks.org/parks/kimlau-square, bounded by Park Row/Chatham Square/Bowery, Oliver Street, and East Broadway (Walk 5)

McCarthy Square nycgovparks.org/parks/mccarthy-square, bounded by Seventh Avenue South, Charles Street, and Waverly Place (Walk 10)

McKenna Square nycgovparks.org/parks/mckenna-square, West 165th Street between Audubon and Amsterdam Avenues (Walk 28)

Mitchel Square Park nycgovparks.org/parks/mitchel-square, bounded by Broadway, St. Nicholas Avenue, West 166th Street, and West 167th Street (Walk 28)

9/11 Memorial (National September 11 Memorial & Museum) 911memorial.org, 180 Greenwich St., 212-266-5211 (Walk 3)

9/11 Tribute Center tributewtc.org, 120 Liberty St., 212-393-9160 (Walk 3)

Straus Square nycgovparks.org/parks/straus-square, bounded by Canal Street, Rutgers Street, and East Broadway (Walk 6)

Stuyvesant Square nycgovparks.org/parks/stuyvesant-square, Second Avenue between East 15th and East 17th Streets (Walk 11)

Titanic Memorial Park Fulton Street between Pearl and Water Streets (Walk 4)

Verdi Square nycgovparks.org/parks/verdi-square, bounded by Broadway, Amsterdam Avenue, West 72nd Street, and West 73rd Street (Walk 19)

MUSEUMS, GALLERIES, AND PUBLIC ART

American Museum of Natural History amnh.org, Central Park West and West 79th Street, 212-769-5100 (Walk 21)

Artifact artifactnyc.net, 84 Orchard St., 212-475-0448 (Walk 6)

Brennan & Griffin brennangriffin.com, 55 Delancey St., 212-227-0115 (Walk 6)

Charging Bull **Statue** chargingbull.com, Broadway and Morris Street (Walk 1)

The Cloisters metmuseum.org/visit/visit-the-cloisters, Fort Tryon Park, 212-923-3700 (Walk 29)

Cooper Hewitt, Smithsonian Design Museum cooperhewitt.org, 2 E. 91st St., 212-849-8400 (Walk 20)

Cuchifritos Gallery + Project Space artistsallianceinc.org, 120 Essex St. (Walk 6)

Eldridge Street Synagogue and Museum eldridgestreet.org, 12 Eldridge St., 212-219-0888 (Walk 6)

4th Street Photo Gallery tinyurl.com/4thstreetphotogallery, 67 E. Fourth St., 212-673-1021 (Walk 8)

The Frick Collection frick.org, 1 E. 70th St., 212-288-0700 (Walk 20)

Garis & Hahn garisandhahn.com, 263 Bowery, 212-228-8457 (Walk 7)

Grey Art Gallery of NYU nyu.edu/greyart, 100 Washington Square E., 212-998-6780 (Walk 9)

Guggenheim Museum guggenheim.org, 1071 Fifth Ave., 212-423-3500 (Walk 20)

Hester Street Collaborative/Leroy Street Studio hesterstreet.org, 113 Hester St., 917-265-8591 (Walk 6)

International Center of Photography icp.org, 1133 Sixth Ave., 212-857-0000 (Walk 16)

Intrepid Sea, Air & Space Museum intrepidmuseum.org, Pier 86 (West 46th Street and 12th Avenue), 212-245-0072 (Walk 15)

Italian American Museum italianamericanmuseum.org, 155 Mulberry St., 212-965-9000 (Walk 7)

James Fuentes jamesfuentes.com, 55 Delancey St., 212-577-1201 (Walk 6)

Jewish Museum thejewishmuseum.org, 1109 Fifth Ave., 212-423-3200 (Walk 20)

Judith Charles Gallery judithcharlesgallery.com, 196 Bowery, 212-219-4095 (Walk 7)

LMAK Projects lmakprojects.com, 139 Eldridge St., 212-255-9707 (Walk 6)

Louise Nevelson Plaza Bounded by William Street, Maiden Lane, and Liberty Street (Walk 3)

Martin Lane Gallery of Historical Americana historyonhand.com, 205 W. Houston St., 212-206-1004 (Walk 10)

Metropolitan Museum of Art metmuseum.org, 1000 Fifth Ave., 212-535-7710 (Walk 20)

Milton Resnick and Pat Passlof Foundation resnickpasslof.org, 87 Eldridge St., 212-226-1259 (Walk 6)

The Morgan Library & Museum themorgan.org, 225 Madison Ave., 212-685-0008 (Walk 14)

Museum of American Finance mcaf.org, 48 Wall St., 212-908-4110 (Walk 3)

Museum of Modern Art moma.org, 11 W. 53rd St., 212-708-9400 (Walk 17)

National Academy Museum nationalacademy.org, 1083 Fifth Ave., 212-369-4880 (Walk 20)

National Museum of the American Indian/US Custom House nmai.si.edu, 1 Bowling Green, 212-514-3700 (Walk 1)

Neue Galerie New York neuegalerie.org, 1048 Fifth Ave., 212-628-6200 (Walk 20)

New Museum newmuseum.org, 235 Bowery, 212-219-1222 (Walk 7)

New-York Historical Society nyhistory.org, 170 Central Park W., 212-873-3400 (Walk 21)

PS122 Gallery ps122gallery.org, 150 First Ave., 212-477-5829 (Walk 8)

Renee and Chaim Gross Foundation rcgrossfoundation.org, 526 LaGuardia Place, 212-529-4906 (Walk 9)

Shin Gallery shin-gallery.com, 322 Grand St., 212-375-1735 (Walk 6)

Soho Contemporary Art sohocontemporaryart.com, 259 Bowery, 646-719-1316 (Walk 7)

Sotheby's sothebys.com, 1334 York Ave., 212-606-7000 (Walk 23)

South Street Seaport Museum southstreetseaportmuseum.org, 12 Fulton St., 212-748-8600 (Walk 4)

Sperone Westwater speronewestwater.com, 257 Bowery, 212-999-7337 (Walk 7)

Tenement Museum tenement.org, 103 Orchard St., 212-982-8420 (Walk 6)

White Columns whitecolumns.org, 320 W. 13th St. (Horatio at West Fourth), 212-924-4212 (Walk 13)

Whitney Museum of American Art whitney.org, 99 Gansevoort St., 212-570-3600 (Walk 13)

Woodward Gallery woodwardgallery.net, 133 Eldridge St., 212-966-3411 (Walk 6)

NOTABLE STRUCTURES

The Ansonia ansoniarealty.com, 2019 Broadway, 212-877-9800 (Walk 19)

The Beresford 211 Central Park W. (Walk 21)

Broadway Bridge tinyurl.com/broadwaybridge, Broadway between West 220th and West 225th Streets (Walk 30)

Capitale (Old Bowery Savings Bank) capitaleny.com, 130 Bowery, 212-334-5500 (Walk 7)

The Cherokee cherokee-nyc.com, East 77th to East 78th Street east of York Avenue (Walk 23)

Chrysler Building tishmanspeyer.com/properties/chrysler-center, 405 Lexington Ave., 212-682-3070 (Walk 15)

Daily News **Building** 220 E. 42nd St. (Walk 15)

The Dakota 1 W. 72nd St. (Walk 21)

The Dorilton 171 W. 71st St. (Walk 19)

The El Dorado 300 Central Park W. (Walk 21)

Empire State Building esbnyc.com, 350 Fifth Ave., 212-736-3100 (Walk 14)

Flatiron Building 175 Fifth Ave. (Walk 12)

The San Remo 145 Central Park W. (Walk 21)

Forward **Building** 175 E. Broadway (Walk 6)

455 Central Park West Central Park West between West 105th and 106th Streets (Walk 21)

Ghostbusters **Building** 55 Central Park W. (Walk 21)

Grand Central Terminal grandcentralterminal.com, 89 E. 42nd St., 212-340-2583 (Walk 15)

1 World Trade Center onewtc.com, bounded by West, Vesey, Fulton, and Washington Streets (Walk 3)

London Terrace Apartments Bounded by 9th and 10th Avenues and West 23rd and 24th Streets (Walk 12)

Rockefeller Center rockefellercenter.com, Fifth Avenue between West 48th and West 50th Streets, 212-332-6868 (Walk 17)

Trump Tower trumptower.com, 725 Fifth Ave., 212-832-2000 (Walk 17)

Tudor City tudorcity.com, bounded by East 40th and East 43rd Streets and First and Second Avenues, 212-949-6555 (Walk 15)

University Heights Bridge nycroads.com/crossings/university-heights, West 207th Street and Ninth Avenue (Walk 29)

Woolworth Building woolworthtours.com, 233 Broadway, 203-966-9663 (Walk 4)

Parks and Playgrounds

Ancient Playground tinyurl.com/ancientplayground, East 84th Street and Fifth Avenue (Walk 20)

Augustus Saint-Gaudens Playground nycgovparks.org/parks/augustus-st-gaudens-playground, Second Avenue between East 19th and East 20th Streets (Walk 11)

Battery Park nycgovparks.org/parks/battery-park, State Street and Battery Place

Bowling Green nycgovparks.org/parks/bowling-green, Broadway and Whitehall Street

Bryant Park bryantpark.org, West 42nd Street and Sixth Avenue, 212-768-4242 (Walk 15)

Captain Jacob Joseph Playground Henry Street at Rutgers Street (Walk 6)

Carl Schurz Park carlschurzparknyc.org, East End Avenue between East 90th and East 84th Streets, 212-459-4455 (Walk 23)

Central Park centralparknyc.org, bounded by Fifth Avenue, Central Park South/West 59th Street, Central Park West, and Central Park North/West 110th Street, 212-310-6600 (Walk 22)

Christopher Park nycgovparks.org/parks/christopher-park, Christopher Street at Seventh Avenue South (Walk 10)

City Hall Park nycgovparks.org/parks/city-hall-park, Broadway and Park Row at Barclay Street, 212-639-9675 (Walks 4 and 5)

Coenties Slip Park Between Water and Pearl Streets (Walk 1)

Columbus Park nycgovparks.org/parks/columbus-park-m015, bounded by Mulberry Street, Baxter Street, Worth Street, and Bayard Street (Walk 5)

Dr. Gertrude B. Kelly Playground nycgovparks.org/parks/dr-gertrude-b-kelly-playground, bounded by West 16th Street, West 17th Street, Eighth Avenue, and Ninth Avenue (Walk 12)

Duane Park nycgovparks.org/parks/duane-park, between Duane and Hudson Streets (Walk 2)

Fort Tryon Park forttryonparktrust.org, Broadway at Dyckman Street, 212-795-1388 (Walk 29)

Gramercy Park Irving Place at East 20th Street (Walk 11)

Herald Square 34thstreet.org, bounded by Broadway, Sixth Avenue, and West 34th Street (Walk 14)

High Line Park thehighline.org, Gansevoort Street to West 34th Street west of 10th Avenue, 212-500-6035 (Walks 12 and 13)

Highbridge Park nycgovparks.org/parks/highbridge-park, Edgecombe Avenue between West 155th and Dyckman Streets (Walk 28)

Imagination Playground Bounded by John Street, Front Street, and South Street (Walk 4)

Inwood Hill Park nycgovparks.org/parks/inwood-hill-park, West 218th Street at Indian Road, 212-639-9675 (Walk 30)

Isham Park nycgovparks.org/parks/isham-park, bounded by Isham Street, Broadway, Seaman Avenue, and Indian Road (Walk 30)

Jackson Square nycgovparks.org/parks/jackson-square, Eighth Avenue at Greenwich Avenue (Walk 10)

James J. Walker Park nycgovparks.org/parks/james-j-walker-park, Hudson Street at Clarkson Street (Walk 10)

John Jay Park nycgovparks.org/parks/john-jay-park-and-pool, East 76th Street near FDR Drive, 212-794-6566 (Walk 23)

John J. Delury Sr. Plaza Fulton Street between Gold Street and Ryders Alley (Walk 4)

Madison Square Park madisonsquarepark.org, Madison Avenue at East 23rd Street, 212-538-1884 (Walk 12)

Marcus Garvey Park nycgovparks.org/parks/marcus-garvey-park, Mount Morris Park West between West 120th and West 124th Streets (Walk 26)

Morningside Park nycgovparks.org/parks/morningside-park, Manhattan Avenue/Morningside Avenue between West 110th and West 123rd Streets (Walks 24 and 25)

Nelson A. Rockefeller Park River Terrace between Vesey and Chambers Streets (Walk 2)

Pearl Street Playground Fulton and Pearl Streets (Walk 4)

Riverside Park riversideparknyc.org, Riverside Drive between West 72nd Street and St. Clair Place, 212-870-3070 (Walk 24)

Sakura Park nycgovparks.org/parks/sakura-park, Riverside Drive and West 122nd Street (Walk 24)

Seward Park nycgovparks.org/parks/seward-park, bounded by Canal Street, Essex Street, Jefferson Street, and East Broadway (Walk 6)

Silverstein Family Park 7 World Trade Center, bounded by Greenwich Street, West Broadway, and Barclay Street (Walk 2)

Tramway Plaza (Roosevelt Island Tram) East 59th Street at Second Avenue (Walk 18)

Union Square Park nycgovparks.org/parks/union-square-park, East 14th Street at Broadway (Walk 11)

Washington Market Park washingtonmarketpark.org, Greenwich Street between Chambers and Duane Streets (Walk 2)

Washington Square Park nycgovparks.org/parks/washington-square-park, bounded by Waverly Place, University Place, West Fourth Street, and MacDougal Street (Walk 9)

Zuccotti Park Broadway at Liberty Street (Walk 3)

SHOPPING

American Girl Place americangirl.com/retailstore/new-york, 609 Fifth Ave., 877-247-5223 (Walk 17)

B&H bhphotovideo.com, 420 Ninth Ave., 212-444-6615 (Walk 13)

Bergdorf Goodman bergdorfgoodman.com, 754 Fifth Ave., 212-753-7300 (Walk 17)

Block Drug Stores blockdrugstores.com, 101 Second Ave., 212-473-1587 (Walk 8)

Bloomingdale's bloomingdales.com, East 59th Street at Lexington Avenue, 212-705-2000 (Walk 18)

Chelsea Market chelseamarket.com, 75 Ninth Ave., 212-652-2110 (Walk 12)

Diamond District diamonddistrict.org, West 47th Street between Fifth and Sixth Avenues, 212-302-5739 (Walks 16 and 17)

Essex Street Market essexstreetmarket.com, 120 Essex St., 212-312-3603 (Walk 6)

House of Oldies houseofoldies.com, 35 Carmine St., 212-243-0500 (Walk 10)

Jack's 99 Cent Store jacksnyc.com, 115 W. 31st St., 212-268-9962 (Walk 14)

Lord & Taylor lordandtaylor.com, 424 Fifth Ave., 212-391-3344 (Walk 14)

9/11 Memorial Museum Store tinyurl.com/911museumstore, 20 Vesey St., 212-267-2047 (Walk 4)

Kelly Guitars kellyguitars.com, 42 Carmine St., 212-691-8400 (Walk 10)

Limelight Shops limelightshops.com, 656 Sixth Ave., 212-255-2144 (Walk 12)

Macy's Herald Square tinyurl.com/macysheraldsquare, 151 W. 34th St., 212-695-4400 (Walk 14)

Malcolm Shabazz Harlem Market 52 W. 116th St., 212-987-8131 (Walk 26)

Mikimoto mikimotoamerica.com, 730 Fifth Ave., 212-457-4600 (Walk 17)

Music Inn musicinn.nyc, 169 W. Fourth St., 212-243-5715 (Walk 10)

St. Mark's Bookshop stmarksbookshop.com, 136 E. Third St., 212-260-7853 (Walk 8)

Saks Fifth Avenue saksfifthavenue.com, 611 Fifth Ave., 212-753-4000 (Walk 17)

South Street Seaport southstreetseaport.com, Fulton Street and South Street, 212-732-8257 (Walk 4)

Three Lives & Company threelives.com, 154 W. 10th St., 212-741-2069 (Walk 10)

Tiffany & Co. tiffany.com, 727 Fifth Ave., 212-755-8000 (Walk 17)

Time Warner Center theshopsatcolumbuscircle.com, 10 Columbus Circle, 212-823-6300 (Walks 19 and 21)

Trash and Vaudeville trashandvaudeville.com, 4 St. Mark's Place, 212-982-3590 (Walk 8)

Van Cleef & Arpels vancleefarpels.com, 744 Fifth Ave., 212-896-9284 (Walk 17)

World Financial Center/Brookfield Place brookfieldplaceny.com, 200 Vesey St., 212-417-7000 (Walk 2)

SPiriTualiTY

All Saints Episcopal Church allsaintsnyc.org, 230 E. 60th St., 212-758-0447 (Walk 18)

Baptist Temple Church 20 W. 116th St., 212-996-0334 (Walk 26)

The Basilica of St. Patrick's Old Cathedral oldcathedral.org, 263 Mulberry St., 212-226-8075 (Walk 7)

Broadway Presbyterian Church bpcnyc.org, 601 W. 114th St., 212-864-6100 (Walk 24)

Brotherhood Synagogue brotherhoodsynagogue.org, 28 Gramercy Park S., 212-674-5750 (Walk 11)

Cathedral of St. John the Divine stjohndivine.org, 1047 Amsterdam Ave., 212-316-7540 (Walk 24)

Central Synagogue centralsynagogue.org, 652 Lexington Ave., 212-838-5122 (Walk 17)

Chinese United Methodist Church cumc-nyc.org, 69 Madison St., 212-267-6464 (Walk 5)

Church of St. Francis of Assisi stfrancisnyc.org, 135 W. 31st St., 212-736-8500 (Walk 14)

Church of St. Francis Xavier sfxavier.org, 46 W. 16th St., 212-627-2100 (Walk 12)

Church of St. Joseph of the Holy Family stjosephoftheholyfamily.org, 405 W. 125th St., 212-662-9125 (Walk 25)

Church of St. Luke in the Fields stlukeinthefields.org, 487 Hudson St., 212-924-0562 (Walk 10)

Church of St. Mary the Virgin stmvirgin.org, 145 W. 46th St., 212-869-5830 (Walk 16)

Church of St. Paul the Apostle stpaultheapostle.org, 405 W. 59th St., 212-265-3495 (Walk 19)

Church of St. Vincent Ferrer csvf.org, 869 Lexington Ave., 212-744-2080 (Walk 18)

Church of Sweden New York svenskakyrken.se/newyork, 5 E. 48th St., 212-832-8443 (Walk 17)

Church of the Annunciation theannunciation.net, 88 Convent Ave., 212-234-1919 (Walk 27)

Church of the Ascension ascensionnyc.org, Fifth Avenue and West Tenth Street, 212-254-8620 (Walk 9)

Church of the Blessed Sacrament 152 W. 71st St., 212-877-3111 (Walk 19)

Church of the Epiphany epiphanynyc.org, 1393 York Ave., 212-737-2720 (Walk 23)

Church of the Good Shepherd goodshepherdnyc.org, 4967 Broadway, 212-567-1300 (Walk 29)

Church of the Guardian Angel guardianangelchurch-nyc.org, 193 10th Ave., 212-929-5966 (Walk 12)

Church of the Intercession intercessionnyc.org, 550 W. 155th St., 212-283-6200 (Walk 28)

Church of the Lord Jesus Christ of the Apostolic Faith tcljc.com, 1421 Fifth Ave., 212-369-3037 (Walk 26)

Church of the Master pcusa.org/congregations/5643, 81 Morningside Ave., 212-666-8200 (Walk 25)

Church of the Most Precious Blood tinyurl.com/mostpreciousblood, 109 Mulberry St., 212-226-6427 (Walk 5)

Church of the Transfiguration transfigurationnyc.org, 29 Mott St., 212-962-5157 (Walk 5)

The Church of the Transfiguration littlechurch.org, 1 E. 29th St., 212-684-6770 (Walk 14)

Congregation Ramath Orah ramathorah.org, 550 W. 110th St., 212-222-2470 (Walk 24)

Congregation Shearith Israel shearithisrael.org, 2 W. 70th St., 212-873-0300 (Walk 21)

Convent Avenue Baptist Church conventchurch.org, 420 W. 145th St., 212-234-6767 (Walk 27)

Eldridge Street Synagogue and Museum eldridgestreet.org, 12 Eldridge St., 212-219-0888 (Walk 6)

Episcopal Church of the Crucifixion churchofthecrucifixion.org, 459 W. 149th St., 212-281-0900 (Walk 27)

The Episcopal Church of the Heavenly Rest heavenlyrest.org, 2 East 90th St., 212-289-3400 (Walk 20)

Episcopal Church of the Incarnation churchoftheincarnation.org, 209 Madison Ave., 212-689-6350 (Walk 14)

Fifth Avenue Presbyterian Church fapc.org, 7 W. 55th St., 212-247-0490 (Walk 17)

First Baptist Church firstnyc.org, 265 W. 79th St., 212-724-5600 (Walk 19)

First Church of Christ, Scientist firstchristiansciencechurchnyc.com, 10 W. 68th St., 212-877-6100 (Walk 21)

First Corinthian Baptist Church fcbnyc.org, 1912 Adam Clayton Powell Jr. Blvd., 212-864-5976 (Walk 26)

Fourth Universalist Society 4thu.org, 160 Central Park W., 212-595-1658 (Walk 21)

Holy Cross Church 329 W. 42nd St., 212-246-4732 (Walk 15)

Holy Trinity Lutheran Church holytrinitynyc.org, 3 W. 65th St., 212-877-6815 (Walk 21)

John Street Church johnstreetchurch.org, 44 John St., 212-269-0014 (Walk 4)

Kehila Kedosha Janina Synagogue and Museum kkjsm.org, 280 Broome St., 212-431-1619 (Walk 6)

Lincoln Square Synagogue lss.org, 180 Amsterdam Ave., 212-874-6100 (Walk 19)

Madison Avenue Baptist Church mabcnyc.org, 30 E. 30th St., 212-685-1377 (Walk 14)

Madison Avenue Presbyterian Church mapc.com, 921 Madison Ave., 212-288-8920 (Walk 18)

Mahayana Temple Buddhist Association mahayana.us, 113 Canal St., 212-925-8787 (Walk 5)

Malcolm Shabazz Mosque masjidmalcolmshabazz.com, 102 W. 116th St., 212-662-2200 (Walk 26)

Marble Collegiate Church marblechurch.org, 1 W. 29th St., 212-686-2770 (Walk 14)

Middle Collegiate Church middlechurch.org, 112 Second Ave., 212-477-0666 (Walk 8)

Mount Morris–Ascension Presbyterian Church pcusa.org/congregations/10770, 16–20 Mt. Morris Park W., 212-831-6800 (Walk 26)

Mount Washington Presbyterian Church 84 Vermilyea Ave., 212-567-0442 (Walk 29)

Mount Zion Evangelical Lutheran Church 421 W. 145th St., 212-862-8680 (Walk 27)

The National Shrine of St. Elizabeth Ann Seton setonheritage.org, 7 State St., 212-269-6865 (Walk 1)

New York Society for Ethical Culture nysec.org, 2 W. 64th St., 212-874-5210 (Walk 21)

Old Broadway Synagogue oldbroadwaysynagogue.blogspot.com, 15 Old Broadway, 212-662-9767 (Walk 27)

Orthodox Cathedral of the Holy Virgin Protection nycathedral.org, 59 E. Second St., 212-677-4664 (Walk 8)

Our Lady of Guadalupe at St. Bernard's 328 W. 14th St., 212-243-0265 (Walk 12)

Our Lady of Pompeii Church ourladyofpompeiinyc.com, 25 Carmine St., 212-989-6805 (Walk 10)

Park East Synagogue parkeastsynagogue.org, 163 E. 67th St., 212-737-6900 (Walk 18)

The Riverside Church theriversidechurchny.org, 490 Riverside Drive, 212-870-6700 (Walk 24)

St. Barbara Greek Orthodox Church stbarbaragoc.com, 27 Forsyth St., 212-226-0499 (Walk 6)

St. George Ukrainian Catholic Church stgeorgeukrainianchurch.org, 30 E. Seventh St., 212-674-1615 (Walk 8)

St. James' Church stjames.org, 865 Madison Ave., 212-774-4200 (Walk 18)

St. John's Lutheran Church stjohnsnyc.org, 81 Christopher St., 212-242-5737 (Walk 10)

St. Luke's Lutheran Church & St. Luke's Theatre stlukesnyc.org/stlukestheatre.com, 308 W. 46th St., 212-246-3540 (church), 212-246-8140 (theater) (Walk 16)

St. Mark's Church-in-the-Bowery stmarksbowery.org, 131 E. 10th St., 212-674-6377 (Walk 8)

St. Mary's Catholic Church of the Byzantine Rite stmarysbyzantinenyc.com, 246 E. 15th St., 212-677-0516 (Walk 11)

St. Patrick's Cathedral saintpatrickscathedral.org, Fifth Avenue at East 50th Street, 212-753-2261 (Walk 17)

St. Peter's Church saintpeters.org, 619 Lexington Ave., 212-935-2200 (Walk 17)

St. Peter's Roman Catholic Church stpetersnyc.org, 22 Barclay St., 212-233-8355 (Walk 4)

St. Rose of Lima Church stroseoflimachurchnyc.org, 510 W. 165th St., 212-568-0091 (Walk 28)

St. Stephen's United Methodist Church 146 W. 228th St., 718-562-8692 (Walk 30)

St. Thomas Episcopal Church saintthomaschurch.org, 1 W. 53rd St., 212-757-7013 (Walk 17)

Salvation and Deliverance Church salvationdeliverancehq.org, 37 W. 116th St., 212-722-5488 (Walk 26)

Shrine Church of St. Anthony of Padua stanthonynyc.org, 155 Sullivan St., 212-777-2755 (Walk 9)

Sixth Street Community Synagogue sixthstreetsynagogue.org, 325 E. Sixth St., 212-473-3665 (Walk 8)

Sung Tak Buddhist Association (Congregation B'nai Israel Kalwarie) 13 Pike St., 212-513-0230 (Walk 6)

Temple Emanu-El emanuelnyc.org, 1 E. 65th St., 212-744-1400 (Walk 20)

Trinity Baptist Church tbcny.org, 250 E. 61st St., 212-838-6844 (Walk 18)

West End Synagogue westendsynagogue.org, 190 Amsterdam Ave., 212-579-0777 (Walk 19)

Sports and Recreation

Armory Track/National Track and Field Hall of Fame armorytrack.com, 216 Fort Washington Ave., 212-923-1803 (Walk 28)

Asphalt Green asphaltgreen.org, 555 E. 90th St., 212-369-8890 (Walk 23)

Baker Athletics Complex, Columbia University gocolumbialions.com, 533 W. 218th St., 889-546-6711 (Walk 30)

Lucky Strike bowlluckystrike.com, 624–660 W. 42nd St., 646-829-0170 (Walk 15)

Tony Dapolito Recreation Center nycgovparks.org/facilities/recreationcenters/M103, Clarkson Street at Seventh Avenue South, 212-242-5418 (Walk 10)

Miscellaneous

The Alhambra Ballroom alhambraballroom.net, 2116 Adam Clayton Powell Jr. Blvd., 212-222-6940 (Walk 26)

The Bowery Mission bowery.org, 227 Bowery, 212-674-3456 (Walk 7)

Circle Line circleline42.com, Pier 83 (West 42nd Street and 12th Avenue), 212-563-3200 (Walk 15)

New York Amsterdam News amsterdamnews.com, 2340 Frederick Douglass Blvd., 212-932-7400 (Walk 26)

New York Stock Exchange nyse.com, 18 Broad St., 212-656-3000 (Walk 3)

125th Street 1 Subway Station West 125th Street at Broadway (Walk 27)

Port Authority Bus Terminal tinyurl.com/portauthoritynyc, 625 Eighth Ave., 212-502-2200 (Walk 15)

207th Street A Station tinyurl.com/207thstsubway, Broadway at Isham Street (Walk 30)

Whitehall Terminal, Staten Island Ferry siferrry.com, 212-344-7220 (Walk 1)

Appendix 3: BIBLIOGRAPHY

BOOKS

Cragoe, Carol Davidson. *How to Read Buildings*. New York: Rizzoli, 2008.

Cudahy, Brian J. *Under the Sidewalks of New York*. Fordham University Press, 1995.

Dunlap, David. *From Abyssinian to Zion: A Guide to Manhattan's Houses of Worship*. New York: Columbia University Press, 2004.

Fischler, Stan. *The Subway and the City*. New York: Frank Merriwell, 2004.

Helmreich, William B. *The New York Nobody Knows*. New York: Princeton University Press, 2013.

Hermes, Will. *Love Goes to Buildings on Fire: Five Years in New York That Changed Music Forever*. New York: Faber and Faber, 2011.

Homberger, Eric. *The Historical Atlas of New York City*. New York: Henry Holt and Company, 1994.

Jackson, Kenneth T., ed. *The Encyclopedia of New York City*. New Haven: Yale University Press, 1995.

Jump, Frank. *Fading Ads of New York City*. Mount Pleasant: The History Press, 2011.

Sasek, Miroslav. *This Is New York*. 1960. New York: Universe, 2007.

Walsh, Kevin. *Forgotten New York*. New York: Collins Reference, 2006.

White, Norval, and Elliot Willensky with Fran Leadon. *AIA Guide to New York City,* 5th ed. New York: Oxford University Press, 2010.

WEBSITES AND BLOGS

City of New York nyc.gov

Corcoran Group Real Estate corcoran.com

(continued)

Curbed NY ny.curbed.com

Daytonian in Manhattan daytoninmanhattan.blogspot.com

Downtown Express downtownexpress.com

Ephemeral New York ephemeralnewyork.wordpress.com

EV Grieve evgrieve.com

Forgotten New York forgotten-ny.com

New York City Department of Buildings nyc.gov/html/dob

New York City Department of Education schools.nyc.gov

New York City Department of Finance www1.nyc.gov/site/finance

New York City Department of Parks and Recreation nycgovparks.org

The New York City Organ Project nycago.org/organs/nyc

New York *Daily News* Archives nydailynews.com/archives

***New York* magazine** nymag.com

New York Songlines nysonglines.com

***The New York Times* Archives** nytimes.com/archives

***The New Yorker* Archive** newyorker.com/archive

NYC & Company nycgo.com

Realtor.com realtor.com

StreetEasy streeteasy.com

Time Out New York timeout.com/newyork

Trulia trulia.com

Wikipedia wikipedia.org

Zillow zillow.com

INDEX

Page references followed by *m* indicate a map; followed by *fig* indicate a photograph.

M *(continued)*

Manhattan walking tours *(continued)*
  Marble Hill and Inwood Hill Park, 276m–281
  Morningside Heights, 222m–233fig
  Rockefeller Center, 158m–167fig
  safety and comfort tips for the, 1, 3
  Times Square/Theater District, 146m–157fig
  Union Square, Gramercy Park, Stuyvesant Square, 100m–107fig
  Upper West Side, 176m–185fig
  Wall Street/Financial District, 18m–23fig
  Washington Heights, 260m–267fig
  West Village, 90m–99fig
  Yorkville, 214m–221fig
Manilow, Barry, 152
Manny's Music, 153
Marble Collegiate Church, 129, 133
Marble Hill and Inwood Hill Park
  walking tour
  map of the, 276m
  overview of the, 277–280
  points of interest, 280
  route summary and connecting the walks, 281
Marble Hill Playground, 278
Marcus Garvey Park (a.k.a. Mount Morris Park), 245, 249
Mariner's Gate (Central Park), 201
Mariners' Temple Baptist Church, 39
The Maritime Hotel, 111, 117
The Mark (luxury hotel), 190
The Marlton Hotel (Marlton House), 87
Marquis de Lafayette and George Washington statue (Lafayette Square), 239
Marquis de Lafayette statue (Union Square Park), 103
Marriott Marquis hotel, 148
Martin Lane Gallery of Historical Americana, 91, 97
Martin Luther King Jr. Educational Campus, 180

Mary House, 69
Masonic Hall, 115
Matt Umanov Guitars, 93
Mayne, Thom, 70
Maysles Documentary Center and Cinema, 248, 250
Mean Streets (film), 58
Meatpacking District, 110
Memorial Sloan-Kettering Cancer Center, 203, 218
Mercury Lounge, 75
Mercury statue, 139
Mesivtha Tifereth Jerusalem, 46
MetLife Building, 164
Metro North, 235
Metro North commuter railroad, 243, 277, 278
Metropolitan Museum of Art, 66, 187, 190, 191
Metropolitan Opera House, 180
Meyer Hall (NYU), 82
Middle Collegiate Church, 72, 76
Midtown
  Lower Midtown/Garment District walking tour, 126m–135fig
  Midtown South, 126m–127
  Rockefeller Center walking tour, 158m–167fig
  Times Square/Theater District walking tour, 146m–157fig
Midtown South, 126m–127
Mikimoto, 165, 166
Milan House, 172
Millennium Broadway Hotel, 150
Milligan Place, 85
Milstein Hospital Building, 261
Milton Resnick and Pat Passlof Foundation (art gallery), 49, 52
Minetta Tavern, 82, 86
Minskoff theater, 151
Minuit, Peter, 279
Mitchel, John P., 262
Mitchel Square Park, 262, 266
Modest Rudy's Music Stop, 153
Moishe's Bake Shop, 72, 76

Momofuku Ko (restaurant), 67, 75
Mongolian Mission to the UN, 190
Monroe, James, 68
Moore, Clement Clarke, 113, 365
Moore, Henry, 227
Moore, Marianne, 92, 93
The Morgan Library & Museum, 132–133, 134
Morgan Stanley Children's Hospital, 262
Morning, Present, Evening bas-relief, 154
Morningside Heights walking tour
  map of the, 222
  overview of the, 223–231
  points of interest, 231
  route summary and connecting the walks, 232–233
Morningside Park, 229–230, 231, 238, 240
Morningside Pond, 238
Morris-Jumel Mansion, 261, 266
Moses, Robert, 137, 179
Most Precious Blood Church, 38
Mott Hall School, PS/IS 223, 257
Mount Morris–Ascension Presbyterian Church, 246, 249
Mount Morris Park (a.k.a. Marcus Garvey Park), 246
Mount Morris Park West, 246
Mount Sinai Roosevelt Hospital, 178
Mount Washington Presbyterian Church, 270, 273
Mount Zion Evangelical Lutheran Church, 254, 258
Mount Zion Evangelical Lutheran School, 254
MS 326, 262
Muhlenberg Branch (New York Public Library), 115
Muhlenberg Library, 118
Muhlenberg, William Augustus, 115
Municipal Archives, 34
Municipal Building, 35
Murray's Cheese Shop, 93, 98
Murry Bergtraum High School for Business Careers, 34, 42
Museum Mile, 187

about the author

ELLEN LEVITT is a lifelong resident of Brooklyn, New York, who has written for such publications as *The New York Times,* the New York *Daily News,* and *New York Teacher.* She is also the author of the three books in the series *The Lost Synagogues of New York City* (Avotaynu). A graduate of Barnard College, she has conducted walking, bus, and bicycling tours of New York City and is a veteran public-school teacher.

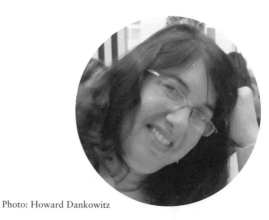

Photo: Howard Dankowitz